PRESCRIPTIONS FOR VIRTUOSITY

Prescriptions for Virtuosity

THE POSTCOLONIAL STRUGGLE OF CHINESE MEDICINE

Eric I. Karchmer

FORDHAM UNIVERSITY PRESS   NEW YORK   2022

Fordham University Press gratefully acknowledges financial assistance and support provided for the publication of this book by Appalachian State University.

Visit us online at www.fordhampress.com.

Library of Congress Cataloging-in-Publication Data available online at https://catalog.loc.gov.

Printed in the United States of America
24 23 22   5 4 3 2 1
First edition

Contents

PRESCRIPTIONS FOR VIRTUOSITY

Introduction

It was a gray and chilly November morning in 2002, two years after my graduation from the Beijing University of Chinese Medicine. I had returned to Dongzhimen Hospital, the main teaching hospital of my alma mater, to spend a few months studying with several senior physicians. I was walking briskly toward the hospital entrance, shortly before the outpatient clinic was to open at 8 A.M. As I approached the hospital, I began to prepare myself for the intense focus I would need for the next four hours. I was going to be shadowing an experienced clinician during his morning shift. It would take my full concentration to follow his clinical work and take good notes as he efficiently worked through his typical caseload of patients, usually two dozen or more before lunch.

I was determined to make the most of this opportunity. I wanted to be a practitioner myself. Although I had completed a five-year medical school degree in Chinese medicine, I still felt distressingly unprepared for the demands of clinical practice. I envied my Chinese classmates, who could continue to develop as doctors within the institutional structure of the hospital, gradually mastering the needed clinical skills as they rose through the ranks of resident, attending physician, and beyond. After graduation, my opportunities for clinical training in China were limited for a couple reasons. First, foreign students like me were welcomed at universities of Chinese medicine, but we were not allowed to work as doctors in China's state-run hospitals. Some of my Korean classmates were working around these restrictions by becoming graduate students, committing to another three to six years of education as a means to also get more clinical training from an advisor. Second, I might have been tempted to follow the lead of my Korean classmates, but I had already started a Ph.D.

degree in Anthropology at the University of North Carolina. It was because of that Ph.D. program that I had originally gone to the Beijing University of Chinese Medicine to conduct my fieldwork. Instead of spending a year or two conducting fieldwork, however, I had stayed for more than five years, learning a whole new discipline in the process. I felt incredibly fortunate to have been able to do so, but I knew I would not be able to write my Ph.D. dissertation unless I reimmersed myself in the academic world of anthropology. Feeling torn by the demands of two professions, frustrated at the challenges of pursuing both, I had decided that I would return to the University of North Carolina to finish my Ph.D. But I was determined to not give up on my dreams of clinical practice. My hope was that through occasional short trips to China, like this one, I would be able to continue refining my clinical skills.

While I fretted about the feasibility of my convoluted career plans, whether I could really learn the clinical craft of Chinese medicine and fulfill the demands of an academic career in the U.S., I knew that many of my Chinese classmates were even more apprehensive about their own futures. A significant number, in fact, wished to *gaihang* or "change professions." I had recently caught up with Chen Shubin, a classmate who had quickly found work after graduation with the multinational medical nutrition company Nutricia in its Beijing office. Chen Shubin did not dislike Chinese medicine. Indeed, like most of our classmates, she had a strong affinity for the profession after having devoted an entire college career to studying it. But she clearly preferred the financial benefits of working for a global pharmaceutical firm over the difficult and poorly compensated work of a doctor of Chinese medicine. She had been very clear minded about this professional choice long before we graduated. Even though some of our teachers had discouraged her from "abandoning her profession," she had persisted in her ambitions. Now that she had settled into her job, she was feeling quite pleased about her career choice and its financial rewards. I caught up with her again in 2008, not long after she had attended a small get-together with many of our classmates. She told me then, about eight years since our graduation, that nearly one-third of our sixty Chinese classmates had now followed in her footsteps and were working as drug representatives for pharmaceutical companies.

Becoming a drug rep was one way out of the profession made possible by the rapid growth of the pharmaceutical industry in China beginning in the mid-1990s (Karchmer, Driver, and Kroeber 1998). I also watched friends pursue more intricate and ambitious paths to other professions. For example, some of the graduate students that I met at the Beijing University of Chinese Medicine were hoping to leverage their graduate training, which often had a strong focus on biomedical research techniques, to become outright biomedical researchers. Huang Yao, the teaching assistant for my biochemistry class, was one such example. She and her husband had both studied Chinese medicine as undergraduates at the Beijing University of Chinese Medicine. Their excellent grades gave them automatic entrance into the graduate programs of their choice at their alma mater. I got to know Huang Yao because she had chosen to get a master's degree in biochemistry, and she had been assigned to be the lab assistant for my biochemistry course. I was struggling in the course, overwhelmed by a whole new vocabulary of chemistry terms in Chinese. I was able to convince Huang Yao to tutor me privately. She patiently and steadfastly guided me through the course textbook, and without her help I could not have passed the course. A little more than a year later, she and her husband had both completed their master's degrees and were moving to New York City. Her husband had been accepted into a Ph.D. program for oncology research at New York University. The last time I caught up with Huang Yao in New York, she was happily working as a computer programmer, having left behind the worlds of Chinese medicine, biochemistry, and perhaps even China. The ambivalence of young doctors like Chen Shubin and Huang Yao about pursuing a career in Chinese medicine was pervasive. As we will see, even those who stayed in the profession to work as doctors often had misgivings about their careers. This ambivalence is one of the defining traits of what I call the "postcolonial condition" of Chinese medicine.[1]

Although I was keenly aware of the mixed emotions of my classmates, I also knew that there were still many excellent physicians working at hospitals of Chinese medicine such as Dongzhimen Hospital, and I was rushing to see one of them in action. I hustled through the waiting room of the outpatient clinic, pulling off my winter jacket and slipping into my white doctor's coat, standard attire for all doctors and hospital technicians, just before striding into the consultation room a few minutes before 8 A.M. On this day, I had arranged to work with Dr. Sun. Three years ago, he had been the main lecturer for our fourth-year medical school class in Chinese Internal Medicine, the key course for that year of medical school. In a pedagogic environment where most professors rarely strayed from the textbooks, Dr. Sun had stood out with his carefully researched lectures, dynamic speaking style, and memorable anecdotes from his own clinical cases. I was hoping that his clinical skills would indeed match his rhetorical talents.

Established in 1958, Dongzhimen Hospital is one of the oldest hospitals of Chinese medicine in China. The hospital consisted of an interconnecting series of well-trod concrete buildings. Despite its dour appearance, I had developed a deep fondness for this complex and the clinical excitement that transpired within its walls. Dr. Sun's consultation hours were being held in a small, narrow room on the second floor, where the internal medicine out-patient clinic was located. The room had almost certainly been converted from some other use to a consultation space, and I didn't remember ever entering it as a student. Dr. Sun sat at a yellow desk, the same basic wooden work desk found in all the consultation rooms, positioned halfway between the hallway door and a tiny window on the far wall. A stack of stools, a small cabinet, and a dusty examination table had been pushed to this far end under-neath the window. The room was so narrow that when Dr. Sun sat at his desk, I would have to awkwardly squeeze between the wall and his chair to get past him. Unlike most of my own experiences as a patient in the U.S., where the clinical exam is centered on the examination table, the desk was always the site of the clinical encounter for an herbal medicine consultation. Dr. Sun would spend the entire morning seated in front of it, conducting consultations and writing prescriptions, too busy on most days to even stand up for a break. The patient would enter from his left and take a seat at a small, three-legged stool at the side of the desk nearest the entrance. Students like me would sit to his right, huddling around the far side of the desk as we took notes.

On this morning, I was sharing the far end of the desk with another medical student, who turned out to be a distant cousin of Dr. Sun. We were participat-ing in the time-honored tradition of "copying prescriptions" (*chao fangzi*), in which a student follows a senior doctor, making notes about the consultation

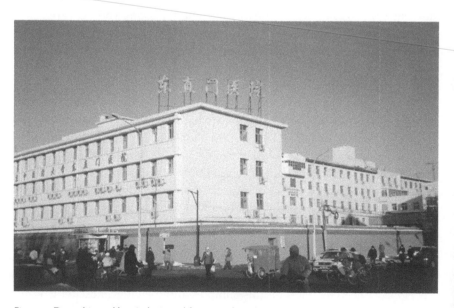

Figure 1. Dongzhimen Hospital, viewed from nearby street, 2002.

and recording the doctor's prescription for later study. As this expression suggests, the prescription lies at the heart of this training method. Far more than a record of the doctor's treatment for an individual patient, the prescription is a condensation of the doctor's therapeutic strategy, both with respect to a specific disorder and his overall clinical style. Unlike Western medicine prescriptions, Chinese medicine prescriptions often contain a dozen or more herbs that the patient usually cooks together in water to make a decoction. Doctors of Chinese medicine assert that the clinical efficacy of a prescription depends not so much on the properties of any single item but on the collective action of the herbs. Moreover, prescriptions are not standardized for medical conditions. Indeed, physicians generally try to individualize the prescription, tailoring it to the patient's unique presentation to the greatest degree possible. Writing a prescription is therefore an art. Some doctors celebrate this fact by writing them out with graceful penmanship. The prescription brings together the physician's skill at identifying the patient's underlying condition, a mastery of hundreds of Chinese medicinal herbs and their multiple clinical uses, and a command of centuries of formulary scholarship about how to best combine the herbs. By copying a doctor's prescriptions, the student hopes to inscribe and ultimately embody the teacher's virtuosity.

A Clinical Encounter

On most days, the rush of patients is so overwhelming that doctors and students have little opportunity to discuss prescriptions and treatment strategies. Outpatient clinics work on a first-come-first-serve basis in China. On a typical day, the waiting room and hallways of the outpatient clinic of a major hospital are filled with patients milling about, anxiously waiting their turn for a consultation.

But on this day, a light drizzle had begun, thinning out the usual morning crowd, giving us occasional opportunities to talk. Around 9:30 A.M., an eighty-four-year-old woman shuffled into the room, her daughter supporting her as she took a seat. The daughter opened her purse and pulled out her mother's outpatient record book, a worn and folded yellow notebook, the size of an elongated index card. Dr. Sun took the notebook and placed it on the desk, pushing aside the blood pressure cuff he had used for the last consultation. He scanned the notes from previous consultations and then looked at the patient: "What's bothering you today?" "My whole body aches," she said in the Beijing patois, putting her hand to her chest, as if to suggest that it was the greatest source of discomfort.

While she and her daughter took turns speaking, Dr. Sun began opening the laboratory tests and other exam results that had been folded and stapled into the record book, adding considerably to its bulk. They included an electrocardiogram from a month ago with a depressed ST section, indicating mild cardiac ischemia. Blood work from a visit two weeks ago showed that her white blood cell count had been high (14.3 x 10^9 cells/liter) and her neutrophil distribution elevated (84 percent), both signs of infection. A biochemical panel did not indicate conclusively any one problem, but Dr. Sun declared it "chaotic," with eight abnormal results. The daughter handed Dr. Sun a recent chest X-ray. Holding it up to the light and angling it toward us, the students, Dr. Sun pointed out cobweb-like interstitial markings caused by a pulmonary infection and drew our attention to the increased spacing of the ribs, a sign of emphysematous changes. He put down the X-ray and then showed us the notes from her last hospital visit, in which a different doctor had diagnosed her with coronary heart disease, chronic nephritis, and interstitial pneumonia.

Turning to a fresh page in the record book, Dr. Sun began writing today's entry, asking the patient questions as he wrote. He quickly jotted down additional complaints about heart palpitations and back pain and then asked her to stick out her tongue. The tongue exam is one of the distinctive features of the Chinese medicine exam. Doctors consider it one of the most important and reliable ways to assess the patient's overall condition. Dr. Sun carefully noted the shape and color of the tongue, as well as the texture and color of the tongue coating. Next, he gestured toward the patient's wrist to begin the pulse exam, another distinctive feature of a Chinese medicine consultation. She extended her arm, palm up. Dr. Sun put three fingers on her radial artery, letting his fingertips gently roll over the artery, sensing its resilience as he varied the pressure. He repeated this process with the other wrist. In Chinese medicine pulse taking, doctors feel for the overall presentation of the pulse and record its texture according to twenty-eight basic pulse forms. Several pulse presentations may present simultaneously, and they can also vary across the three positions on each wrist. Like the tongue exam, the pulse is considered an excellent indicator of the patient's overall condition and an essential part of any consultation (Kuriyama 1999; Farquhar 2014). The pulse exam is so iconic to Chinese medicine clinical work that patients sometimes turn it into a test of a doctor's clinical skills. I observed more than a few patients begin their consultations by silently extending their wrist, with the expectation that the physician would be able to state the patient's symptoms based on the pulse alone.

Having completed his exam, Dr. Sun looked up from his notes and addressed the two women. He recommended that the patient be admitted to the hospital. Her condition was too complicated and unstable to be treated

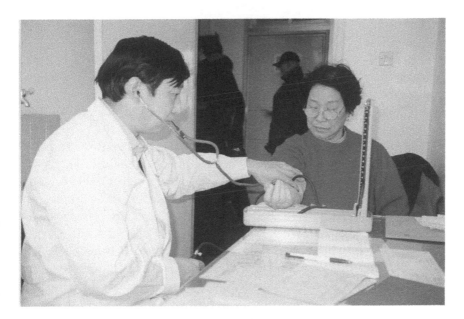

Figure 2. Sun Pei checking the blood pressure of a patient, 2002.

on an outpatient basis. Since Dr. Sun has recently joined the nephrology department, he suggested that the patient be admitted to this ward. It would be permissible with her chronic nephritis, and he could personally care for her in that department. They quickly agreed to this plan, and the daughter gathered up the record book, the X-rays, and other belongings and escorted her mother out of the room to begin the admissions process.

The next patient did not enter right away, so Dr. Sun turned toward his two students to discuss this case with the excitement that only a devoted teacher might have. "What formula would you use for that patient?" he quizzed. Dr. Sun's cousin and I looked back at him blankly. I felt overwhelmed by the complexity of the case. Could a single formula address the patient's heart, lung, and kidney problems? Each one alone would be difficult to treat. "First of all," Dr. Sun said, breaking the silence, "the patient should be diagnosed as having Chest Blockage (胸痹), due to cold and phlegm. In the sixth edition of the *Chinese Internal Medicine* (中医内科学) textbook, Chest Blockage was misleadingly renamed Chest Blockage and Heart Pain (胸痹心痛). But interstitial pneumonia corresponds perfectly to Chest Blockage, which can also account for the patient's mild cardiac ischemia. The proper formula should be Trichosanthes Fruit, Chinese Garlic, and Pinellia Decoction (*Gua Lou Xie Bai Ban Xia Tang*) to 'invigorate chest yang' (*zhenfen xiongyang*)."

I was instantly intrigued by this explanation for several reasons. First, Dr. Sun had sorted the patient's acute and most dangerous symptoms from her chronic and less concerning ones. Moments earlier, the patient's complicated symptoms, test results, and biomedical diagnoses had been a confusing morass for me. Dr. Sun had now laid out a clear strategy for intervening. Treat the pneumonia and Chest Blockage first and then address more long-term problems later.

Second, Dr. Sun's diagnosis of Chest Blockage was unusual, and as he subsequently explained, he intended it as a critique of the sixth edition of the *Chinese Internal Medicine* (中医内科学) textbook, the very textbook he had taught to me a few years earlier. The term "Chest Blockage" originates in the second-century canon the *Essentials of the Golden Casket* (*Jingui Yaolue*; 金匮要略), written by Zhang Zhongjing (張仲景) (150 C.E.–219 C.E.). In contemporary practice, Chest Blockage has become widely associated with the biomedical diagnosis of coronary heart disease. In fact, the sixth-edition textbook makes this statement explicitly: "The disorder of Chest Blockage and Heart Pain corresponds to angina pectoris due to coronary heart disease" (Wang Yongyan, Li Mingfu, and Dai Ximeng 1997, 108). To emphasize this correspondence, the textbook took the additional step of calling this condition "Chest Blockage and Heart Pain," rather than just Chest Blockage, as had been the convention in earlier editions of *Chinese Internal Medicine*. Heart Pain is a traditional nosological term, actually discussed in the same chapter of the *Essentials of the Golden Casket* as Chest Blockage, but this name change suggested modern congruences that Dr. Sun wanted to challenge.[2]

When I was a student, many of my teachers had been critical of the sixth-edition textbooks, which had just been introduced to college curriculums, for going too far in incorporating elements of Western medicine. Here was a clear example of the danger of this trend. A junior doctor, such as Dr. Sun's cousin or I, would probably never think to apply Chest Blockage to a case of interstitial pneumonia because we had already been trained, in part by these textbooks, to understand the term more narrowly as the equivalent of coronary heart disease. I thought back to the patient clutching her chest at the beginning of the consultation. Dr. Sun's insight gave me a tangible new insight into a dimension of this Chinese medicine term that I had never envisioned before.

Third, Dr. Sun's analysis also illuminated new uses of a classic formula. *Essentials of the Golden Casket*, like the other major work by Zhang Zhongjing, the *Treatise on Cold Damage* (*Shanghan Lun*; 傷寒論), are two of the earliest and most revered clinical texts in Chinese medicine scholarship. Many of the 262 unique formulas of *Essentials* and 112 formulas of the *Treatise* are still commonly used today (Li Keguang and Zhang Jiali 1993, 1; Nanjing College of Chinese Medicine 1992 [1959], 1). But it is often not apparent to students how the pithy descriptions in these works can be applied to actual clinical situations. The chapter on Chest Blockage contains several well-known formulas, so I was excited to hear Dr. Sun explain his choice of Trichosanthes Fruit, Chinese Garlic, and Pinellia Decoction in the following manner. "This formula is an excellent choice for this patient. Antibiotics are generally not very effective in treating interstitial pneumonia. In Western medicine, one might also consider steroids. But this approach compromises the immune system and could exacerbate the infection. In a similar fashion, we must not use the related formula Unripe Bitter Orange, Chinese Garlic, and Cinnamon Twig Decoction (*Zhi Shi Xie Bai Gui Zhi Tang*), because Cinnamon Twig (*Gui Zhi*) is too warming and might also worsen the infection. We could consider replacing it with Ephedra (*Ma Huang*), which is also warming but won't intensify the infection because of its strong Lung dispersing properties."

Lastly, I was fascinated that Dr. Sun was calibrating his choice of Chinese medicine formula based on how he thought it would affect the patient's biomedical pathology. Whereas in the previous statement, Dr. Sun had resisted conflating the diagnostic term of Chest Blockage with the modern notion of coronary heart disease, here he shifted tactics to embrace the biomedical pathophysiology of infection, a concept that has no equivalent in Chinese medicine. He compared common Western medicine treatments for infections—antibiotics and steroids—with possible Chinese medicine formulas: Trichosanthes Fruit, Chinese Garlic, and Pinellia Decoction and Unripe Bitter Orange, Chinese Garlic, and Cinnamon Twig Decoction. These two formulas are classically understood to "unblock the yang, dissipate clumps, expel phlegm, and direct the qi downwards" (Scheid et al. 2009 [1990], 514), and it had never occurred to me that these properties would also make them effective in resolving an infection of any sort. Dr. Sun's point was more nuanced than this, since one formula was clearly superior to the other in this case of interstitial pneumonia. The latter formula could only work with some modifications, such as substituting the "dispersing" Ephedra for the "warming" Cinnamon Twig.

I was delighted with this explanation and the way that Dr. Sun seamlessly wove together knowledge of the body and its diseases with a mastery of possible therapeutic interventions. But it was striking not only for this display of clinical virtuosity, but also for Dr. Sun's embrace of hybridity. Throughout the consultation, Dr. Sun was continually tacking back and forth between the worlds of Chinese medicine and Western medicine: reviewing EKGs, X-rays, and blood work, conducting the tongue and pulse exam, comparing diagnoses in the two medical systems, and lastly adjudicating between the merits of various Western medicine and Chinese medicine therapies. I was dazzled by the speed and surety of his intellectual oscillations, at one moment critiquing colleagues who too easily assumed equivalences between Chinese medicine and Western medicine, at another moment leveraging a different congruence between the two medical systems to finalize his therapeutic decision. Although Dr. Sun struck me as particularly adept at these hybrid maneuverings, I also knew he was not doing anything unusual. Doctors of Chinese medicine in China are expected to be fully competent in both Chinese medicine and Western medicine, even though their biomedical counterparts would never be expected to go beyond the field of biomedicine in their clinical work. As we will see, this kind of hybridity is an inescapable feature of every clinical encounter at an institution of Chinese medicine in China.

The clinical encounter just described challenges us with a very basic question: "What is Chinese medicine?" The answer is not obvious. The hybridity, the entanglements of Chinese medicine and Western medicine, are profound and visible to even the casual visitor to a hospital of Chinese medicine. As Dr. Li Chengwei, now a professor at the Beijing University of Chinese medicine, once told me when he was a graduate student, "Chinese medicine today cannot exist without Western medicine." Yet this hybridity is surrounded by an element of mystery. Even as doctors blend elements of Chinese medicine and Western medicine in nearly every clinical counter, they rarely discuss how or why. The curriculums for Chinese medicine programs are carefully designed to give students equal amounts of training in Chinese medicine and Western medicine. But there is no course, no textbook, no official protocol about how doctors should use the two medical systems together. Hybridity seems to just happen with little or no apparent justification in most clinical situations. Dr. Sun's brief comments in the previous case were striking because they were almost effusive compared to what I was used to. As reticent as doctors tend to be about how to blend medical systems, they can be surprisingly vocal and vigilant about policing the boundaries between the two. Dr. Sun's critique of the sixth-edition textbooks was one small example. He delighted in explaining his own hybrid innovations on how to treat the biomedical condition of interstitial pneumonia with Chinese medicine therapies, but he made sure to critique the textbook editors who were irresponsibly, in his mind, drawing congruences between Chest Blockage and coronary heart disease. Scholars and doctors insist that Chinese medicine is its own unique system of medicine. They vigorously defend it against the equivalences with Western medicine that they perceive as devaluing, even as they must continuously translate between the two medical systems.

A Postcolonial Framework

In order to explore the complexities of the contemporary clinical practice of Chinese medicine as exemplified by Dr. Sun's case, it is essential to understand it within the broader social context, including the decisions of many of my classmates to pursue careers outside of Chinese medicine. I believe these trends reflect a set of power inequalities that are most productively understood as part of the "postcolonial condition" of contemporary Chinese society. In postcolonial studies, scholars such as Dipesh Chakrabarty have defined the "postcolonial condition" as a state in which the West continues to exercise a cultural dominance over the formerly colonized, making the West the necessary point of reference for any historical, sociological, or scientific claim made about the East (Chakrabarty 2000). In other words, postcolonial scholars have argued that the power inequalities of European colonization have persisted in the contemporary period, even though the vast majority of formerly colonized societies achieved political independence by the 1960s. Instead of overt political domination, these societies struggle with colonial-like power inequalities that take subtle, cultural forms.

The concept of postcolonialism helps to situate the predicament of contemporary doctors of Chinese medicine at the intersection of local historical forces and the massive global transformations that have remade the world since the end of World War II. I have insisted on this analytic framework even though postcolonialism is a concept that originated among South Asian scholars and has been notably absent from the field of China studies. To avoid confusion, I want to clarify the reasons for this choice. One common dismissal of the concept of postcolonialism, widely shared among Chinese intellectuals, is that it is inappropriate to the unique historical circumstances of China (Chen Houcheng 1996). In contrast to the subcontinent of India, which was under direct administrative control of the British, China was never subject to full political control by a European power. For roughly a century, beginning with the Opium War of 1840, European and later Japanese imperial powers operated through smaller colonial concessions, primarily "treaty ports," leaving much of the nation under the control of the Qing court up to 1911 and a weak Republican state from 1911 to 1949. The conventional designation for this period of intensifying imperial encroachment is that it was a period of "semi-colonialism." In addition to these historical distinctions, Chinese intellectuals have not shared the critical, antiessentialist proclivities of their South

Asian counterparts (X. Zhang 1997, 88–99). As Prasenjit Duara, an Indian scholar of Chinese history, writes:

> The preoccupation with the utopia of modernity in the Chinese narrative of History, its role as the only standard of value, closed off . . . much that its older histories, narratives, and popular cultures had to offer. Chinese intellectuals, by and large, have not challenged the Enlightenment project to the same extent as postmodern and post-colonial intellectuals (Duara 1995, 49).

Many China studies scholars have also been wary of the concept of postcolonialism for methodological reasons. Tani Barlow has argued that the post–World War II rise of the area studies paradigm and a focus on the problems of modernization in China led to an avoidance of uncomfortable questions about colonization (Barlow 1997, 373–411). Early postwar scholarship on China, exemplified by the work of John Fairbanks, elided questions of political domination in the nineteenth and twentieth centuries by focusing on how China-West relations contributed to the modernization of China. Fairbanks's model, known as "China's response to the West," eventually fell out of favor for its assumption of a static and passive Chinese society. Beginning in the 1980s with Paul Cohen's "China-centered approach," scholars began to give more dynamic and nuanced accounts of China's late imperial and early modern history (Cohen 1984). But these carefully researched histories, not unlike the Fairbanks's program, did not critically address the problem of colonialism and its impact. "China" and the "West" continued to be taken-for-granted, naturalized entities in this scholarship. Thus, it is perhaps not surprising that the field of postcolonial studies, emerging in the 1980s and 1990s with strong poststructuralist affinities, was slow to attract followers in the world of China studies.

This book has intentionally departed from these long-standing trends in China studies and builds on more recent scholarship that has sought to bring China into the field of colonial studies. Instead of emphasizing the differences with British India, this new scholarship highlights the commonalities between European imperial projects throughout the world and the specific forms it took in China. Instead of relying on naturalized and unquestioned assumptions about what constitutes "China" and "the West," this scholarship emphasizes how these terms were produced through the emergent and messy nature of European and Japanese imperialism. This scholarship has shown that colonial domination did not follow a blueprint but worked through techniques of administration that were often shared across disparate colonial regimes (Yang 2019). James Hevia has argued most emphatically against the distinctions between the semicolonialism of China and colonial projects elsewhere in the world.

> Colonization was not . . . a simple matter of conquest and administration; all colonial settings were informed by a dynamic interaction between colonizer and colonized. . . . As a result, it is difficult to posit any pure form of colonization or any complete model that could fix our understanding of colonial processes.
>
> Instead, we might consider all the entities produced in the age of empires as forms of semicolonialism — especially that patchwork of patchworks, British India, notwithstanding its canonical status as the colony of colonies. . . . From this perspective, therefore, China was not outside the "real" colonial world. Rather, it was a variation on forms that were both present and incomplete in Africa, South America, and South and Southeast Asia (Hevia 2003, 26).

Refusing to distinguish China from other colonial projects by the "incomplete penetration" of the British, Hevia reframes China's "semicolonial" status as emblematic of all imperial projects in the age of empires.

I consider my analysis to be a continuation of this work to integrate China into colonial studies. Just as China was not isolated from the empire building projects of Europe and Japan, it has not been disconnected from the postcolonial forces that have shaped so-called developing nations since the end of World War II. In fact, I consider the story of Chinese medicine to be emblematic of these processes. A postcolonial framework does not erase the unique historical context of China and Chinese medicine, but it makes visible important transnational connections, such as what Warwick Anderson has called "the postcolonial worldliness of biomedicine" (Anderson 2014).[3] In *Encountering Development: The Making and Unmaking of the Third World*, Arturo Escobar has argued that development is "a historically singular experience, the creation of a domain of thought and action" that emerged in the early post–World War II era and continues to the present. He has claimed that the discourse of development constructed formerly colonized regions of the world as the "Third World" and shaped interventions in these areas, often with dire consequences, through foundational concepts such as overpopulation, famine, poverty, and illiteracy (Escobar 1995, 10–12). The story of contemporary Chinese medicine is unique in many ways to China's historical conditions in the twentieth century, but it is also inseparable from global processes, such as those that Escobar has traced in the context of development discourse.

Double Truths

Like the problems of development, the postcolonial predicament of Chinese medicine operates through institutional, discursive, and cultural processes. The defining feature of this predicament is the unquestioned prestige of biomedicine in China. Whether we are considering the career choices of my classmates or the clinical decisions of Dr. Sun, their actions are reminiscent of Frantz Fanon's analysis of how settler values were privileged over native ones in colonial Africa (Fanon 1963). Fanon summarizes the psychology of the colonized in the following manner:

> All colonized people . . . position themselves in relation to the civilizing language, i.e., the metropolitan culture. The more the colonized has assimilated the cultural values of the metropolis, the more he will have escaped the bush (Fanon 2008 [1952], 2).

Just as many of my classmates were eager, if not desperate, to escape the confines of the Chinese medicine profession, skilled physicians like Dr. Sun must position themselves in relation to the "civilizing language" of biomedicine.

The postcolonial predicament of Chinese medicine has been institutionalized in the asymmetries of the national healthcare system, which contains two parallel but unequal systems of medicine. There are state-run schools, hospitals, and research institutions for both Western medicine and Chinese medicine, but the former are more numerous, more respected, and more authoritative and are considered more scientific than the latter. The hegemonic place of Western medicine in contemporary Chinese society, its status as a "civilizing language," produces numerous other asymmetries. For example, with regard to medical training, students of Western medicine are generally required to take a semester-long introduction to Chinese medicine. But this training is irrelevant to the doctor's professional advancement. By contrast, students of Chinese medicine have a curriculum that devotes nearly 50 percent of allotted course time to topics in Western medicine. Doctors of Western medicine can choose to incorporate some Chinese medicine into their clinical work, although most do not; doctors of Chinese medicine, however, must be skilled practitioners of biomedicine. As we will explore in Chapter 5, one key reason for these different professional burdens is that hospitals of Chinese medicine require that medical records for all admitted patients contain a "double diagnosis," diagnoses in both Chinese medicine and Western medicine. There is no such requirement for biomedical institutions.

As doctors of Chinese medicine work between two medical systems, they must innovate and find ways to negotiate the differences between these two practices. There is much to celebrate about the hybrid interventions that emerge through this process. But it is important to recognize that this clinical work requires navigating an epistemological quandary: what is the truth status of Chinese medicine claims about the body, illness, and healing? The answer is fraught. Chinese medicine is defined by its difference from Western medicine; difference marks its "Chinese-ness." At the same time, this difference is inherently problematic. Any deviation from the standards of Western medicine can be interpreted as error, as evidence that Chinese medicine is not scientific. Doctors of Chinese medicine resolve this postcolonial dilemma by embracing a position of "double truths." As many doctors have reminded me, "Western medicine is scientific, but Chinese medicine is scientific, too." By insisting on this adverb "too," the all-important supplement that makes this claim work, doctors are implicitly recognizing the power inequalities between Western medicine and Chinese medicine. Chinese medicine is true, but it is always in juxtaposition to, and secondary to, the claims of Western medicine. As we will see, this subaltern status means that Chinese medicine has also become a profoundly hybrid practice, one that incorporates or blends significant elements of Western medicine. These adaptions, however, do not mean that it is necessarily an impoverished medicine. As the vignette about Dr. Sun suggests, this hybridity can be enacted with great virtuosity.

In One Hundred Years . . .

A postcolonial framework not only helps to understand the power inequalities that exist between the two medical systems, but it also helps orient us to the deeply conflicted attitudes that exist toward Chinese medicine in China. These attitudes range from extreme dislike and skepticism to nationalist embrace and celebration, but they all share an acute awareness of the geopolitical weakness of this healing practice. These complex sentiments contribute to the unique social context that doctors of Chinese medicine must navigate in carrying out their clinical work.

I personally was unprepared for the intense attitudes about Chinese medicine that I encountered during my research. Perhaps typical of a young anthropologist, I was full of romance for this seemingly exotic medical practice. I believed that, even if my initial enthusiasm was naïve, it was not ungrounded. I had been inspired by exciting new developments in the field of science studies. The foundations of Chinese medicine, its immanent philosophy of yin and yang, the deep relationality of the five phases, the organ system, and the meridian pathways struck me as a perfect example of the feminist science of partial perspectives that Donna Haraway eloquently called for in her 1988 manifesto "Situated Knowledge." In this essay, Haraway asserted that the problems of race, class, and gender—"White Capitalist Patriarchy"—were inextricably linked to unexamined, totalizing claims about objectivity in modern science. By embracing alternative views, becoming open to the "partial perspectives" of historically disadvantaged groups, science could become more inclusive and the power inequalities that were so pervasive in the world of late capitalism might be challenged (Haraway 1988). When I began my research, I had expected to find a robust politics of resistance within the Chinese medicine community, even if practitioners lacked Haraway's language to articulate their work. I assumed that I was joining an alternative collective of doctors and scholars who were committed to creating a more diverse world.

Instead, I encountered widespread ambivalence from my new colleagues in the field of Chinese medicine. My classmates and teachers were not radicals; they were mostly unconcerned with "White Capitalist Patriarchy." Many classmates speculated that the language, concepts, and principles of Chinese medicine might be as foreign to them as they were to me. Their high school education was focused on what is colloquially called *shulihua*, or "mathematics, physics, and chemistry"—a common reference to the foundations of the modern science—not on history, philosophy, and literature, disciplines that might be equally or more pertinent to the study of Chinese medicine.[4] To my surprise, even the best students were often not particularly enthusiastic about Chinese medicine. One classmate, who graduated third in our class, an important honor that earned her automatic admission to the master's program of her choosing at the university, told me quite unabashedly after our graduation that she preferred the straightforward logic of Western medicine because she couldn't "grasp the Chinese medicine way of thinking."

Sometimes, ambivalence slid into deep pessimism. One friend, Lai Lili, a recent graduate of the Beijing University of Chinese Medicine, had been radicalized by her experience. She was quite open with me about her disappointment with Chinese medicine. She felt like she had been "deceived" (*bei pian le*) by the university and was eager to *gaihang*, to switch professions, perhaps to anthropology. Although she felt a certain gratitude for her training, particularly when it came to managing her own personal health, she had decided that she would never practice clinical medicine.[5] During my earlier years at the Beijing University of Chinese Medicine, I remember many conversations about the future of Chinese medicine with Lai Lili and her former classmates. These discussions were almost always gloomy affairs. To this young group of graduates, the very future of Chinese medicine was in doubt. The profession was standing still, if not regressing. The field was oriented to the past, to the classic texts and great doctors of long ago, but science and medicine were advancing at an inexorable pace. Younger doctors were focused on staying abreast of the latest developments in Western medicine, rather than mastering the craft of Chinese medicine. Or like this group, they simply wanted to leave the profession altogether. Under these conditions, how could Chinese medicine hope to compete with the global institutions of biomedicine?

A few years later, in 2001, a health magazine published a lengthy and well-researched article called "The Lonely Century of Chinese Medicine" that captured the apocalyptic spirit of those conversations. I have reproduced some of the section headings from this article to help capture the pessimism that I frequently encountered during my research. I heard each of these statements on numerous occasions.

In one hundred years, will Chinese medicine still exist?

We have not trained any true doctors of Chinese medicine in the last few decades.

For those who want to study Chinese medicine, there is truly no door to enter, no path to follow.

We [the old doctors] are the final generation [of Chinese medicine doctors].

The textbooks are getting worse and worse.

The teachers don't believe in Chinese medicine themselves.

The better one is at math, physics, and chemistry, the harder it is to accept Chinese medicine.

In the name of "scientization," Chinese medicine is destroying itself (Hao Guangming 2001).

The author had interviewed many leading doctors in the field (some of whom I later had the honor of interviewing myself) and had indeed captured the apprehensions of the Chinese medicine community. If the twentieth-century advances of biomedicine continued in the twenty-first century—and why shouldn't they?—Chinese medicine would be eliminated as a clinical practice through a Darwinian process of selection. In one hundred years, it would become obsolete.

Although I never directly discussed the ethical virtues of Haraway's "situated knowledges" with these friends, I had no doubt about how it would have been received. It was precisely the "situated-ness" of Chinese medicine that was so concerning to them. These young graduates had grown up in a world where the supposedly universal knowledge of modern science was considered essential to fulfilling a collective aspiration to modernize Chinese society and create a great nation. As I saw again and again, doctors of Chinese medicine desired the supposed objectivity, rationality, and universality of science because they perceived these qualities to be lacking in Chinese medicine. Doctors yearned for strength. They did not reject Western medicine; they embraced it. They were not interested in critiques of science; rather, they wanted to emulate science. It was essential to show that "Chinese medicine was scientific, too" or to abandon it altogether.

Since the 2010s, there has been an interesting surge in the popularity of Chinese medicine, but the same anxiety about geopolitical weakness also shapes these new sparks of enthusiasm. This shift is related to President Xi Jinping, who came to power in 2013 and is clearly a supporter of Chinese medicine. He often incorporates expressions from Chinese medicine into his public speeches, turning classical references to illness and therapies into a homespun analysis of social ills and the policies needed to correct them.[6] Whereas previous administrations had an ambiguous relationship with Chinese medicine, the current one is eager to use Chinese medicine as part of its "soft power" agenda to extend China's international influence alongside new investment programs, such as the Belt and Road Initiative, also known as the New Silk Road.

I got to witness some of this new interest in Chinese medicine in June 2018, when I was invited to speak at a conference called the "International Conference on the Dissemination of Traditional Chinese Medicine Culture," hosted by the People's Medical Publishing House (*Renmin Weisheng Chubanshe*). The participants were a mix of local Chinese scholars and officials, Chinese medicine doctors living and working abroad, and a small number of foreign scholars of Chinese medicine. Many Chinese participants spoke in great detail about the spread of Chinese medicine to various regions of the world, sharing their experience as teachers and practitioners in those areas. This was not surprising, given the theme of the conference, but I was caught off guard by the strongly nationalist tone of these talks. Most Chinese participants clearly saw their work as part of a larger global strategy—a New Silk Road, as several of them mentioned—to spread Chinese influence abroad. Some of them openly spoke in the idiom of "conquest." For the publishing house, this conference presented a mix of business and political opportunities. They generously hosted the conference, covering the travel expenses for all seventeen international participants. The two-day conference opened with a twenty-minute speech from a board member of the publishing house, the signing of two memorandums of agreements with Chinese medicine associations in Switzerland and Argentina, and a dramatic presentation of new publications of translated Chinese medicine texts, the latter two events accompanied by stirring music, a swarm of photographers, and a supporting cast of elegantly dressed employees from the press!

This display of official enthusiasm for Chinese medicine was unimaginable while I was a student in the 1990s. It is too early to know what effect it will have on the profession or public opinion. But it is also clear that sentiments about Chinese medicine, both positive and negative, remain intimately tied to the China's geopolitical status in the current world order, while the truth status of Chinese medicine remains troubled and unresolved. It's important to remember that this epistemological quandary is also rooted in decades of far less enthusiastic state policies that preceded the Xi Jinping era. Kim Taylor has argued that Chinese medicine was never part of the larger Communist agenda to transform China into a modern, socialist country, and that its current, fairly sizeable role in the national healthcare system is primarily the result of a series of fortuitous events and energetic efforts by its supporters rather than the whole-hearted embrace of China's political leaders (Taylor 2004). This long history of ambiguous state support was publicly on display as recently as 2006, when vocal critics of Chinese medicine, such as Zhang Gongyao (张功耀) and Fang Zhouzi (方舟子), organized a public campaign in China's nascent online community to have Chinese medicine removed from the national healthcare system. For these opponents, Chinese medicine is a pseudo-science, a blemish on the healthcare system and an insult to national pride. There was little to no official government response to this campaign for months, until the leaders began collecting signatures for a formal petition. Only then did the government act to ban the online petition and curtail the growing online interest in this campaign (Zhang Gongyao 2006; Fang Zhouzi 2007).

Although I began my research in Chinese medicine with the hope of experiencing a liberating, feminist science, I discovered instead a troubled but perhaps more important phenomenon: a collective of doctors and scholars grappling with their own postcolonial predicament. This book offers no easy solutions to the problem of postcoloniality. But if there is to be an embrace of traditional knowledges in our rapidly globalizing world, if there are to be ways to move beyond the power inequalities of a world still trapped in the legacy of centuries of empire building, then the struggles of contemporary doctors of Chinese medicine and their quest for virtuosity will be an invaluable guide to that future.

Two Names

This work is dedicated to outlining the postcolonial predicament confronting Chinese medicine practitioners and the innovations they have developed in response. It is not a simple story of domination, because the forces of inequality have also produced hybridity and change. To explain how both processes—domination and change—operate within the postcolonial predicament of Chinese medicine, it is essential to begin with a distinction that might seem too obvious to merit the attention that it deserves—the names. China has two main forms of medical practice, which are known in China as "Chinese medicine" (*zhongyi*; 中医) and "Western medicine" (*xiyi*; 西医). These two names emerged in the early twentieth century as European medical practices spread to China, and they were established as the official names of these two medical practices in the Communist era.

It is significant that China's two main medical practices are currently distinguished by geographical markers. Prior to the nineteenth century, there was only one term for medicine (*yi*; 醫) in China, and it broadly referred to medical practices derived from or related to a literate tradition that could be traced to the Han (206 B.C.E.–220 C.E.) and pre-Han (before 206 B.C.E.) medical writings of early China. Historically, *yi* has been qualified in various ways, such as by the social status of the practitioner, to describe "Confucian doctors" (*ruyi*), "imperial physicians" (*taiyi*), or "generational doctors" (*shiyi*)—that is, part of a family lineage of doctors, and so on (see Andrews 2014, 9). In the late imperial era, the concept of *yi* could be modified by general geographic distinctions. "Eastern medicine" (*dongyi*), for instance, might refer to styles of practice in Korea or Japan (Suh 2017). Certain medical lineages became associated with a specific locale, such as the emergence of Menghe medicine (*Menghe yixue*) in the late Qing and Republican periods (Scheid 2007). In all these expressions, however, medicine or *yi* still referred to a shared genealogy of texts and traditions, a family of practices (Wittgenstein 2009 [1953]).

In Communist China, the terms "Chinese medicine" and "Western medicine" mark a bifurcation in China's world of medical practices.[7] Each term represents both a profound reduction in the diversity of healing practices that once existed in China and an intensified divide between two forms of medical practice.[8] To help understand the transformation symbolized by these two names, it is helpful to look at the excellent scholarship of Bridie Andrews and Sean Lei on medical practices in the Republican era (1911–49) just prior to this shift. Drawing on the observations of Qiu Jisheng, a well-known early twentieth-century doctor of Chinese medicine, Bridie Andrews has described a medical pluralism that existed in the city of Shaoxing circa 1915 that would be unimaginable in contemporary China. One of the main groups that Qiu Jisheng identified was doctors of "Chinese medicine" (*zhongyi*), which he subdivided into roughly a dozen specializations. They were contrasted with a number of different "spirit doctors" (*shenyi*), including blind "diviners" (*wenbu*), "ghost-seers" (*guiyan*), and "enlightened grannies" (*wupo*), to name a few. Other religious and ritual practices were also featured in the many activities listed under "family medicine" (*jiayi*). Qiu further distinguished itinerant healers, known as "river and lake doctors" (*jianghu yi*). These included "street healers" (*guolu langzhong*), "market healers" (*haitan langzhong*), "tooth worm removers" (*xiao yachong*), "drug peddlers" (*caoyao dan*), "tiger skin merchants" (*hupi ke*), and others. Qiu described the doctors, mostly Chinese medicine physicians, associated with government and charitable institutions as various "official" and "semi-official" doctors, respectively. Doctors of "Western medicine" (*xiyi*) were also mentioned in Qiu's account. They ran one- or two-person clinics, located primarily in the city, treating "external" or minor surgical conditions. A few Western-style doctors trained in Japan were identified as doctors of "Eastern medicine" (*dongyi*) (Andrews 2014; Qiu Shiting 2006, 8–18).

Sean Lei has described an even more complex mix of medical practices in Shanghai, drawing on the 1933 publication of Pang Jingzhou, a well-known doctor of Western medicine. Pang's description included a fascinating visual diagram that included forty-three different styles and associations of medical practitioners. Not surprisingly, given Shanghai's colonial history, the role of Western medicine was much more prominent than in Qiu's earlier account. Lei has pointed out that the term "Chinese medicine" did not appear in this diagram, and "Western medicine" was used only once to identify the "Association of Western Medicine" (*xiyi gonghui*), whose members treated primarily venereal disease and paradoxically relied on Chinese herbal medicine. Lei used the curious absence of these terms in Pang's account to astutely argue that "there was really no such thing as a unified medical system, whether biomedical or Chinese" at this moment in history (Lei 2014, 123).

Pang described a highly fragmented terrain of medical practices where boundaries were often permeable, and it would have been nearly impossible to guess that two relatively unified medical professions would emerge from it two decades later. Within the nascent world of Western medicine, there were foreign doctors, as well as Chinese doctors trained in the various national styles, which Pang grouped as (1) China, England, and the U.S.; (2) Germany and Japan; (3) France and Holland; and (4) Belgium, Austria, and Switzerland. Despite their internal divides, these groups sought collectively to distinguish themselves from lesser trained practitioners, who may have learned as assistants in missionary hospitals or other venues. Pang's description of indigenous healing practices captures even more complexity. A great number of practices were lumped under the domain of "chaotic medicine and pharmacy" (*huntun yiyao*), including exorcist shamans, Daoist temples, divination, altars for spirit mediums, talismans, and so on. Among Shanghai's more than 5,000 licensed traditional practitioners at the time, Lei believed they probably fell into some of Pang's somewhat more respectable categories, such as "faction of awakened young practitioners of Old Medicine," the "conservative faction," "neo-Confucian medicine," the "Communication faction of Old Medicine," and so on (Lei 2014, 121–40). As Lei has shown, the politics of these names had become very contentious in this period. Biomedical doctors were branding themselves as doctors of "scientific medicine," "modern medicine," or "new medicine," while dismissing traditional doctors for practicing "old medicine." Conversely, traditional doctors were quite successfully building political support for their practice by renaming it as "national medicine" (*guoyi*) (Lei 2014, 109–11).

In Chapter 1, we will look more closely at the social changes that produced the new medical professions of Chinese medicine and Western medicine out of these fragmented beginnings. Although the names "Chinese medicine" and "Western medicine" are imperfect in many respects, I use them extensively in this book for two reasons. One, they are the standardized names for the two main forms of institutionalized medicine in China today and remind us of the local perceptions of these medical practices. Two, I hope the reader will see them as heuristic reminders of the postcolonial context in which the two medicines emerged, in particular of the "imaginative geography" described in Edward Said's classic work *Orientalism*. It is not an accident that these names allude to a geopolitical divide—between East and West, Orient and Occident—that has informed colonial discourses for centuries and was uncritically adopted in the field of China studies. Notice how Said understands this notion of "imaginative geography" to operate within colonial, or what he calls Orientalist, discourse.

> [Orientalism] is rather a *distribution* of geopolitical awareness into aesthetic, scholarly, economic, sociological, historical, and philological texts; it is an *elaboration* not only of a basic geographical distinction (the world is made up of two unequal halves, Orient and Occident) but also of a whole series of "interests" which . . . it not only creates but also maintains (Said 1978, 12).

I consider the opposition of East and West to lie at the heart of the postcolonial power inequalities that doctors of Chinese medicine confront. The terms "Chinese medicine" and "Western medicine" echo the unequal opposition between "China" and the "West" that has been part of the legacy of Orientalism.

Said's imaginative geography is important for understanding the postcolonial dynamics confronting Chinese medicine doctors, but it only tells half the story. It does not offer us any theoretical tools for grasping the hybridity of clinical practices that have been proliferating in conjunction with the Orientalist opposition of East and West. The phenomenon of hybridity has been an important theme among postcolonial scholars in South Asia (Bhabha 1994; Gupta 1998; Langford 2002). But it has generally not been explored with the same critical edge as the postcolonial power inequalities themselves. As a result, I have turned to the work of Bruno Latour, where the concept of hybridity is central to his examination of both science and modernity (Latour 1987, 1993). In conventional understandings of science, philosophers have assumed a radical divide between the world and our linguistic representation of it. Truth claims require logical assurances about the accuracy of any scientific statement about nature (Latour 1999, 24). In the Western philosophical tradition, this divide between world and word has been reproduced in other stubborn dualisms, such as the dichotomies of subject-object, mind-body, reason-passion, and nature-culture. Like other scholars, Latour is critical of the manner in which these dualisms inevitably privilege one term over the other (Gordon 1988; Grosz 1994). The West's claim to modernity, he argues, begins with the presumption of a superior command of science and then extends the inequalities of dualistic thought to the relations between the West and the Rest, between so-called moderns and nonmoderns.

Latour is not alone in rejecting these dualisms, but he is unique in relating them to practices of hybridization. He argues that the dichotomies of Western thought, or purifications, as he calls them, are only made possible by hidden practices of hybridization. For example, Latour argues that the practice of science proceeds through repeated transformations between matter and form, thing and sign. These hybrid mediations are forgotten, however, when a scientific claim is made, leaving behind only two purified realms of language and nature (Latour 1999, 69–74). Latour advances a parallel argument in his discussion of what he calls the Modern Constitution. Modern societies insist on their superiority to nonmodern peoples based on their supposed ability to separate Nature from Culture, to investigate the natural world free from cultural influences. These divides between Us and Them, Nature and Culture, however, are made possible by a proliferation of hybrid networks. For Latour, these hybrid blendings of human and nonhuman are found in all communities, as the anthropology of non-Western societies has shown so clearly. But only moderns are driven by the work of purification to conceal them, in the process imposing dualisms—and inequalities—on their relations to the world. Latour argues that it is only through greater attention to the process of hybridization that the so-called Great Divide between the West and the Rest will begin to disappear, and we will come to understand that "we have never been modern" (Latour 1993).

Latour's claim that the work of purification is only made possible by the work of hybridization in the Modern Constitution has striking parallels to the postcolonial dynamics of Chinese medicine. Doctors of Chinese medicine tend to make claims about the nature of Chinese medicine through acts of purification, asserting Orientalist distinctions with Western medicine. The two medical practices are often described as if they are mirror images of each other: the strength of one will often be presented as precisely the weakness of the other. At the same time, physicians like Dr. Sun translate and move between these two practices with incredible dexterity. These hybrid processes are not repressed, as in Latour's account. Many doctors enthusiastically embrace them. But their significance in constituting the contemporary practice of Chinese medicine is rarely recognized. It will be necessary to grasp how the processes of purification and hybridization work together to understand the postcolonial condition of Chinese medicine.[9]

Three Dualisms

To tell the story of the postcolonial transformation of Chinese medicine, I have organized the book around three dualisms that capture key dynamics of contemporary Chinese medicine theory and practice. Each dualism is taken from a popular expression about the relative strengths of Western medicine and Chinese medicine with regard to the speed of therapeutic action, the nature of the body, and the method of diagnosis. These are not the only comparisons one hears, but I consider them to be the most important.[10] They are common in everyday conversation amongst laypersons, but also are widely shared between doctors. They are not arbitrary opinions about the two medical practices. Rather, they are the pillars of a discursive formation that organizes the relationship between Chinese medicine and Western, particularly in the absence of an accepted theory to guide this intellectual work. Each dualism operates according to the two processes of Latour's Modern Constitution, both as an axis of purification that divides Chinese medicine from Western medicine and as a device for translation that facilitates hybrid blendings of the two medical practices.

One extremely important feature of these dualisms is that they are all recent inventions of the Communist era. There is no historiographic evidence that these comparisons existed in the Republican era (1911–49) or earlier. To help the reader better understand the postcolonial transformation of contemporary Chinese medicine, I have organized each dualism as a distinct story that allows me to combine both historical and ethnographic materials to explain the emergence of contemporary Chinese medicine. Each story begins in the Republican period, when Chinese medicine and Western medicine were not considered incommensurate forms of medical practice. Then I trace the emergence of the dualisms around the issues of therapy, bodies, and diagnosis in the Communist period, demonstrating how they produced new ontological divides and concomitant hybridities.

I believe there are several advantages to this organizational structure. First, it allows me to explore the complexities of the postcolonial transformation of Chinese medicine by traversing the same epistemic and clinical transitions from three unique but complementary perspectives. By teasing apart these different dimensions of the postcolonial transformation of Chinese medicine, I can begin with dualisms that are simpler for the lay reader to follow and gradually progress to the more technical ones that are at the heart of contemporary clinical practice. Second, this approach allows me to integrate my ethnographic research with a significant amount of historical research that I was able to conduct after my graduation from the Beijing University of Chinese Medicine.[11] In doing so, I hope to bridge a concerning divide in the scholarship on Chinese medicine in which historical research has often been divorced from the contemporary concerns of clinical practice and ethnographic research mistakes recent innovations for timeless, ahistorical traditions. Third, this approach will also show that the most intense period of domination—and change—within the profession of Chinese medicine took place during the postcolonial moment, after the establishment of the People's Republic of China in 1949, rather than the early twentieth century as some historians of medicine have argued.

Although all three dualisms share a similar historical trajectory and reflect a shared postcolonial dynamic, they are some important differences. The first two comparisons—what I call the acute-chronic and structure-function dualisms—are simpler stories. Each can be told in the space of a single book chapter. In Chapter 1, I examine the prejudice that Chinese medicine is only suitable for treating chronic illnesses, as expressed in the phrase that "Western medicine treats acute illnesses; Chinese medicine treats chronic illnesses" (*xiyi zhi jixingbing; zhongyi zhi manxingbing*). I show that doctors of Chinese medicine were widely recognized for their skill in treating acute conditions during the Republican era. However, the efforts of the Communist state to build a national healthcare system in the 1950s dramatically affected this perception and resulted in a major clinical shift toward the treatment of chronic conditions. In Chapter 2, I argue that the popular expression "Western medicine treats structural pathologies; Chinese medicine treats functional pathologies" (*xiyi zhi qizhixing bingbian; zhongyi zhi gongnengxing bingbian*) is also a Communist-era development. The structure-function dualism tends to constrain clinicians, limiting them to less serious "functional" conditions and reserving the more serious "structural" ones for doctors of Western medicine.

The third comparison—what I call the disease-pattern dichotomy—is the most complex of the three dualisms, because the concepts of disease and pattern are essential to everyday clinical practice. I have devoted four chapters to discussing this dualism; two chapters are focused on the historical emergence of key concepts and two others on exploring their implications for clinical practice. This part of the book is inspired by the popular expression that "Western medicine diagnoses disease; Chinese medicine diagnoses patterns of disharmony" (*xiyi bianbing; zhongyi bianzheng*) and makes an in-depth exploration of the key clinical methodology of Chinese medicine, known as "pattern discrimination and treatment determination" (*bianzheng lunzhi*). In Chapter 3, I argue that this dualism did not yet exist in the Republican period, although key innovations around the practice of diagnosis set the stage for its emergence in the Communist era. In Chapter 4, I highlight the importance of the new institutions of Chinese medicine, in particular the development of standardized, national textbooks in the early 1960s. This is when "pattern discrimination and treatment determination" was defined as the key methodology of Chinese medicine. In Chapter 5, I turn toward the specifics of clinical medicine. Following a medical case in detail, I show how the disease-pattern dualism makes possible a truly hybrid form of institutionalized medicine through the use of "pattern discrimination and treatment determination." Although this methodology should be recognized as the greatest innovation of the contemporary Chinese medicine profession, the quintessential technology for navigating the postcolonial predicament of Chinese medicine, I argue that it can easily succumb to the power inequalities of contemporary practice. It may even inadvertently marginalize Chinese medicine therapies in everyday hospital work. In Chapter 6, I turn to another clinical case, recounted by Dr. Sun, that offers an alternative look at "pattern discrimination and treatment determination." We see that in the hands of a virtuoso physician this methodology can be the basis for innovation and a reinvigoration of the discipline.

Two Audiences

As a medical student at the Beijing University of Chinese Medicine in the 1990s, I was one of only a handful of students from outside East Asia in the entire school. Both my classmates and teachers were curious about why I had chosen to study Chinese medicine. To my surprise, I found it very difficult to answer this question. At first, I thought that the problem must be my Chinese language skills. I would explain that I came as an anthropology graduate student, interested in doing research on Chinese medicine for my Ph.D. dissertation, but that I was now also hoping to become a doctor of Chinese medicine. I knew that anthropology, especially cultural anthropology, was a relatively unknown academic field in China, so I would typically give a brief introduction to the field as well.[12] These crude explanations were inevitably met with baffled expressions. More than a few individuals came to the exact same conclusion: "So your Ph.D. research has actually nothing to do with your study of Chinese medicine."

After many such exasperating conversations, I eventually realized that something more profound than my non-native language skills was at the root of our miscommunication. What these friends wanted to know was not why an anthropologist was studying Chinese medicine, but what *was the relevance of anthropological research* to the study of Chinese medicine? To be interested in doing research on Chinese medicine was perfectly understandable. Professors, doctors, and graduate students at Chinese medicine institutions across the country are engaged in research on Chinese medicine. But their methodologies, usually clinical trials and laboratory research, are borrowed from biomedical research protocols. Unfamiliar with the anthropological study of medicine, these individuals wanted to know, quite reasonably, what kind of outcomes could be expected from this different type of research. When I had finally grasped the source of these misunderstandings, I was dismayed to realize that I had no answer to this question. In fact, I had been trained to ponder it in the inverse: what is the relevance of Chinese medicine to anthropology? At the most empirical level, I believed that my research would add to the ethnographic record on Chinese medicine, a record that remains relatively thin today. At the theoretical level, a successful project might provide insights into the nature of indigenous healing systems, offer critical perspectives on Western medicine, or perhaps even contribute new approaches to the field of medical anthropology. Regardless of its ultimate impact, I knew that my research could only constitute itself as anthropology by orienting itself toward the academic discipline of anthropology, a field that was for better or worse centered on the academic institutions of the West. The vector of this scholarship had to begin with the community of the research subjects and end with the community of anthropologists.

My Chinese medicine classmates and teachers were confused because they had assumed the opposite directionality to my research. They wanted to know how the world of anthropology could contribute to Chinese medicine. How might anthropological methodologies expand Chinese medicine research protocols? Could it provide better criteria for evaluating clinical efficacy? Could it provide evidence for the scientific basis of Chinese medicine? How could it help Chinese medicine attain more international recognition? Since my research did not seem to address any pressing concerns such as these, they naturally just assumed that it had "nothing" to do with Chinese medicine.

When I began my studies at the Beijing University of Chinese Medicine, I was an anthropologist in search of a research topic. When I finished five years later, I was a doctor of Chinese medicine, still pursuing my ethnographic research interests but also deeply interested in practicing clinical medicine. One of my important motivations in writing this book has been to search for an answer to those persistent questions about the relevance of anthropology to the study of Chinese medicine, not just for all those friends who couldn't understand my garbled explanations the first time around, but for myself as well. Does my research as an anthropologist have relevance to my practice as a doctor? Can it help me, or more importantly, my classmates, teachers, and other colleagues of Chinese medicine, who have never studied anthropology, become better doctors or scholars? I hope that it will. I have written this book for (at least) two audiences: readers interested in anthropology *and* doctors of Chinese medicine. One of my struggles in trying to write for these two readerships that know so little about each other has been to find a language and a narrative structure that both groups can understand and find meaningful. If, after reading this book, anthropologists can appreciate the richness, the clinical potentialities, and the significance of Chinese medicine practice for a postcolonial world, and if doctors and scholars of Chinese medicine can better understand the social, historical, and political terrain of their practice, then I will have achieved my goal. The story of contemporary Chinese medicine is too significant for audiences around the world to not know it better. The perspectives of anthropology, history, and other humanities are too important, I believe, for doctors of Chinese medicine not to understand them more deeply.

1
Efficacies of the State

For many observers outside China, the efficacy of Chinese medicine remains in doubt or is only now just tentatively being confirmed by double-blind clinical trials for a few specific interventions. Inside China, the picture is more complicated. Although there is no shortage of detractors who reject Chinese medicine as a superstitious practice with little clinical merit, many people believe that the efficacy of Chinese medicine is already well established for a very wide range of conditions. But these supporters, including doctors of Chinese medicine, also recognize limits to its effectiveness. One of the most notable limitations is that Chinese medicine is considered slow acting, making it more suitable for chronic diseases, where speed is not a requirement of the therapeutic intervention. This claim is almost always made in comparison to the efficacy of Western medicine, which is considered to be fast acting and more appropriate for acute conditions. Thus, one of the most commonly heard claims about the two medical systems is that "Western medicine treats acute diseases; Chinese medicine treats chronic diseases" (*xiyi zhi jixingbing; zhongyi zhi manxingbing*). To laypersons and doctors alike, this maxim expresses one of the fundamental differences between the two medical systems and their therapeutic potentials. It is the basis for what I call the "acute-chronic dualism," one of the key postcolonial formulations that contributed to the transformation of Chinese medicine in the second half of the twentieth century.

Expressions like this one are much more than an innocent comparison of Chinese medicine and Western medicine. These perceptions of efficacy shape patients' health-seeking behaviors, doctors' clinical decisions, and the organization of the hospital itself. In today's hospitals of Chinese medicine,

Chinese medicine therapies are favored in the outpatient clinic, where patients tend to have less acute conditions, while Western medicine predominates in the inpatient wards and is used almost exclusively in the Emergency Care Department. The acute-chronic dualism has become one important way that doctors negotiate the relationship between Chinese medicine and Western medicine. Behind its veil of linguistic symmetry, it inscribes unequal power relations: Western medicine is essential for the treatment of acute, critical conditions; Chinese medicine is only appropriate for chronic, less severe illnesses.

Scholars and administrators have recognized that this perceived lack of efficacy in the treatment of acute conditions is a problem for the Chinese medicine profession. In the early 1980s, the Chinese Medicine Department at the Ministry of Health began organizing training courses in Chinese Emergency Medicine. Huang Xingyuan (黄星垣), a widely respected doctor and important contributor to some of the early editions of the national textbooks (see Chapter 4), was entrusted with bringing together the materials from these courses into one of the first texts devoted to this topic (Huang Xingyuan 1985).[1] Projects such as this one eventually led to the development of a new textbook in 1997 (a new volume for the sixth- edition national textbooks of Chinese medicine) called *Chinese Emergency Medicine* (中医急诊学). I happened to be a fourth-year medical student at the Beijing University of Chinese Medicine when this textbook was first introduced to Chinese medical school curriculums across the country. Although this course was allotted a relatively small number of hours compared to the major courses such as Chinese Internal Medicine, Chinese Gynecology, (Western) Internal Medicine, and Surgery, the teaching staff repeatedly reminded us of its importance. Typically, minor specialization courses such as this one would have been taught by junior faculty instructors. For the Chinese Emergency Medicine class, however, many of the most respected clinicians from Dongzhimen Hospital were invited to lecture to the class.

But the energy of this experimental new class did not carry over into our clinical training. When I began my clerkship in the Emergency Medicine Department, a required part of our clinical training, it was immediately apparent that doctors in this department rarely used Chinese medicine therapies. Unlike the outpatient services or inpatient wards, where Chinese medicine is usually part of the treatment even though patients may also receive biomedical therapies, few patients in the Emergency Medicine Department received any Chinese medicine treatments at all. At the time, my clinical teacher, Li Li, was particularly focused on mastering the department's new ventilator; her skill in intubating patients and operating this machine would be decisive in saving lives. Likewise, her colleagues prided themselves on their command of other life-saving Western medicine interventions.

The absence of Chinese medicine in the Emergency Room was not openly discussed—it was too routinized to merit this kind of attention—but it clearly reflected more than the preferences of a few doctors. Structurally, the department was not set up to use Chinese medicine to provide acute emergency medical care. When I asked doctors why they did not use more Chinese medicine therapies, they often pointed to various logistical hurdles, such as the challenge of preparing herbal medicine prescriptions. In Chinese medicine hospitals, herbal medicine represents the dominant therapeutic modality. Herbal prescriptions consist of a combination of herbs, often a dozen or more that must be weighed, assembled, and decocted before they can be administered. Outpatient visitors will need to wait one to two hours for the hospital pharmacy to fill a prescription of raw, uncooked herbs. Admitted patients typically wait about four to five hours because their prescriptions must also be cooked and delivered to the patient's room. Thus, if an attending physician orders a new herbal prescription for an admitted patient following the morning rounds, the patient will not receive the actual decoction until the midafternoon. In addition to these logistical delays, which complicate the timely delivery of herbal prescriptions to emergency room patients, there was an additional obstacle that functionally precluded the use of herbal medicine by Emergency Medicine doctors when I was doing my rotation—the Chinese medicine pharmacy closed at five P.M. every day. Only the Western medicine pharmacy was open in the evenings, when a majority of admissions to the Emergency Medicine Department were being made.

None of these obstacles should have been insurmountable, and doctors were certainly thinking about solutions. When I was a student in the 1990s, many of my teachers were calling for the development of new drug forms (ji-xing) so that the cumbersome decoction preparation process could be circumvented. One such example that I saw being used in the Emergency Medicine Department was herbal medicine infusions, such as Qing Kai Ling (Clearing and Opening Infusion), based on the famous traditional bolus known as Calming the Palace Bovine Bezoar Pill (An Gong Niu Huang Wan). This formula was often given intravenously for cases of acute strokes or high fevers but almost always used in combination with other Western medicine therapies.[2] Other than a handful of such infusions, however, Chinese medicine interventions were so infrequent during my clerkship in the Emergency Room that I clearly remember one day when all the medical students came running to watch a doctor attempt an acupuncture treatment. The patient had suffered a stroke. He was unconscious, breathing with difficulty, and febrile, perhaps because of an infection that had not been identified yet. The admitting doctor had already initiated several Western medicine interventions, and one of the residents decided to try an acupuncture treatment to help lower the patient's fever. He pricked the patient at the ten fingertips, known as the *shi xuan* acupuncture points, squeezing a couple drops of blood from each finger. A half dozen students crowded around one side of the bed as the resident worked to squeeze out drops of blood, one fingertip at a time. To our delight, the treatment worked, and the patient's temperature began to inch downward, until it had fallen about one degree Celsius in fifteen minutes.

Not all medical emergencies take place in a hospital Emergency Medicine Department. I witnessed quite a few critical situations during my inpatient clerkships. But no matter where they occurred, the medical response I witnessed was consistent with what I observed in the Emergency Medicine Department. Doctors of Chinese medicine turned to Western medicine when acute and urgent medical conditions arose. Chinese medicine was too slow-acting, it seemed, to be effective in emergency situations. As I had heard on so many occasions, it seemed as if Western medicine was required for acute conditions and Chinese medicine was best reserved for chronic ones. I would have never thought twice about this seemingly unassailable claim until I was fortunate enough to get funding for an oral history project in which I interviewed over forty senior physicians who had studied and practiced Chinese medicine in the Republican period (1911–49). These conversations were among some of the most scintillating that I have ever had about Chinese medicine, and I felt honored to have been welcomed into the homes, offices, and clinics of these doctors. Through these interviews, I learned, to my surprise, that in the early twentieth century, doctors and patients alike celebrated the speed of Chinese medicine and considered it essential for the treatment of acute illnesses. Western medicine, by contrast, was considered to be clinically limited in its applications.

How did the perceptions of Chinese medicine and Western medicine change so dramatically in such a short period of time? If these doctors were correct in their recollections, how could one of the clinical strengths of Chinese medicine be forgotten so quickly? To answer these questions, we must reassess many of the assumptions about the twentieth-century history of Chinese medicine. But before embarking on this task, it will be essential to first reflect more broadly about how one assesses clinical efficacy in general. This issue will be decisive in understanding how the clinical practice of Chinese medicine underwent a major therapeutic reorientation in the Communist era.

The Authority to Judge

"Does it work?"

This is the question that I have been asked most frequently about Chinese medicine. I almost always stumble in response. Of course, it works, I usually say, but not in every instance. It may depend on the skill of the doctor, the patient's condition, how the treatment is given. My compulsion to articulate these caveats, which only reinforce the doubts of the interlocutor, remind us how rarely the question is asked of Western medicine. Western medicine therapies are widely assumed to work, even if many specific therapies fail or work imperfectly. If one were pressed to explain this belief in the efficacy of Western medicine, then one might point to a vast body of research, based on randomized control trials. This form of epistemological authority, however, is a relatively recent invention that only dates to the 1950s. Joseph Dumit has argued that clinical trials are profoundly shaped by the commercial imperatives of the pharmaceutical companies that run them and are far from transparent, unambiguous arbiters of therapeutic efficacy (Dumit 2012). Yet despite the critical work of Dumit and other scholars, the efficacy of biomedicine is generally not questioned, either in the West or in China. By contrast, the efficacy of Chinese medicine may be doubted, as it generally has been in the West, or it may be tentatively granted for certain clinical situations, as is sometimes the case in China.

How does one assess the efficacy of Chinese medicine? There have been countless clinical trials and other studies of Chinese medicine. These sorts of biomedically inspired studies are an important part of contemporary research agendas and often essential to the career trajectories of doctors and professors. While they serve important institutional needs, doctors generally do not reference them in their clinical work. During all my months of clinical training and the countless hours I spent "copying prescriptions" with senior doctors, it was rare to hear a doctor reference "the latest study" when designing a treatment. On occasion, doctors might mention a recent pharmacological study on an individual herb as a rationale for including it in a prescription. But treatment principles, key formulas, and the rationale for a particular intervention were not justified by clinical studies. The major reason for this general disinterest is that Chinese medicine therapies are not designed to treat modern biomedical disease categories, which is an essential feature of a randomized clinical trial. As we will see later in the book, Chinese medicine therapies are crafted around a different diagnostic concept known as *zheng* (证), which is usually translated as "pattern" or "pattern of disharmonies" (Kaptchuk 2000). Moreover, treatments do not contain an isolated pharmacological compound that targets a specific disease or even a specific *zheng*. Instead, herbal medicine formulas consist of *combinations* of medicinal herbs that are designed to address the underlying pattern of disharmony, to help patients achieve an equilibrium in their bodies, but not to interrupt a pathological process as it would be understood in Western medicine. Senior doctors often scoff at the whole enterprise of biomedically inspired research protocols as an exercise in getting the "rats to nod in agreement" (*haozi dian tou*). Younger doctors often must engage in this sort of research for the sake of their career trajectories, but when they seek to improve their clinical craft, their primary interest is in an opportunity to "copy prescriptions" with a senior doctor.

In the absence of clinical trials to authorize therapeutic decisions, Judith Farquhar has shown that doctors of Chinese medicine value "experience" (*jingyan*) above all else, as a guide to clinical action (Farquhar 1994). But as the following vignette shows, "experience" is epistemologically weak, not only in relation to the knowledge claims of Western medicine, but also against the agendas of state authorities (Lei 2002). It was only during the Communist era that the interests of the state and the claims of Western medicine merged in such a way as to devalue the practices of Chinese medicine. The following vignette was recounted to me by Wang Juyi (王居易), a much-admired Beijing acupuncturist and the first doctor that I interviewed for my oral history project. It was only after I had completed this project that I realized this story answered one of the questions that became central to these interviews—how Chinese medicine became efficacious only for chronic diseases. This story takes place around 1961 and shows that in the early 1960s the authority to assess the clinical efficacy of Chinese medicine had shifted decisively into the hands of the Western medicine profession. While it does not discuss the acute-chronic dualism directly, it does capture the historical moment and the new conditions of clinical practice that led to the emergence of this dualism.

When I met Wang Juyi in 2008, he had already retired from his original work unit, the Beijing Hospital of Chinese Medicine, where he had worked for more than forty years. He used to treat dozens of patients each day, sometimes as many as 120 individuals in a day, at this well-known hospital in the center of Beijing. I visited with him at his small private clinic in the southwest of Beijing, one of the sleepier corners of the city. He enjoyed the slow pace of his own clinic, accepting only patients who came to him through personal introductions. He gave himself plenty of time to treat each patient carefully and then perhaps step into another room for a cigarette break. I had the good fortune to listen to some of his thoughtful lectures on meridian theory in the fall of 2008, shortly after I had arrived in Beijing to begin my oral history project. After we finished the weeklong course, I asked Wang Juyi if he would agree to be interviewed. Wang Juyi was born in 1937 and had been a member of the first class of students to matriculate at the Beijing College of Chinese Medicine (now called the Beijing University of Chinese Medicine). He was younger than some of the other doctors I would be interviewing later, but I knew he would have many insights about Chinese medicine in the early years of the People's Republic, when today's institutions were just being established.

Wang Juyi's memories of his student years were rich and included many fond anecdotes about his teachers, who would become revered figures in the contemporary world of Chinese medicine. But his most remarkable story concerned a treatment that he personally witnessed by the famous bonesetter Liu Shoushan (刘寿山). He often told this story to his students to encourage them and show them what was possible in the hands of a clinical virtuoso. I share it here as an example of the new standards of truth and clinical efficacy that were quickly becoming hegemonic in the early Communist period.

Liu Shoushan lived from 1901 to 1980, and his career spanned the great social and political upheavals of both the Republican and Communist eras. He managed to become an excellent doctor despite the enormous challenges that he faced as a young man. He was recruited to join the Bonesetting Unit (*Zhenggu Zhuanke*) in the Chinese External Medicine Department (*Zhongyi Waike*) at the Dongzhimen Hospital in 1959, one year after the establishment of the hospital. According to the hospital gazette, the unique skills of Liu Shoushan (and his student Xi Da) transformed the Bonesetting Unit from an unremarkable division of a half dozen doctors with few patients to a dynamic subspecialty with 80–100 outpatient visits per day (Dongzhimen Hospital Gazette Office 1997, 67). In 1962, Dongzhimen hospital formed an independent Orthopedics Department out of the Bonesetting Unit, with Liu Shoushan as the chief.

Because Dongzhimen Hospital was the main affiliated hospital of the Beijing College of Chinese Medicine, Wang Juyi got the chance to work closely with Liu Shoushan during his medical training. One of the striking things that he noted about his teacher, beyond his impressive clinical skills, was the fact that he was illiterate. In today's institutionalized healthcare system, a bachelor's degree in medicine is the minimum requirement to work as a doctor in a Beijing hospital, and beginning in the 1990s doctors found it difficult to progress professionally without a master's or Ph.D. But during the Republican era, there were few legal barriers to practicing medicine, making it possible, albeit still very difficult, for someone as poor and disadvantaged as Liu Shoushan to become a doctor. Liu Shoushan grew up in the countryside of Hebei Province and never learned to read or write. He came to Beijing as a teenager to work in a small restaurant run by a distant relative near Longfu Temple. One of the frequent patrons of this small restaurant happened to be a famous bonesetter, Wen Peiting. Liu Shoushan was a particularly attentive waiter, often putting aside a portion of the doctor's favorite dishes so that he could still enjoy them even if he arrived after the restaurant had sold out of these items. Eventually, the doctor become aware of the special service and thanked the owner of the restaurant, only then learning that it was Liu Shoushan who had been saving the dishes for him. According to Wang Juyi, the doctor was so struck by this young teenager's thoughtfulness, he asked the owner if he could take him on as a disciple. The owner immediately brought Liu Shoushan over to the doctor and told him to kowtow to his new teacher. Liu Shoushan then moved in with his teacher, and like a typical disciple, began by helping with chores around the house and clinic as he learned his new trade. Every day, he practiced martial arts and the other physical skills needed in bonesetting. Because he was illiterate, his teacher would read important passages from medical texts out loud so that Liu Shoushan would commit them to memory. He supposedly was able to memorize entire books in this fashion.

Despite his impressive clinical skills, Liu Shoushan represented a problem for Dongzhimen Hospital and for the profession in general. How could an illiterate bonesetter be regarded as a doctor in modern China? How can doctors of Chinese medicine work in institutionalized settings without an education in modern medicine? These conundrums came to a head one day with a clinical case that Wang Juyi happened to witness. On this day, a group of Western medicine doctors were also with Liu Shoushan in his outpatient clinic. These doctors were participants in the experimental new program to train doctors of Western medicine in Chinese medicine (*xiyi xuexi zhongyi*). Launched in 1955 by enthusiastic Communist party leaders, and later endorsed by Mao Zedong, this program was designed to produce a new kind of doctor with systematic training in both medical systems. Mao Zedong predicted that they would create a "new medicine (*xinyi*)" that would dialectically supersede its predecessors. Unfortunately, most of the participants were far less enthusiastic than these party leaders. Many joined the program under pressure from local leaders; some were even scornful of Chinese medicine and considered their enrollment in this program as a form of punishment.

The patient was a young boy from the countryside who had broken his tibia and fibula. The bones had not been set, and they had healed together in a malunion that prevented the boy from properly supporting his weight with this leg. His father had already taken him to numerous doctors, who had all told him that it was too late to reset the fracture and there was nothing that could be done. In desperation, he had brought his son to Liu Shoushan. While Liu Shoushan examined the boy, the Western medicine doctors looked at his X-ray and immediately concluded that there was indeed no treatment. The surgical techniques and spatial frames that are now used in Western medicine to treat such problems did not exist at this time. The condescension of these Western medicine doctors toward Liu Shoushan, who had never studied anatomy and knew little about reading X-rays, was palpable. Deferring to their expertise, Liu Shoushan turned to the boy and father and said, "I can't treat this." The father began to beg. "We've come to you because all the Western medicine doctors said it can't be treated. My son lives in the countryside. If his leg is crippled, he can't work. He can't survive. In the countryside, we need to do physical labor to survive. Please save us." "Save you?" Liu Shoushan said dismissively. "There is nothing that can be done. If Western medicine doctors already say that there is nothing that can be done, there is even less than can be done with Chinese medicine." The father dropped down to his knees and pleaded, "Doctor, you must save me, save our family." Touched by this display of emotion, Liu Shoushan helped the father up. "Don't be like that. Take your son outside, and we will discuss it."

In the discussion that followed, the Western medicine doctors remained adamant that there was nothing to be done for this child. Once fractures heal, the new bone is just as strong as the original bone, making it impossible rebreak it at the original site for a proper setting. Any attempt would only produce a new fracture, further compounding the boy's problem. Perhaps moved more by the father's pleas than the doctors' pessimism, Liu Shoushan called the father back in. "I'm willing to give it try. If it works, you're in luck. If it doesn't, then it just means I don't have the talent." "Please just give it try," the father pleaded. "It doesn't matter if it doesn't work." "Okay, but don't tell your son." Liu Shoushan sent the father out to bring in the son, and while he waited, he walked across the room several times, carefully measuring his steps. After the son came in, he did a second examination and said to him, "We can't treat this problem right now. I'm going to give you some medicine to wash your leg. It might help a little. When you walk, stand up straight. Don't always walk so bent over." The boy said, "So you can't fix it." "I am going to give you some medicine. That will help." It seemed that after a second exam, Liu Shoushan had reconsidered his intentions. The boy said, "Thank you, grandfather." The father started to lead him out, but just as they got to the door, Liu Shoushan leapt forward, delivering a swift kick to the boy's leg. The boy shrieked and crumpled to the ground. The doctors immediately carried him to the X-ray room. Sure enough, Liu Shoushan had broken the leg at the exact point of the original fracture. He reset the fracture, and the boy was on his way toward a full recovery.[3]

From the perspective of contemporary medical practice, the striking thing about this medical case is that Liu Shoushan's treatment "worked." Mei Zhan has argued that in contemporary Chinese society a successful Chinese medicine treatment has the aura of a miracle, as if the doctor has somehow defied the laws of nature (Zhan 2009, 93). Wang Juyi certainly saw this case as almost "miraculous" (hen shen). It taught him that Chinese medicine "contains profound practical experience, experience that is extremely valuable. . . . Its value cannot be denied." But part of the miraculous aura of this event was that Liu Shoushan's clinical virtuosity was witnessed by a group of Western medicine doctors. He had treated the very condition they had declared untreatable. It was only after completing my oral history project that I understood two other essential elements of this medical case. First, it almost never happened. If it hadn't been for the desperation of the father, Liu Shoushan would have simply followed the recommendations of the Western medicine doctors and turned the patient away. Second, the timing of this case, its historical moment, provided the conditions for the treatment to proceed despite the objections of the Western medicine observers. The early 1960s was the historical moment when doctors of Western medicine and Chinese medicine were first brought together within a single institution. As I will discuss in more detail, doctors of Western medicine were involved in the setup and operation of all hospitals of Chinese medicine in the Communist era. Very few doctors of Chinese medicine had worked in an institutional setting prior to 1949. In the intimacy of this new encounter between the two professions, it was imperative to establish new ways of evaluating the efficacy of Chinese medicine. When Liu Shoushan initially declined to treat the child, he was showing deference to the new, emerging standards of clinical care that were being articulated by doctors of Western medicine, who in turn represented one of the most important policies of the Chinese state to reform Chinese medicine. When Liu Shoushan changed his mind and decided to treat the child, he was invoking a different kind of clinical authority: his experience (jingyan), honed through years of clinical practice. Although he won this contest for epistemological authority, it is not hard to imagine that lesser physicians would have never questioned these new standards. When it came to the treatment of acute illnesses in the early Communist era, the authority of the Chinese state would prevail over the experience of Chinese medicine doctors.

Acute Illness in the Republican Period

When I began my oral history project, I had little doubt that Chinese medicine was too slow to be effective for most acute conditions. Thus, I was surprised—in fact incredulous at first—when my interviewees recounted story after story about treating acute, infectious diseases during the early days of their careers. These accounts diverged so radically from my own observations of contemporary clinical practice and from the standard historical accounts of early twentieth-century medicine in China that they were instrumental in helping me formulate the central thesis of this book—that Chinese medicine underwent a postcolonial transformation in the Communist era. As we see subsequently, Chinese medicine was not considered slow-acting during the Republican period, nor was Western medicine assumed to be fast-acting. There was no acute-chronic dualism, and despite some of the polemical rhetoric of this era, doctors of Chinese medicine did not believe there was a fundamental, ontological chasm separating the two medical practices. These perceptions would only take hold in the Communist era.

My interviewees' accounts of treating acute illness were numerous. Zhou Zhongying (周仲瑛) of Nanjing recalled assisting his father in successfully treating many cases of smallpox during epidemics in 1946, 1947, and 1948.[4] He also remembered his father saving the lives of cholera patients in another 1946 epidemic, often using formulas like Poria Five Powder (*Wu Ling San*) to open up yang and transform qi (*tongyang huaqi*) (Wang Zhiying et al. 2008, 16–18). Zhu Liangchun (朱良春), from Nantong, told me how he first made a name for himself during a dengue fever epidemic in 1940.[5] Drawing on his apprenticeship experience with two different teachers, he was able to cure most of his patients from this disease in just three days (Cao Dongyi 2008, 92–97). Shen Fengge (沈凤阁), who grew up in Chongmingdao, not far from Shanghai, remembered accompanying his teacher as he made home visits to the sickest patients. "They all had acute illnesses with fevers . . . such as pneumonia, typhoid, dysentery, malaria. . . . His results were very good . . . and he was a very prestigious man."[6]

A close reading of scholarship on this period also corroborates the importance of treating acute illness. For example, many of the famous physicians of the Menghe current, renowned for a clinical style that emphasized "harmonization and gentleness" and catering to a well-heeled clientele that preferred mild therapies, established their reputations by curing acute, infectious diseases with fast-acting herbs. Chao Shaofang (1896–1950) was famous for treating meningitis and other infectious diseases (Scheid 2007, 150). Ding Ganren, one of the best-known doctors and reformers of the early Republican period, struggled to establish himself as a young doctor in Shanghai, until he acquired fame for his successful treatments during a scarlet fever (*lan hou sha*) outbreak in 1896 (Scheid 2007, 228). As Zhang Qi (张琪), the senior physician from Harbin explained to me, doctors not only commonly treated acute conditions in the Republican period, but "they became famous as doctors of Chinese medicine because they were famous for treating acute diseases (*zhongyi cheng-ming de ren dou shi zhiliao jixing bing chengming de*)."

The recollections of this last generation of doctors who personally studied and practiced during the Republican period painted a picture of clinical prac-tice that was so divergent from contemporary clinical work that it rasied a host of new questions. How could Chinese medical practice change so quickly in a matter of a few decades? How could a fast-acting medicine, indispens-able to the care of acute illnesses, become an impotent bystander in today's emergency rooms? Had Western medicine raced ahead, leapfrogging over its competitor by virtue of its numerous technological developments? It should be acknowledged that many, if not most, of the Western medicine therapies that are central to emergency medicine today—from antibiotics to fight acute infections and catecholamines to maintain blood pressure during shock, to ventilators to assist breathing and CTs to make rapid diagnostic assessments—were only developed in the last half of the twentieth century. But these de-velopments do not fully explain the almost categorical nature of the claims about Chinese medicine today. Doctors and patients alike think of Chinese medicine as not just relatively slow-acting but absolutely so, inherently so. As I will show in the remainder of this chapter, the apparent slowness of Chi-nese medicine is part of a broader transformation of this medical system that includes, among other things, a loss of knowledge and a collective amnesia about how to treat acute conditions.

This failure of medical transmission is captured most emphatically for me by a story told by one of my clinical teachers. In the fall of 1999, prior to my stint in the Emergency Medicine Department, I was doing a clerkship in the Gerontology Department at Dongzhimen Hospital. I noticed that all ad-mitted patients were being treated with antibiotics whenever they had signs of an infection. One day, I asked one of the attending physicians, Hu Yuning, whether it was possible to rely on Chinese medicine alone to handle these infections. At first, she said she wasn't sure. Department policy was to always use antibiotics when indicated. But she mused some more and recalled one of her own medical cases that she had treated outside the hospital. She had been asked to treat a family friend, an elderly woman, who had contracted a case of bacterial pneumonia. The woman was trying to avoid a stay in the hospital and asked Dr. Hu to write her a prescription. She quickly wrote her a prescription for antibiotics, but the woman refused it and demanded a Chinese medicine prescription. Dr. Hu was taken aback. Pneumonia is a serious condition in the elderly, with a high mortality rate, and not something to be trifled with. Her eyes widening, Hu Yuning looked straight at me as she delivered the final lines of her story. "This woman had lobar pneumonia and refused to take antibiotics. I thought she had a death wish. But she insisted, and I had no choice but to write her a Chinese medicine prescription. To my surprise, she got better!"

Dr. Hu had been shocked by her own success. At the time, neither she nor I saw her account as evidence that Chinese medicine might be useful for a whole array of acute illnesses. The collective amnesia highlighted by this story, along with the unknown stories of my interviewees, gestures to a deep epistemic shift in the contemporary practice of Chinese medicine. That doctors, scholars, or laypersons are generally unaware of the "slowing down" of Chinese medicine is perhaps best understood through the work of Thomas Kuhn, Michel Foucault, and other scholars of historical epistemology, who have argued that rapid epistemic changes typically operate through erasures, through obfuscations that tend to minimize these transformations or place them within grander narratives of progressive knowledge accumulation (Kuhn 1970; Foucault 1971; Davidson 2001). I will explore the implications of this epistemic shift for the theoretical foundations of Chinese medicine in Chapter 4. In this chapter, I want to first outline the social conditions that made it seem inconceivable to Dr. Hu—and to countless other doctors of Chinese medicine—that she could cure a case of acute pneumonia with Chinese medicine alone. But first, we must reexamine the dominant narrative through which medicine in the Republican period has been studied: as a clash between the rapidly growing, modernizing profession of Western medicine and the traditional, out-of-step-with-the-times practitioners of Chinese medicine. Once we recognize the limitations of this narrative, we can explore the more powerful social and demographic forces that were transforming the field of medicine.

Contested Histories

One of the focal points of Republican-era medical history has been the struggle between the two professions of Western medicine and Chinese medicine. My interviewees' perspectives on this struggle would turn out to be a second key revelation from my oral history project. Historians generally agree that both professions were only just emerging in the early twentieth century. Zhao Hongjun has marked 1915 as the moment when Western medicine became an identifiable profession in China, because two professional associations of Western medicine were formed that year. He estimates that there may have only been 500–600 doctors of Western medicine in the whole country at that time, and among them perhaps only 300 who had received a formal and systematic education (Zhao Hongjun 1982, 115). While Chinese practitioners of Western-style medicine were too few to constitute a profession before this moment, doctors of Chinese medicine may have been too numerous and fragmented. Nonetheless, beginning at roughly the same time, Chinese medicine practitioners gradually began to develop some of the institutions associated with a modern medical profession—medical schools, journals, associations, and so on. Historians have observed the greatest growth in new medical institutions in the 1920s and 1930s (Zhao Hongjun 1982; Scheid 2007; Deng Tietao 1999; Andrews 2014).

These two emerging professions became deeply entangled in the complicated politics of this period. Doctors of Chinese medicine were becoming anxious about the political might of their new rivals. In the journals of Chinese medicine that proliferated during the 1920s and '30s, it is easy to find polemical pieces defending the value of Chinese medicine and denouncing the discrimination of government officials or other public figures. Doctors of Chinese medicine generally found political support among more conservative politicians. By contrast, doctors of Western medicine often became allied with the left-leaning and more radical political factions. Zhou Zuoren, younger brother of the great writer Lu Xun and a leading intellectual of this period in his own right, gave a relatively straightforward account of how the two new medical professions were becoming entangled in the larger political debates of this era. Writing in 1929, he explained his support for Western medicine, while acknowledging that he was a "complete outsider with regards to medicine."

> Why [do I support Western medicine]? To be honest, what I fear is the reactionary [forces] that seek a return to the ancients (*fugu*). China is currently in the midst of a reactionary trend. The debates between Chinese medicine and Western medicine are an expression of the resistance of the old forces to the new forces. . . . The return to the ancients [policies] have already been successful in many aspects. In politics or ethics, whatever is new is left or red and can be considered as a criminal act and punished as such. Only the new forces in medicine have not been categorized in such a way as to facilitate their repression, hence the clashes. . . . The fate of this isolated brigade will be closely followed (Fang Zhouzi 2007, 188).

The date of this excerpt from Zhou Zuoren is significant for medical histori-ans. In this same year, the Western-style doctor and political activist Yu Yunxiu (余雲岫) proposed a legislative bill to ban Chinese medicine. Although this bill failed to pass, it has come to symbolize the prejudice that has confronted the Chinese medicine profession for most of the twentieth century. In most scholarly accounts of this period, the existential threat posed by this event has been a central ingredient to the narrative that the two professions were embroiled in a life-and-death struggle.

Broadly speaking, historians have focused on two features of the Republican-era clash between the two professions. First, scholars such as Ralph Croizier and Zhao Hongjun have examined the intellectual debate about the value of Chinese medicine. Fueled by the radicalism of the May Fourth Move-ment, many Chinese intellectuals beginning in the 1920s called for the urgent dissemination of scientific knowledge. They perceived Chinese medicine as an obstacle to their aspirations to modernize Chinese society and attacked it as a remnant of the old society, an unscientific practice that perpetuated superstitious beliefs. Writers such as Lu Xun, Ba Jin, Lao She, and Zhou Zuoren mocked the ignorance of old-style doctors (Croizier 1968, 72–77). Liang Qichao famously lamented, "Yinyang and Five Phases doctrines have been the general headquarters for more than the two thousand years of super-stition. . . . The very medicine upon which the lives of our generation depend is the product of this type of concept" (Zhao Hongjun 1982, 225). The distaste for Chinese medicine was captured by the well-known historian Fu Sinian in a 1934 essay that he wrote for the *Ta Kung Pao*, one of the leading newspapers of this period.

> The most shameful, the most detestable, the most disheartening thing
> in China now . . . is this so-called debate between Chinese medicine
> and Western medicine. . . . Only the debate between Chinese medi-
> cine and Western medicine can fully expose the deep-rooted flaws of
> the Chinese people. How can the result of forty years of developing
> [modern] schools be that [the fate of] Chinese medicine is still a
> question! Individuals with modern education still accept the Chinese
> medicine nonsense about the Five Phases and Six Qi! Self-declared
> proponents of modernization are still using their political or social
> connections to protect Chinese medicine! Does this not demon-
> strate clearly that the minds of Chinese people have a fundamental
> problem? . . . That today we are still debating Chinese medicine and
> Western medicine demonstrates to the whole world that we are a
> different race of people. That we can't escape this medieval stage [of

development] after forty years of [modern] schools makes people feel
that [modern] education is futile (Fang Zhouzi 2007, 191).

Second, scholars such as Sean Lei and Bridie Andrews have addressed
some of the political struggles and institutional developments that paralleled
these intellectual debates. Both authors demonstrate that there was nothing
natural or inevitable about the development of Western medicine in China.
Doctors of Western medicine were quite effective in aligning themselves
with the biopolitical goals of the state and using their political power to their
advantage (Lei 2014; Andrews 2014). With the formation of the Nationalist
government in 1928 by the Kuomingtang (KMT), the two medical camps
became engaged in a bitter struggle for state resources and support. Following
the proposed bill to outlaw Chinese medicine in 1929, the Chinese medicine
profession effectively organized to stop this bill. By recruiting allies within
the KMT government, the Chinese medicine profession achieved a tenuous
but formal legal parity with Western medicine by the mid-1930s (Deng Tietao
1999, 177). The Republican-era clash between the two medical professions
was an important catalyst for change within the Chinese medicine community, further spurring the development of medical schools and journals, while
giving new urgency to reformist visions of Chinese medicine (Deng Tietao
1999, 176). Sean Lei has argued that these important changes were driven by
the "encounter with the state." By foregrounding the new role of the Chinese
state, made possible by the KMT's unification of the country through the new
Nationalist government, Lei was also able to explain why Western medicine
had been present in Chinese society for decades, promoted primarily by Western missionaries since the mid-nineteenth century, without having a major
impact on the practice of Chinese medicine (Lei 2014, 4–5).

Given the scholarly consensus around the "life-and-death struggle" narrative, the second surprising finding from my oral history interviews was that my
interviewees were either indifferent toward or more often just unaware that
such a struggle was even going on. Li Zhenhua (李振华) of Tianjin began
studying medicine with his grandfather in his home village in Hebei Province as a teenager in the 1930s. When I asked him why he would want to
study Chinese medicine, given the political climate and the prejudices against
Chinese medicine, he remarked, "I was young at the time, I didn't even know
there were two types of medicine." It was only later, after the death of his
grandfather, when he went to Beijing to continue his studies at a Republican-
era private school, the Beiping College of National Medicine (北平國醫學
院), several years later that he encountered the practice of Western medicine.
Another well-known doctor of the same name, Li Zhenhua (李振华), from

Luoning County in Henan Province, told me that he only learned of the Republican-era conflict after the establishment of the People's Republic in 1949. He Ren (何任), the famous physician from Hangzhou who attended the Shanghai New China College of Medicine (上海新中國醫學院) in 1938, explained that he was the third generation to study medicine in his family. "We never thought about why we would study Chinese medicine. This is what my father did, so this is what I was going to do. . . . At that time, [doctors of] Chinese medicine and Western medicine were engaged in a furious debate, but we were not aware of it."

Of the doctors that I interviewed, only two doctors seemed to be aware of this clash. Deng Tietao (邓铁涛), who was born in 1916, remembered following the debates in the Guangzhou newspapers as a young teenager, indignantly reading claims that ginseng had the clinical potency of a turnip. Later as a student at the Guangzhou Technical College of Chinese Medicine (廣州市中醫專門學校), his awareness of this struggle was invigorated by his teachers, some of whom had petitioned to stop the passage of the abolition bill. Deng Tietao has passionately defended the scientific value of Chinese medicine throughout his long career. I was not surprised that he had followed these debates closely—only that other doctors had not.

The only other doctor among my interviewees that followed this clash of medical professions was Gan Zuwang (干祖望). Born in 1912, he was a key figure in later helping to create the Ears, Nose, and Throat specialization within Chinese medicine. His response surprised me because it was so mischievous. He told me that he had great admiration for Yu Yunxiu and considered his book *Deliberations on the Divine Pivot and Simple Questions* (靈素商兑) to be one of the most important books on Chinese medicine. Prior to his proposed bill to abolish Chinese medicine, Yu's book, published in 1916, was one of the sharpest and most cogent attacks on Chinese medicine. He argued that the *Yellow Emperor's Inner Canon* (*Huangdi Neijing*; 皇帝內經), the most important ancient medical text in China, was "filled with innumerable mistakes" and based on "a crude anatomy, vague and empty discourse, and dim nothingness" (Yu Yunxiu 1932 [1928], 1). Relishing the irony of his views, Gan Zuwang told me that Yu Yunxiu "had insulted Chinese medicine, but he was right!"

Since we know that the clash between the two medical professions, in particular the abolition proposal, produced a strong political response by the Chinese medicine community, the question becomes, why were so many of my interview subjects ambivalent or even unaware of these events? They were certainly a bit too young to participate in the heady events of 1929 and its aftermath. But I had expected them to more like Deng Tietao—namely, to have been steeped in a political consciousness that would have shaped the rest of their medical careers. I think there are two reasons for their general lack of awareness. First, for all the polemics and scholarly attention that it has received, the struggle between the two professions was highly circumscribed. As the historian Zhao Hongjun has pointed out, the conflict was undoubtedly an urban phenomenon with its center in Shanghai. He notes that there were some sharp exchanges in Beijing and Tianjin, but many doctors in these cities on both sides advocated for the integration of the two medical systems (Zhao Hongjun 1982, 98–101). The textual documentation for this struggle has been easy to locate in the journals and other publications from this period, but scholars have mistakenly assumed that these documents represented the profession as a whole. The reflections of my interviewees will demonstrate the narrowness of that archival record—or perhaps that scholars have just read it too narrowly. My oral history project was also a circumscribed endeavor. The doctors that I interviewed were among the most successful young doctors to emerge out of the transition to the Communist period. Indeed, it was their contemporary fame that allowed me to find them. Yet as we will see, their own backgrounds were quite diverse, reminding us how complex the field of medical practice was during the Republican period.

Second, it is likely that doctors and scholars alike have all been shaped by the political agenda of the Chinese Communist Party (CCP), perhaps far more deeply than we have realized. Despite its own ambivalent record toward Chinese medicine, the CCP was eager to portray their adversaries as enemies of Chinese medicine. I remember clearly in my History of Medicine in China class at the Beijing University of Chinese Medicine that we were taught that Yu Yunxiu had "extreme prejudices" against Chinese medicine and that the KMT was determined to undermine the profession. It was only the determined action of the Chinese medicine community that was able to stave off the worst excesses of the Nationalist government. In the end, our textbook claimed that "the [Nationalist government] was unable to achieve their goal of eliminating Chinese medicine, [but] they did cause serious devastation to the medicine of the motherland" (Zhen Zhiya and Fu Weikang 1984, 131–32). This one-sided portrayal of the KMT ignores the sharp divisions within the party. Many members were strong supporters of Chinese medicine, and policy on Chinese medicine became a means for attacks against one's own enemies within the party. Zhao Hongjun has pointed out that the party leader, Chiang Kai-shek, never made a single public comment about Chinese medicine, demonstrating his utter indifference on this issue (Zhao Hongjun 1982, 138).

I cannot claim that my interviewees were ideal spokespersons for the sentiments of this era—they were the surviving few who were healthy enough and willing to be interviewed—but I suspect they did give a reasonable reflection of the urban parameters of this clash.[7] As we will see, other recollections from these doctors will continue to displace the centrality of the clash of medical professions' narrative, at least as far as clinical practice is concerned. Their memories of the demographics, the clinical institutions, and the nature of medical transmission in the late Republican and early Communist eras suggest an alternative history of this period that will help us understand how Chinese medicine became "slow medicine" after 1949.

The Numbers

One of the key facts of the Republican period, and perhaps the main reason that most doctors were unaffected by the clash between the two medical professions, is that doctors of Chinese doctors vastly outnumbered doctors of Western medicine. Almost all my interviewees reported that there were few, if any, doctors of Western medicine working in their vicinity. Li Jiren (李济人), born in 1931 in She County in Anhui Province, said there were no doctors of Western medicine near his home village when he was growing up. "In the countryside [at that time], you could say that 99 percent of the doctors were Chinese medicine doctors." Guo Zhongyuan, who was born in 1924 in Miyun County, outside of Beijing, recalled that there were four doctors of Chinese medicine in his small village of Daxingzhuang but only a couple doctors of Western medicine in the entire county. "They had worked as a nurse for a bit in the army, then came home and started a clinic. . . . Their technical skills weren't good . . . and they didn't have any equipment, not like modern hospitals. They would just listen with a stethoscope. . . . They couldn't treat much, much less than a Chinese medicine doctor."

In urban areas, doctors of Western medicine would have been more numerous, but still considerably fewer than their Chinese medicine counterparts. Clustered in hospital facilities or running private clinics, their services and treatments were often beyond the financial reach of most people (Deng Tietao 1999, 15; Croizier 1968, 52). Government documents estimate that there were approximately 9,000 registered physicians of Western medicine in the country in 1937 at the outbreak of the Sino-Japanese war, when most of my interviewees were just beginning their studies or their professional careers (Croizier 1968, 54–55). About 22 percent of them were concentrated in Shanghai, making their numbers in other cities even more scarce (Scheid 2007, 182). Although there aren't official statistics for the number of traditional physicians at this time, it is likely that there were about 500,000 doctors of Chinese medicine. This figure is the estimate found in internal Communist party documents for the number of doctors of Chinese medicine in 1954, and we can use it as a rough guide to the number of doctors in the Republican era (Editorial Department for the Compilation of Chinese Medicine Work Documents 1985, 44).

This sharp disparity in the number of Chinese medicine and Western medicine doctors is captured by Zhang Xichun (張錫純), a famous advocate for blending the two medical systems. In a 1929 journal article responding to the abolition proposal, he summarized the demographic distribution of the two medical professions and its implications for health care for China at this time.

> I've recently learned about the Central Ministry of Health meeting, in which the leaders have favored the opinions of Western medicine doctors to abolish Chinese medicine and Chinese herbs. [They made this decision] because the leaders are not members of the medical profession and don't know the actual circumstances concerning Chinese medicine and Western medicine. Looking at today's situation, in big cities and commercial areas, no more than one out of ten patients see a doctor of Western medicine. In the average prefecture and county, no more than one or two out of a hundred patients visit a doctor of Western medicine. Western medicine has been in China for many years. If it was so obviously superior to Chinese medicine, why are there so few believers? This is clear evidence. The Divine Farmer and the Yellow Emperor created Chinese medicine to protect our yellow race. Whenever there have been epidemics, there have also always been efficacious herbs and formulas to save lives. This is why the population of the yellow race is, in fact, greater than other races. The abolition of Chinese medicine would greatly affect the livelihood of the people and the wealth of the nation.

This general picture of the relative sizes of the two medical professions in 1929 would have changed to a small degree by 1949 with the continued growth of the Western medicine profession. Official PRC statistics show that there were 38,000 doctors of Western medicine in 1949. But in terms of clinical efficacy none of my interviewees seemed to think of Western medicine doctors as competitors. He Ren remembers two major hospitals in Hangzhou during the Republican era, the French Shen'ai Hospital and the British Guangji Hospital. Although he recalled that they seemed to be well run, "most people held Chinese medicine in higher regard," he told me.[8] Deng Tietao remarked that in the age before antibiotics, the clinical efficacy of Chinese medicine to treat acute infectious diseases was in high regard, even by doctors of Western medicine. Deng recalled curing a young boy with a high fever whose father had a clinic of Western medicine right next to his on Great Peace South Road (*Taiping Nanlu*) (now People's South Road [*Renmin Nanlu*]) in the late 1940s. That the doctor had turned to his Chinese medicine competitor for help was emblematic for Deng of the relative clinical strengths of the two professions at this time.[9] Zhang Jin (张缙), the well-known acupuncturist from Harbin, began his career as a doctor of Western medicine, graduating from the Shenyang China Medical University (瀋陽中國醫科大學) in 1951. But when he began working as a clinician, he discovered that "Western medicine had very few methods for curing disease. At the time, some people would joke that we were 'three sector doctors (*sanduan daifu*).' The head was one sector. If the head hurt, we used aspirin. The middle, the gastrointestinal tract, was the next sector. If the stomach hurt, we would use Stomach Powder (*Wei San*) [a compound probably containing calcium carbonate]. . . . And last, if the legs and arms hurt, we would use acetophenetidin."[10] Yang Zemin (楊則民), the Marxist thinker and scholar of Chinese medicine from the Republican era, tried to give a more philosophical explanation to this situation: "Chinese medicine can cure illness and not know the patient's disease. Western medicine may know the site of the disease and not have a therapy. This is why Chinese medicine disease names are chaotic and Western medicine lacks therapies" (Zhao Hongjun 1982, 239–40; Deng Tietao and Cheng Zhifan 2000, 192).

The Private Clinic

The second key fact about medical practice in the Republican era is that the locus of clinical care was the private clinic. Almost all hospitals were hospitals of Western medicine. They were relatively few and limited to urban areas. Some of the new private schools of Chinese medicine also established small hospitals and used them as sites for clinical training (Scheid 2007, 196). But many colleges were unable to resolve the finances of building and running a hospital (Deng Tietao 1999, 175). As a result, even my interviewees who attended colleges of Chinese medicine—about one-third of the total—received their clinical training in the private clinics of their teachers rather than in a hospital of Chinese medicine. Most doctors had clinics in their home, although some doctors in urban areas rented a consultation space. Doctors in rural areas, where access to herbs might be more limited, were more likely to have a pharmacy attached to their clinic. Doctors in urban areas typically just offered consultation services but sometimes did acupuncture, as well. Mornings were generally for walk-in consultations (*menzhen*), afternoons for house calls (*chuzhen*), either to those too infirm to visit the clinic or to those wealthy enough to pay an additional fee for the home visit.

Because medical practice was private and patients paid for services out of pocket, economics played an important role in shaping clinical work. Many of my interviewees commented that the average patient could only afford to see a doctor for urgent medical issues. That meant that nagging, chronic conditions, which would require a long course of treatment, or minor afflictions, which might get better on their own, went untreated. Only the wealthy had the resources to deal with these sorts of discomforts. The average patient therefore only sought medical help for acute illnesses and expected results in just a couple of doses. Jin Shiyuan (金世元), the well-known Chinese medicine pharmacist who apprenticed at the Fuyou Pharmacy in the early 1940s, recalled, "It was unheard of to fill a prescription for ten doses [like one often does today]. The biggest prescriptions that we filled were for two to three doses, and usually it was just one dose."[11] As a teenager, Lou Duofeng (娄多峰) of Yuanyang County in Henan studied with his grandfather, a specialist in Warm Disorders therapies. "He never needed more than the three doses to cure a patient, and usually the problem was resolved in one or two doses."[12] Li Jinyong (李今庸), who grew up in Zaoyang County, a mountainous region of Hubei Province, pointed out that the privations of war (caused by marauding Japanese and KMT armies) made it impossible for peasants to address anything but the most urgent problems, while at the same time creating the conditions for epidemic disease. "At the time, during the Sino-Japanese war, life in the countryside was so hard. Peasants could only [afford to] take one or two doses of medicine. We treated only acute diseases. If you didn't get results in one or two doses, they didn't come back."[13] A few of my interviewees, such as Li Bingnan (黎炳南), originally from Huizhou City in Guangdong, and Zhou Xinyou (周信有), originally from Andong (now Dandong) in Liaoning, commented that they saw a considerable number of patients with chronic illnesses. It is possible that the first instance reflects the greater affluence of southern China, while the second instance was determined by Japanese colonial policy, which required acute, infectious illnesses to be treated at biomedical hospitals (M. S. Liu 2009).

Medical Training

The third key fact about medical practice in the Republican era was that medical training, in spite of the rapid spread of a modern school-based educational system in China, remained centered on apprenticeships and the classics. Approximately two-thirds of my interviewees studied medicine through apprenticeships, usually with a relative or local teacher. The remaining one-third attended a school of Chinese medicine, one of the new developments of the Republican era.[14] But almost all these individuals later had an apprenticeship or similar relationship with a clinical teacher after they had finished their coursework. Yan Runming (阎润茗) graduated from Huabei College of National Medicine (華北國醫學院) in Beijing and then did a five-year apprenticeship with Zhao Shuping (趙樹屏) while also studying acupuncture closely with a Buddhist monk, Li Chunxian (李春仙).[15] For his final year of clinical training at the Shanghai New China Medical College (上海新中國學院), He Ren returned home to study with his father.

There were some differences in the texts used by apprentices and students, but they were probably only minor when compared with the curriculum of contemporary students. For apprenticeships, the key texts remained relatively unchanged from the standards of the nineteenth century, a combination of introductory books (*qimeng shu*), such as *Drug Properties Verses* (藥性賦), *Essentials of Materia Medica* (本草備藥), *Formulas in Rhyme* (湯頭歌), and the classics, with greater emphasis on the latter by the most literate teachers. The canonical text for most of my interviewees from northern China was the Qing dynasty text *The Golden Mirror of Medical Orthodoxy* (醫宗金鑒). In southern China, apprentices studied the four classics (*si bu jingdian*), which meant a greater focus on the Warm Disorders approach. Rote memorization of these texts was central to apprenticeship training, and my interviewees still had impressive recall of passages they had first memorized more than seventy years ago. In the new medical colleges, student used textbooks that were written by their teachers. Although the intricacies of textbook writing are beyond the scope of this chapter, we can broadly generalize that they were lightly edited versions of the classics and popular introductory books, especially when compared to the standardized textbooks of today's Chinese medicine universities.

Perhaps most importantly, my interviewees had little or no training in Western medicine at this time. This absence stands in sharp contrast to contemporary doctors of Chinese medicine, who have not only studied Western medicine intensively but are competent practitioners of it. In the Republican period, knowledge of Western medicine was valued by a small group of doctors, such as Zhang Xichun, Yun Tieqiao, Lu Yuanlei, Shi Jinmo, and others, who were eager to reform Chinese medicine. But its importance within these elite circles did not necessarily translate into educational reforms. The recently established medical colleges all offered some courses in Western medicine, but these usually did not go beyond the basics of anatomy and physiology. My interviewees who attended these private schools all agreed that these courses were very rudimentary. The rest of my interviewees, who learned medicine as apprentices, had almost no exposure to Western medicine, except perhaps through the late Qing physician Tang Zonghai, whose popular writings incorporated some basic Western anatomy (see Chapter 2). What these recollections demonstrate is that, in stark contrast to today's doctors of Chinese medicine, the average doctor in the Republican era did not need to know Western medicine.

Here, the exceptions help prove the rule. With the start of the Sino-Japanese War, Zhu Liangchun came to Shanghai to complete his medical training with Zhang Cigong (章次公). He recalled that his teacher and re-spected clinician Zhang Cigong would send patients to get blood chemistries at nearby laboratories and promoted the practice of "double diagnosis, single treatment" (*shuang chong zhenduan, yi chong zhiliao*)—that is, making a di-agnosis in both Chinese medicine and Western medicine but treating with Chinese medicine alone. Zhu Liangchun traced his own commitment to in-tegrated medicine back to Zhang Cigong. He fondly remembered the feeling of learning from a teacher on the cutting edge of a new trend in medicine. But he also recalled that most doctors saw his teacher as a traitor to Chinese medicine for his hybrid approach. "It is not that I want to be a traitor to Chi-nese medicine," Zhang Cigong would respond. "The times have made me be a traitor." Xu Jiqun (许济群), known for being one of the chief editors of the highly regarded fifth edition of the Chinese Medicine Formulary text-book, also wistfully remembered learning a little Western medicine in his

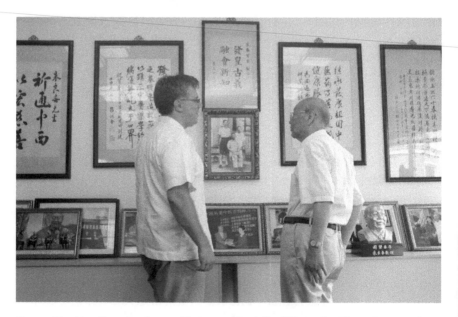

Figure 3. Zhu Liangchun showing an old picture of himself and his teacher Zhang Cigong to the author, 2011. Photo by Wang Xiaobin.

early days in Shanghai. He took a special course on the "three routine labs" (*san changgui*) so he could incorporate blood, urine, and phlegm analysis into his practice in the 1940s. He proudly told me how he once used these skills to diagnose a case of malignant malaria and successfully treated it with quinine. I asked him if he felt like he was "betraying" Chinese medicine with this use of Western medicine. He dismissed that notion with a wave of his hand. The Shanghai medical market was extremely competitive at that time, he recalled, and it was important to stay one step ahead to succeed. These anomalies, the incorporation of Western medicine into one's clinical practice, were to become the norm after 1949.

Encountering the State

The three aspects of Chinese medicine practice in the Republican era summarized earlier—the numerical preponderance of Chinese medicine doctors, the small number of hospitals (and near absence of Chinese medicine hospitals), and the minimal exposure to Western medicine—changed rapidly during the Communist era as the state began building a national healthcare infrastructure. As these social conditions changed, so did the nature of clinical work in Chinese medicine. In the 1950s, doctors of Chinese medicine did play a prominent role in the control of some epidemics, most notably two outbreaks of Japanese B encephalitis, in Shijiazhuang in 1955 and in Beijing in 1956 (China Academy of Chinese Medicine 2003, 43, 48, 59). Indeed, the second outbreak helped establish Pu Fuzhou (蒲辅周) as one of the leading Chinese medicine physicians of his times. Recognizing that treatment strategies for the Shijiazhuang outbreak were not working as effectively in Beijing, Pu quickly drafted a brief treatise on eight different strategies and sixty-six formulas for treating Japanese B encephalitis that not only improved clinical outcomes but also seamlessly blended approaches from the Cold Damage and the Warm Disorders currents, two camps that had been bitterly opposed to each other in the Republican period, as we will see in Chapter 3 (Pu Fuzhou and Gao Huiyuan 1960, 51–64). But despite these accomplishments, prejudice against Chinese medicine was hardening, and Li Zhizheng (李志正) recalls that it was soon common to hear the claim that "Chinese medicine cannot treat infectious diseases" (China Academy of Chinese Medicine 2003, 43). According to Deng Tietao, by the end of the 1950s, just ten years after the revolution, doctors of Chinese medicine had begun turning their attention away from acute disease toward the treatment of chronic illnesses.[16]

One of the surprising aspects of this new direction for clinical practice is that it happened at a moment when state support for Chinese medicine was greater than it had ever been. The Communist Party has often portrayed its policies toward the Chinese medicine profession as a reversal of the repressive policies of the KMT. Today the Communist Party can boast that it has established thirty colleges of Chinese medicine, built 2,500 hospitals of Chinese medicine, and trained hundreds of thousands of Chinese medicine doctors (Editorial Committee of the China Medical Yearbook 2001, 454–55, 499). Compared to the Nationalist era, when private individuals, not the state, took most of the initiatives to develop modern institutions of Chinese medicine, these sound like impressive achievements. Yet since the 1950s, the status of Chinese medicine doctors has declined, and the range of their clinical work has eroded. How can we explain these developments? To borrow a phrase from Sean Lei, I argue that the 1950s was the moment when Chinese medicine "encountered the state." As my interviewees have shown, Lei's intriguing thesis that the 1929 proposal to abolish Chinese medicine decisively pulled doctors of Chinese medicine into the political arena needs to be reformulated when we consider the realm of clinical practice. The Nationalist state under the KMT was too divided and weak, even during the Nanjing Decade (1928–37), the height of its political power, to seriously alter the nature of clinical medicine in China. Under the highly centralized government of the Communist era, however, Chinese medicine underwent a profound transformation. Perhaps Zhou Xinyou's comments about the difference between his life as a doctor in Manchukuo, the Japanese puppet state (1932–45) that privileged Western medicine, and as a doctor in Communist-controlled Liaoning Province, can help illuminate what the new role of the Communist state was. "[Before Liberation] there was no meddling between doctors of Chinese medicine and Western medicine. Even though the [Manchukuo] state didn't support Chinese medicine, it allowed you to run a practice. Later [after Liberation], there was meddling. Western medicine was 'exercising leadership' over Chinese medicine."

This "exercise of leadership" took several forms. First, in the early years of the People's Republic, far greater resources were devoted to building Western medicine institutions. According to official Ministry of Health statistics, the number of doctors of Western medicine grew very quickly after the establishment of the People's Republic in 1949. Starting at 38,000 doctors in 1949, this workforce nearly doubled in eight years to 73,600 in 1957 and then grew by two and a half times over the next eight years to 188,700 in 1965 (Editorial Committee of the China Medical Yearbook 2001, 455). The cost of this remarkable growth may have been lower-quality doctors; some observers noted that medical school classes had swelled to 400–600 students (Sidel 1973, 156).

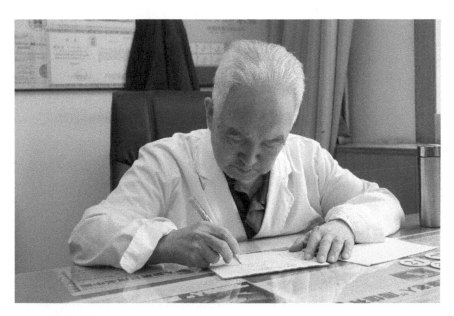
Figure 4. Zhou Xinyou writing a prescription in his private clinic, 2011.

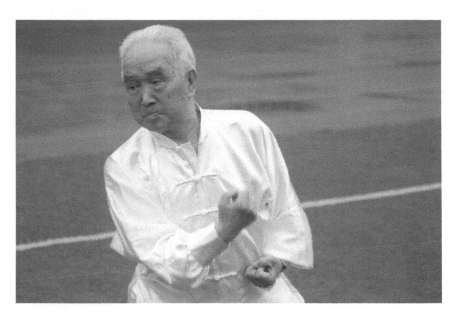
Figure 5. Zhou Xinyou, a prize-winning martial artist in his youth, giving a performance in 2011 at age ninety-one.

By comparison, the official number of Chinese medicine doctors was 337,000 in 1957. This drop from the earlier estimate of 500,000 was probably because of the new licensing requirements (Taylor 2004, 37–41). In 1957, the pharmacist Jin Shiyuan also participated in one of the licensing exams. He recalled that of the more than 1,900 people who took the licensing exam in 1957, only 150 passed. He saw this high failure rate as a more or less accurate reflection of the skill levels of the participants and not as an attempt to curtail the profession. In the early 1950s, Chinese medicine was still a way to make a living for someone who had some education. Anyone who could read a few ancient medical texts could pass himself off as a doctor, Jin claimed. Regardless of the political motivations behind the exams, the result was that professional development in Western medicine was racing ahead while a winnowing process was still going on within the Chinese medicine community.

At the same time, institution building for the Chinese medicine profession proceeded far more cautiously, especially in the early 1950s. Up to 1954, policy toward Chinese medicine focused on "scientizing Chinese medicine" (*zhongyi kexuehua*), which meant retraining doctors, not developing new institutions. Beginning in 1950 and continuing until the late 1950s, doctors were strongly encouraged to attend "Chinese medicine improvement classes" (*zhongyi jinxiuban*), which focused on providing a foundation in Western medicine (Taylor 2004, 38–41). Classes were usually held in the afternoon or evenings to accommodate doctors' work schedules and lasted for six months to a year. In addition to this Western medicine training, doctors were also encouraged to study Marxism and Maoist thought, sometimes in formal classes. Although most of my interviewees complained about the prejudicial attitudes of bureaucrats toward Chinese medicine during this period, they were generally appreciative of the opportunities to study Western medicine and Marxism. Li Zhenhua of Henan studied dialectical materialism on his own and excitedly told me, "It was the key to understanding the *Inner Canon*." During this period, doctors of Chinese medicine did not work in hospitals, but they were encouraged to form "united clinics" (*lianhe zhensuo*), creating small group practices with usually less than a dozen doctors. Most of my interviewees found this situation to be professionally rewarding, because it encouraged intellectual exchange and reduced the financial stress of working on one's own.

Beginning in 1954, after the purges of several high-ranking officials in the Ministry of Health, government policy shifted and institution building for Chinese medicine began in earnest (Lampton 1977; Taylor 2004). But the emphasis on scientizing Chinese medicine continued in new forms. One new approach was to "integrate Chinese medicine and Western medicine" (*zhongxiyi jiehe*) by training doctors of Western medicine in Chinese medicine (*xiyi xuexi zhongyi*) to create doctors with expertise in both medical systems capable of finding their points of integration. Three-year training courses were inaugurated in 1955 and soon earned the enthusiastic support of Mao Zedong. Although many Western medicine physicians were reluctant participants in these experimental courses, some of them went on to become leading figures in the Chinese medicine community. A second approach to reforming Chinese medicine was adopted by the new colleges of Chinese medicine. All but one of the original private schools opened during the Republican era had failed to survive the financial challenges of operating during the Sino-Japanese war and the reinvigorated KMT opposition after the war. In 1956, the central government established four colleges of Chinese medicine in Beijing, Shanghai, Guangzhou, and Chengdu, rapidly expanding to other major provincial capitals, until there were twenty-one colleges in 1965. Training in Western medicine became a central component of the curriculum for these new colleges, making up nearly 50 percent of the required course hours. Although most educators accepted the necessity of some Western medicine training, the proper proportion of Chinese medicine courses to Western medicine courses was an important area of debate that prompted a famous letter to the Ministry of Health by leading professors at the new colleges of Chinese medicine. The five authors complained that the one-to-one ratio of Chinese medicine to Western medicine courses was causing a major pedagogical problem. In trying to master two types of medicines, the students had not achieved proficiency in either (see Chapter 4) (Ren Yingqiu 1984, 3).

Coinciding with the development of these medical schools was the creation of Chinese medicine hospitals, building on the "united clinic" experience of the early 1950s and drawing on the operational model of the biomedical hospital. Considerably larger and better financed than their private Republican-era predecessors, these institutions also distinguished themselves by incorporating a significant amount of Western medicine expertise into standard hospital work. As Deng Tietao recalled, all patients had to receive a Western medicine diagnosis in those early days. A small number of Western medicine physicians assigned to these hospitals assisted with this task. The presence of Western medicine in the new Chinese medicine hospitals continued to grow in other ways, as Zhu Fangshou (诸方受), a well-known Chinese medicine orthopedic specialist, explained to me. Zhu Fangshou had been a participant in a one-time experiment at the Beijing Medical College (1952–57) to give Chinese medicine doctors comprehensive training in Western medicine. These graduates brought additional Western medicine skills to the new hospitals. The next year, the first graduates of the "doctors of Western medicine studying Chinese medicine programs" arrived, followed by new graduates each year. In 1962, the first class of graduates from the new colleges of Chinese medicine began to work in these hospitals, bringing with them their considerable knowledge in Western medicine.

The creation of Chinese medicine colleges and hospitals during the Communist era were important achievements for the Chinese medicine profession, accomplishments that were probably unimaginable for Republican-era doctors. But these institutional gains also intensified the encounter with Western medicine, making biomedicine integral to the everyday clinical practice of Chinese medicine (Scheid 2002; Karchmer 2010). While a new hybrid medical practice emerged in the urban medical institutions, a similar push to bring Western medicine into rural areas had a far more detrimental effect on the practice of Chinese medicine in the countryside. Although rural doctors were strongly encouraged to join "union clinics" during the 1950s, the conditions of their work did not change too dramatically at first. But eventually it became hard for union clinics to find or cultivate new doctors, because other CCP policies in the countryside were undermining the apprenticeship form of medical training. Prior to 1949, well-off rural families had the means to educate their children and might encourage them to pursue a medical apprenticeship. In the 1950s, these wealthy families were typically the objects of CCP class struggle campaigns and may not have been able to finance a medical apprenticeship for their children.[17] Because of limited success in training new doctors of Chinese medicine, union clinics gradually brought in new members with some professional training in Western medicine. Xiaoping Fang reports that for Hangzhou Prefecture, this trend meant that the number of Chinese medicine doctors in union clinics was less than 50 percent of the total by the early 1960s (Fang 2012, 63). With the advent of the Cultural Revolution (1966–76), this trend was accelerated by the barefoot doctor program. This new program, intended to address the general scarcity of medical services in the countryside, required the recruitment of large numbers of participants. Contrary to the propaganda about this program, Xiaoping Fang argues that most barefoot doctors in Hangzhou Prefecture were trained primarily in Western medicine, usually outside their local communities, and saw themselves as practitioners of Western medicine first and foremost (Fang 2012, 53–66). These new training procedures together with the increasing availability of pharmaceuticals in the countryside meant that by the end of the Cultural Revolution, Western medicine had become the dominant form of medical practice in the Chinese countryside.

The end of the Cultural Revolution may have represented the nadir of the Chinese medicine profession, eroded by three decades of policy that supported Chinese medicine in name but curtailed it in practice or shoe-horned it into the integrated medicine model at the institutional level. Historians have yet to fully understand what this "encounter with the state" has fully meant for the Chinese medicine profession. But perhaps Lu Bingkui (吕炳奎), a doctor of Chinese medicine and a high-ranking government official who passionately advocated for his profession throughout his political career, can help us sense the impact of the social and political changes of the Maoist period on the practice of Chinese medicine. Writing shortly after the fall of the Gang of Four when it became possible to make critical statements about the Cultural Revolution, the period he refers to as the "ten lost years," Lu Bingkui painted a bleak picture of the field.

> At the end of the "ten lost years," there were only 240,000 [doctors of Chinese medicine], and today there are 250,000. Compared to Liberation, this is a loss of about one half. Western medicine has grown by more than a factor of 10; Chinese medicine has shrunk in half. This "half" is according to official statistics, but the reality is worse. According to our surveys, only 20–30 percent of these 200,000 plus doctors have systematically studied Chinese medicine. . . . With this dearth of Chinese medicine personnel, Chinese medicine institutions are also pathetically few. There are almost 2 million hospital beds in the entire country. Chinese medicine has only 50,000 beds. But of these 50,000 beds, there are no more than 5,000 that are being managed with Chinese medicine. . . . Chinese medicine doctors can now only do a little outpatient work, treating a few common illnesses. Under these conditions, . . . how can the profession advance? It's impossible (Cui Yueli 1993).

Despite Lu's bleak account, there has been a significant rejuvenation of the Chinese medicine ranks since the 1980s. Many of my interviewees in the 2000s felt that the prospects for the profession were brighter than they could ever remember. Nonetheless, the Chinese medicine profession that has rebuilt itself since the 1980s is a significantly different form of medical practice. One of the most significant aspects of that transformation is that it has become "slow medicine."

Why exactly did the social and political changes of the Maoist period push Chinese medicine doctors toward the treatment of chronic illnesses? According to Deng Tietao, the overall effect was to "take away the stage" for Chinese medicine doctors to treat acute diseases. He pointed out that the rapid growth of Western medicine hospitals in the early 1950s and the inauguration of a new health insurance system (*gongfei yiliao*) in 1951, which only provided reimbursement for hospital services, pulled patients with insurance coverage

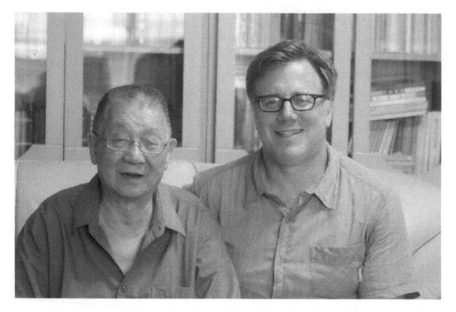

Figure 6. Li Jinyong, age eighty-six, meeting with the author in 2011 to discuss his decades of medical practice and teaching. Photo by Wang Xiaobin.

into the hospitals. Impressed with hospital technology—the laboratory exams, X-rays, and other medical devices—these new visitors gradually developed a preference for Western medicine in the management of acute illnesses.[18] Li Jinyong pointed out that hospital administrators played a central role in pushing this transition in Wuhan. Because administrators usually had a background in Western medicine and were sensitive, and probably sympathetic, to the Western medicine bias of their superiors in the Ministry of Health, they were able to curtail the work of Chinese medicine doctors according to their own prejudices.

We can see precisely this same complaint being voiced during the Japanese B encephalitis outbreak in the 1950s, when Chinese medicine doctors were demonstrating the ability to contribute to urgent state matters of public health. In the introduction to a brief manual published in 1956 by the Hebei Province Association of Public Health Work about the Chinese medicine treatments for this disease, Duan Huixuan (段慧轩), the head of the association and director of the Hebei Bureau of Public Health, praised the contributions of Chinese medicine doctors in the treatment of Japanese B encephalitis and complained about the obstruction of Western medicine hospitals to their work.

One aspect of the problem is publicizing the experience of Chinese medicine therapies, but an even more important aspect is the close cooperation with [Western medicine] hospitals, which will allow a better implementation of the successful experience of Chinese medicine doctors. . . . Some hospitals have not cooperated enough, affecting the use of Chinese medicine therapies. Some hospitals have over-emphasized the primacy of Western medicine diagnosis before allowing Chinese medicine treatments, causing unnecessary delays [in patient care]. This is inappropriate. Now that it has been shown that Chinese medicine has superb results in the treatment of encephalitis, I hope that all localities will act in accordance with the spirit of revolutionary humanism, putting the lives of the patients first, working together as closely as possible, to help Chinese medicine doctors be as efficacious as possible (Hebei Province Association of Public Health Work 1956, 3).

Unfortunately, Duan Huixuan's call for hospitals to cooperate with Chinese medicine professionals was not heeded. Countervailing social and political forces overwhelmed his enthusiasm for Chinese medicine to contribute to the treatment of acute infectious diseases in the Communist era. As Li Jinyong explained, the clinical virtuosity demonstrated so strikingly in the Japanese B encephalitis outbreaks was never passed on to the next generations of doctors.

Why do the clinical skills [of younger doctors] today not match those of the old doctors? The old doctors accumulated years of experience, coming from the old society where they saw a lot. But . . . beginning with the very first class of college graduates that went to the hospitals to work, whenever there was a patient with an acute febrile disease, the patient was immediately sent for Western medicine care. Chinese medicine doctors were not allowed to participate. . . . As a result, the old doctors couldn't use their skills in treating acute diseases, and young doctors couldn't learn them.[19]

In general, my interviewees did not have grand explanations for the transition that they witnessed. They pointed to small factors—the emphasis on Western medicine in the new hospitals of Chinese medicine, the effects of the new health insurance system, the prejudices of hospital administrators. But when we view these comments against Wang Juyi's story of his teacher, Liu Shoushan, the illiterate bonesetter, we can see a unifying theme: the Chinese state through its new institutions and policies had become the arbiters for the efficacy of Chinese medicine by the late 1950s. Perhaps the most skilled doctors, like Liu Shoushan, could defy these new institutional constraints in certain situations, but subsequent generations of doctors could not. In a relatively short period of time, a collective amnesia would set in; doctors of Chinese medicine would not even know that their predecessors were once skilled physicians in the treatment of acute illnesses.

Acute and Chronic in the Communist Era

In 2011, I had the good fortune to visit with Deng Tietao at the Guangzhou University of Chinese Medicine. I had already interviewed him on two other occasions. As he had gradually come to understand my research interests, his welcome grew with each visit. He was already ninety-four and less energetic than he had been on my previous visits. On this occasion, he arranged for me to meet his disciples, tour the hospital where he had worked for decades, and talk with the doctors and scholars who were carrying on his remarkable legacy of clinical work and historical research at his university. His personal assistant, Chen Anlin, was eager for me to give a talk to the medical students about the oral history project of 2008–9, particularly since Deng Tietao had been one of the key informants for that project. I hastily put together a few thoughts and called the talk "Slow Medicine: How Chinese Medicine Became Effective for Only Treating Chronic Illnesses."[20] I was nervous that I would not be at my most articulate on such short notice. I knew that most students of Chinese medicine had almost no knowledge of the social and clinical changes that I learned about through my interviews. Would they believe me? Would my message be lost in translation? At the end of the talk, Liu Wenbin (刘文斌), one of Deng Tietao's main disciples, came up to me and politely complimented me. I had really understood the essence of Chinese medicine, he said. "It truly is a slow medicine." I was crestfallen. Even one of Deng Xiaoping's closest disciples had not understand my talk.

I later learned that Liu Wenbin had not been present for most of the talk. But even as his tried to be a gracious host and offer a few complimentary remarks, it was revealing that he had misunderstood the title of my talk. Just the day before he had been taking me on a tour of the university's affiliated hospital. We had spent quite a while with one of his patients, who was suffering from Guillain-Barre syndrome. This rare condition causes muscle weakness and can develop into a devastating total paralysis, sometimes severely impairing respiratory function. From the biomedical perspective, this syndrome develops when one's immune system attacks the body's nervous system. The

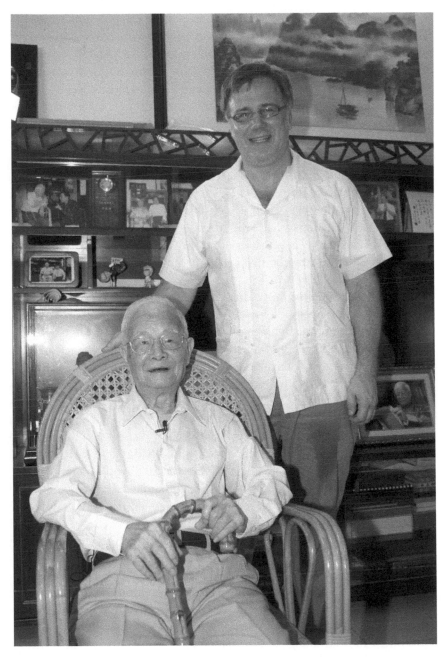

Figure 7. The author visiting with Deng Tietao, age ninety-four, in his home in 2011. Photo by Wang Xiaobin.

exact cause is not known, and biomedical treatments can only ease symptoms. Roughly 70 percent of patients will recover on their own, but the process can take years, and complete function may not return. Deng Tietao was famous at the hospital for pioneering Chinese medicine treatments for this condition. He had argued that this syndrome, like other diseases of muscle weakness such as myasthenia gravis, should focus on treating the Spleen, because the "Spleen rules the muscles" (*pi zhu jirou*). Deng was known for using modifications of the thirteenth-century formula Supplement the Middle and Augment the Qi Decoction (*Bu Zhong Yi Qi Tang*) to treat this difficult condition. As soon as we stepped into the room, the patient could not stop singing the praises of Liu Wenbin. He insisted on getting out of bed to show us that he could now walk around the perimeter of his bed while supporting himself with one arm on the bed frame. Liu Wenbin had misunderstood the title of my talk because he knew Deng Tietao only as a master of treating chronic illnesses. Those were the clinical skills he had inherited from him and were clearly on display that afternoon.

In terms of the acute-chronic dualism that I proposed at the beginning of this chapter, contemporary Chinese medicine has been noticeably affected along the axis of purification in this dualism. Patients and doctors alike believe that Chinese medicine is only suitable for chronic illnesses. But even as this deeply engrained conviction has limited the practice of Chinese medicine, it has also spurred innovations along the axis of hybridization. Doctors frequently use both medical practices to navigate the temporal dimensions of complex clinical situations. For example, it is common to use Western medicine to manage the acute presentations of a disease and then turn to Chinese medicine to deal with long-term, underlying pathologies. During the summer of 2002, I got a chance to observe a skilled Chinese medicine dermatologist at Guang'anmen Hospital use this approach quite nimbly. He was well known for his treatments of lupus erythematosus, the auto-immune disorder that typically presents with a "butterfly rash" on the face. He treated most lupus patients with Chinese herbal remedies exclusively. But during acute flare-ups, this disease can have systemic ramifications that cause devastating injuries to the kidneys, heart, and lungs. In these situations, this doctor would turn to corticosteroids to quickly bring the inflammation under control and then return to his exclusive Chinese herbal therapies to manage the underlying auto-immune causes of this disease. He explained to me that this strategy took advantage of the relative strengths of each medical system. Indeed, we can use this hybrid logic to understand the operations of Chinese medicine hospitals as a whole. This point was made to me most succinctly by my teacher Li Li from the Emergency Medicine Department at Dongzhimen

Hospital. During one of our discussions about the near absence of Chinese medicine treatments in her unit, she reminded me to think holistically about the patient's care. "Do not forget. After our patients leave the Emergency Room, they usually transfer to an inpatient ward or will continue to be treated in the outpatient clinic. Those are the places where they can receive the most benefit from Chinese medicine treatments."

Within the realm of chronic illnesses, hybridity is also ever present. As China's medical landscape began to change after 1949, doctors of Chinese medicine had little choice but to reorient this clinical expertise. Many of my interviewees traveled this path with great success, becoming masters of certain chronic conditions. But in each instance, they had to learn to apply their clinical skills to the treatment of biomedical diseases, thinking creatively across the two medical systems. Zhang Qi, who had explained to me the necessity of treating acute illnesses in the Republican era, was best known for his treatments of kidney failure in the Communist period. Zhu Liangchun, who had first earned acclaim for dengue fever treatments in the Republican period, was renowned in his later life for his treatments of rheumatoid arthritis and cancer. When I had the good fortune to visit with him at his home in Nantong in 2012, his children took me on a tour of the private medical center they had established in his name, the Liangchun Chinese Medicine Clinical Research Center (良春中医药临床研究所). This small private hospital, where his children work as doctors of Chinese medicine, now employs nearly fifty individuals and is dedicated to using Zhu Liangchun's innovative treatments for rheumatological diseases and cancer. During a tour of the hospital, his daughter, Zhu Jianhua, who had trained under her father, proudly introduced me to a young man with severe kyphosis (rounding) of his upper back caused by ankylosing spondylitis. "He made the mistake of treating this condition with steroids when he was a teenager, and it stunted his growth. Now he is here and doing well. He knows our treatments are better and safer." Later in the day, I had the chance to speak with this patient when he got up to walk the hospital grounds. The strong curve in the upper back of this petite man meant that he had to crane his neck upward to speak with me when we were standing. He expressed regrets for the poor decisions of his youth — the steroids were so easy to take — and thankfulness for the care he was now receiving. In the same year, I also visited with Li Jiren, who generously offered to let me observe his clinical practice one morning. On that day, two young boys with Duchenne-type muscular dystrophy came for treatment. I had grown up watching the Jerry Lewis telethons and remembered well the teenage boys who were wheelchair-bound and rarely lived beyond their early twenties. I was surprised to see patients with such a rare genetic condition at his clinic. Li

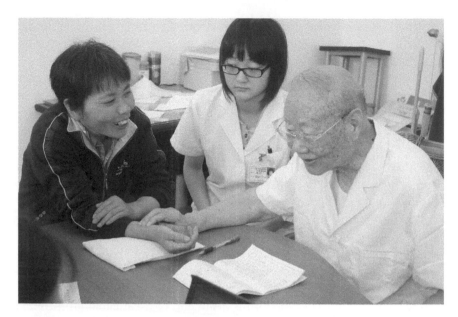

Figure 8. Zhu Liangchun treating a patient at age ninety-three. Nantong Hospital of Chinese Medicine, 2011.

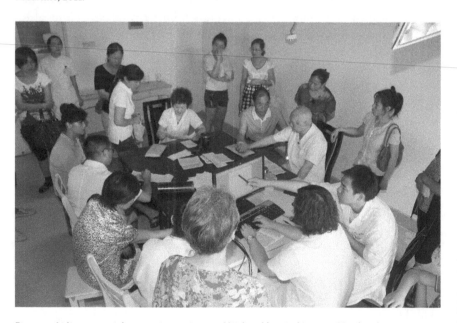

Figure 9. Li Jiren, age eighty, treating patients at Yijishan Hospital in 2011. His daughter sits to his right and makes an entry into the medical record book before Li Jiren consults with the patient. Two junior doctors sit to his left, making a digital record of the consultation. Patients wait their turn.

Jiren said, "They know Chinese medicine can help. Of course, it is extremely difficult to treat, but I have had some patients who have lived into their forties, even fifties, and were able to have families of their own."

A Turning Point?

Of the three dualisms explored in this book, the acute-chronic dualism has perhaps led to the greatest changes in clinical practice. It has generally resulted in a reductionist narrowing of the clinical applications of Chinese medicine. But perhaps these postcolonial shifts are not as total and irreversible as they might seem. In early 2003, the SARS epidemic swept across China and many parts of the globe. As healthcare institutions in China struggled to treat patients who had contracted this unknown, contagious, and virulent disease, some doctors of Chinese medicine ultimately played a role in containing the outbreak. Marta Hanson has noted how the positive role of Chinese medicine doctors in managing this epidemic almost entirely escaped the attention of the Western media (Hanson 2010). In the middle of the crisis, however, Chinese officials were not clear what role doctors of Chinese medicine should play. Li Jinyong told me administrators at the affiliated hospital of the Hubei University of Chinese Medicine were desperate not to admit a single SARS patient for fear that the hospital could not handle it.[21] But in Guangzhou, the capital of the province where the epidemic originated, Chinese medicine is probably more popular than in any other part of the country. Perhaps it was the greater respect accorded doctors of Chinese medicine in this region that allowed them to participate in the treatment of SARS patients from the beginning.

Deng Tietao, one of the most revered doctors in the city, proudly told me that the mortality rate for SARS was lower in Guangzhou than the rest of the country precisely because of the contribution of Chinese medicine. In a review of the 103 SARS patients admitted to the Guangdong Provincial Hospital of Chinese Medicine from January to April 2003, researchers found that seven died, a mortality rate of 6.79 percent that compares quite favorably to other epidemic areas, where the rate was as high as 15 percent (Lin Lin, Yang Zhimin, and Deng Tietao 2004). Deng Tietao pointed out to me that these statistics omitted all the patients with high fevers who were cured by timely herbal medicine treatments before the disease progressed to a stage where it could be positively identified. In addition, he noted that there were no cases of SARS among hospital staff, who all took Chinese herbal medicine prophylactically, thus highlighting another presumed advantage of Chinese medicine—its preventive emphasis.[22] The treatments at Guangdong Provincial Hospital of Chinese Medicine used a combination of Western medicine and Chinese medicine therapies. But the main Western medicine therapies (aside from standard emergency and critical care inventions) were massive doses of corticosteroids, which proved to be of only limited benefit and sometimes resulted in devastating side effects. In the absence of effective Western medicine therapies, these doctors rediscovered an entire theoretical apparatus within Chinese medicine designed for the treatment of acute illness. The successes of Chinese medicine doctors in Guangzhou were eventually recognized in other outbreak areas. Beijing officials lifted a ban on the use of Chinese medicine for the treatment of SARS on May 8, 2003. Deng Tietao told me that doctors of Chinese medicine had finally learned they could treat acute illnesses again.[23]

Despite Deng Tietao's passionate account of Chinese medicine during the SARS epidemic, the larger social impact of this event was far more modest. Nonetheless, a body of Chinese medicine literature around the SARS experience began to accumulate in the subsequent years (Zhong Jiaxi et al. 2005; Liu Bichen 2006; Zhu Jiayong and Zhu Shengshan 2003; Cao Lijuan and Wang Ti 2014). At the same time, some meaningful shifts in policy regarding Chinese medicine were occurring in the late 2000s and early 2010s, which some scholars have attributed to the clinical successes during SARS (Cao Lijuan and Wang Ti 2014). As we will see in the Epilogue, these changes enabled a much larger role for Chinese medicine practitioners in China's next major epidemic, the COVID-19 pandemic of 2020.

2

Geographies of the Body

To anyone who has encountered both Western medicine and Chinese medicine, it quickly becomes apparent that the two medical systems are based on very different assumptions about the body. Or so I assumed for many years. Prior to my fieldwork, I was already familiar with Western scholars who had written thoughtfully about these differences. I knew that Chinese medicine was not based on detailed knowledge of the anatomical body. For example, Manfred Porkert had argued that the Chinese term *zang* (臟) does not refer to "organ" as the term has been typically translated. He proposed the alternate term "orb" because *zang* refers to both "a bodily substratum with ill-defined material and spatial contours" and "a physiological function associated with the substratum and qualitatively defined in time with precision and subtlety" (Porkert 1974, 107). Thus, he argued that "the Chinese word *fei*" (肺) calls to mind only coincidentally and vaguely the modern anatomical concept of "the lungs." Instead, *fei* "designates primarily and predominantly an orb of function" (Porkert 1974, 107). I had learned similar lessons from the famous historian of Chinese science and medicine Nathan Sivin. In his translation of an important twentieth-century Chinese medicine textbook, Sivin noted the limited role of anatomy in the history of Chinese medicine.

> It is plain that traditional [Chinese] anatomy from first to last lacked
> the detailed and systematic character that we find even in Galen
> of Pergamon (second century A.D.), and many aspects of the body's
> content were not studied at all. . . . In traditional [Chinese] medicine
> the tissues and internal structures of the body are unimportant by
> comparison with metabolic processes. That is why they receive so little

attention. . . . The goal of this effort was not a perfected description of the body, but an understanding of the function and dysfunction that could guide therapy (Sivin 1987, 118–23).

My early encounters with the two medical systems as a student at the Bei-jing University of Chinese Medicine reaffirmed the basic assessments of these two famous scholars. Our training emphasized that the body of Chinese med-icine was not an impoverished version of modern anatomy but rather its own unique interpretation of the human physical form. Comparisons between the two bodies were inevitable, since we were studying anatomy and physiology at roughly the same time as the basic principles of Chinese medicine. But these comparisons seemed to naturally emphasize the distinctiveness of each medical system. In *Basic Theory of Chinese Medicine* (中医基础理论), we learned that the Brain was a minor organ in the Chinese medicine body (Wu Dunxu, Liu Yanchi, and Li Dexin 1995; Farquhar 1998). By contrast, anatomy class showed us that the brain was situated at the apex of a vast network of neurons; an intimate understanding of the brain and nervous system would be essential for making sense of countless clinical situations in Western medicine (Yan Zhenguo, Zhu Peichun, and Wei Dajin 1995). An organ of considerable importance in Chinese medicine is the Spleen, which scholars recognize as the "seat of acquired essence" (*houtian zhi ben*), the organ responsible for the "transportation and transformation" (*pi zhu yunhua*) of nutrients and fluids, and central to innumerable clinical considerations (Wu Dunxu, Liu Yanchi, and Li Dexin 1995). In Western medicine, however, the spleen is classified as part of the lymphatic system and attributed relatively minor immunological functions.

For many years, I embraced this perspective, emphasizing differences, not similarities, in the bodies of Chinese medicine and Western medicine. But as my research progressed, I gradually began to doubt whether there was such a yawning ontological gap. Could ancient Chinese doctors have been truly uninterested in the inner structures of the body but finely attuned to its func-tional subtleties, as Porkert and Sivin had suggested? In clinical practice, doc-tors always found ways to make translations between these two bodies. Some-times a teacher would remind students to think of the Spleen and Stomach of Chinese medicine as a rough equivalent to the digestive system in Western medicine. A discussion of the Heart Spirit might be clarified by a reference to the brain and the modern idea of consciousness. Moreover, whenever I com-pared the two medical systems to the healing practices that I learned about in my medical anthropology training, the sharp divides seemed to fade. For example, both medical systems are relatively devoid of spiritual or religious content, at least in their contemporary forms, and primarily concerned with the physical body of the individual patient. Classic ethnographic accounts of non-Western healing systems, however, are populated with lineage groups, ancestral spirits, religious rituals, and various nonhuman actors that make Chinese medicine seem surprisingly materialist by comparison (Janzen 1978; Kleinman 1981; Finkler 1985). The anthropological analysis of these other healing systems also suggested therapeutic principles that seemed very foreign to Chinese medicine. In his classic essay on Ndembu healing, Victor Turner concludes "that the Ndembu 'doctor' sees his task less as curing an individual patient than as remedying the ills of a corporate group" (Turner 1967, 392). The collective nature of this healing ritual seemed to be totally absent from the Chinese medicine clinical encounters that I was observing.[1]

While I had the luxury of musing about these comparisons, doctors of Chinese medicine do not. They are deeply anxious about the relationship between the bodies of Western medicine and Chinese medicine. The epistemological status of Chinese medicine, its claim to be a science, seems to hinge on how one understands the body of Chinese medicine. Urgent clinical decisions seem to be hopelessly entangled with the truth status of a body based on philosophical premises and not anatomical dissections.

In this chapter, I argue that doctors have resolved this quandary through the second postcolonial dualism of this book: the structure-function dualism. Doctors today assert that the body of Chinese medicine is "true" and therefore constitutes a valid theoretical foundation to the medical system because it describes the body's functional operations, not its structural makeup. Although this claim can take many forms, I encountered it most frequently in the popular maxim "Western medicine treats structural pathologies, and Chinese medicine treats functional pathologies" (*xiyi zhi qizhixing bingbian; zhongyi zhi gongnengxing bingbian*). But unlike Manfred Porkert and Nathan Sivin, who were almost certainly influenced by contemporary Chinese scholars in developing their claims, I stress that this understanding is a uniquely postcolonial phenomenon. It needs to be analyzed crticially, and one must not impose the structure-function dualism on any historical context other than the post-1949 period. New historical research by Yi-Li Wu has already helped to demonstrate that late Imperial healers closely examined the structures of the body, even if China lacked the tradition of dissection found in Europe (Wu 2015, 2017). In the early twentieth century, leading doctors of Chinese medicine were careful readers of the new translations of European anatomy texts. But unlike today's doctors, they did not perceive the anatomical descriptions in these texts to be at odds with the body of Chinese medicine. In fact, they used European anatomy as evidence to promote their vision of a reformed

Chinese medicine. It was only in the Communist era, when new social and political conditions recast one medical system as fast acting and the other as slow acting, that a universal body shared by both medical systems became untenable. It was replaced by the structural body of Western medicine and the functional body of Chinese medicine.

Anxiety at the Borders

The structure-function dualism is a means for framing the relationship between the two medical systems, but one that is inherently unstable. The concepts of structure and function are not native to Chinese medicine. They were adopted from Western medicine, where knowledge of bodily structure in the form of anatomy serves as a foundation for understanding questions of function and dysfunction as described in the fields of physiology and pathology, respectively. But when imported into contemporary Chinese medicine, structure and function operate in complex ways. On the one hand, they work as purifying categories, producing the ontological divide that separates the bodies of Western medicine and Chinese medicine. These discursive symmetries have become the conventional way for describing the differences between the two bodies. But structure and function also facilitate points of translation and help doctors navigate between the two medical systems in clinical practice. When doctors treat patients, the differences between the two bodies narrow, or perhaps even disappear. The three ethnographic vignettes that follow give a glimpse into how contemporary doctors anxiously move between these poles of purification and hybridization.

One of my earliest introductions to the delicate politics regarding the relationship between Chinese medicine and Western medicine came during my second year of medical school, in a course on the *Yellow Emperor's Inner Canon* (*Huangdi Neijing*; 皇帝內經). This ancient text, thought to be written by multiple authors and compiled roughly around 100 B.C.E., is considered the oldest extant medical text in China and the source of most of the theoretical claims about the body and cosmos that form the basis of Chinese medicine. It is also an extremely difficult text because of its abstract philosophical ideas, its disjointed and fragmented structure, and its archaic language. I had been eagerly looking forward to this course, which I thought would unlock the essential teachings of Chinese medicine. But much to my disappointment, I found the class dull and the textbook dry. It turned out that the secrets of the *Inner Canon* were often hidden beneath seemingly countless, minute philological questions that stretched the limits of my classical Chinese abilities. To make matters worse, I was not inspired by our teacher, Professor Wang. His lectures were a dry recapitulation of the textbook. His voice was also quiet, making it difficult to follow his lectures. The beauty and magic of this ancient text seemed to recede the more I tried to approach it.

The slow pace of these classes left me totally unprepared when one day Professor Wang stopped lecturing, peered down at the class roll resting on the lecture podium, and randomly called on a student to explain a passage from the *Inner Canon*. A few rows behind me, one of my classmates jumped up from his seat. My heart fluttered. If Professor Wang had called on me, I would have been caught daydreaming. It was proper classroom etiquette for students to stand when they addressed the teacher, but the suddenness of my classmate's movements probably meant that he too had been lost in reverie. I looked back at him. His clothes were rumpled, and his hair was matted to one side. He spoke rapidly and quietly, making it difficult for me to follow his response. But it didn't matter because Professor Wang cut him off. For the first time all semester, he raised his voice and boomed, "You are using Western medicine physiology to explain this passage. The organs of Chinese medicine are not the organs of Western medicine! You must not confuse the two."

Do not conflate! The boundaries between Chinese medicine and Western medicine must be defended. My classmate had transgressed these boundaries by bringing ideas from our Western medicine course on physiology into a Chinese medicine course on medical theory. One could hardly blame him. Our curriculum was a mixture of courses from both medical systems. We shuffled between Chinese medicine and Western medicine courses throughout the day, receiving roughly an equal number of class hours in each type of course. Depending on the semester, we might be simultaneously studying Basic Theory of Chinese Medicine and Anatomy, Histology and Chinese Materia Medica, *Inner Canon* Studies and Physiology, Pathology and Chinese Formulary, *Treatise on Cold Damage* Studies and Biochemistry, or Parasitology and *Essentials of the Golden Casket* Studies. The very structure of the curriculum seemed to invite comparisons, and yet professors rarely made them, at least in class. This reticence was quite understandable for the professors of Western medicine. Many of them had little or no training in Chinese medicine. But the professors of Chinese medicine were well versed in Western medicine. In private, I found they had a great deal to say on this subject. But in the classroom, they kept these two medical systems neatly segregated.

In the third year of medical school, we got our first exposure to clinical care in the form of small group visits to nearby hospitals. My small group was assigned to the Sino-Japanese Hospital, close to the university campus. We worked with an attending physician who would take us to visit patients on his ward of the hospital and let us do mock consultations. Just before he brought us into the room of one elderly male patient, he instructed us to pay special attention to the patient's pulse. The patient sat up as we entered and didn't seem bothered by the onslaught of questions from eager and inexperienced medical students. He cheerfully answered our questions and let our entire group of eight students take turns as we placed three fingers first on one wrist and then the other. Unlike pulse taking in Western medicine, which focuses primarily on the number of beats per minute, the Chinese medicine pulse exam is concerned with the texture and qualities of the pulse at three sites on the wrist (Kuriyama 1999). Both doctors and laypersons alike consider it to be an esoteric art that requires years, even a lifetime, of clinical experience to master. We had learned the twenty-eight basic pulses in our Chinese Medicine Diagnosis course, but we had little confidence that we could relate the sensations under our fingertips to the pulse types crammed into our heads.

After shepherding us back into the hallway, our teacher pulled the patient's door shut and quizzed us: "What kind of pulse was that?" We volunteered different answers: "Slippery." "Wiry." "Tense." "Floating. . . ." The attending physician shook his head. "That was a wiry pulse. Remember that feeling. That was a typical wiry pulse." He then pointed out some of the patient's symptoms that were consistent with this pulse. At the end of this discussion, just before we moved on to the next patient, I interjected with a question: "Does a wiry pulse also indicate high blood pressure?" I had heard other doctors mention a wiry pulse as a common presentation for patients with high blood pressure. The attending physician breathed in quickly, pursed his lips, furrowed his brow, and then unleashed a torrent of words. "You absolutely cannot assume that a wiry pulse indicates high blood pressure! What about the patients with an empty pulse that have high blood pressure. . . ." His voice strained as he tried to impress the gravity of my mistake upon all of us with a litany of counterexamples. My face flushed as I sensed my classmates staring at me.

Of course, I knew that a wiry pulse—the sensation of "pressing on the strings of the zither"—indicated specific Chinese medicine pathologies, such as patterns of Liver and Gall Bladder illness, pain, or phlegm. That was standard textbook knowledge. But was it possible that this pulse might have a correlation to certain Western medicine conditions in addition to its Chinese medicine patterns of disharmony? As I would later learn, a renowned physician of the early twentieth century, Zhang Xichun (張錫純), made just such a claim in his medical treatise of 1909, *Records of Cherishing China and Referencing the West in Medicine* (醫學衷中參西錄). In this modern classic, still popular with doctors today, he argued that patients with hypertension often have a wiry pulse. This was in fact the origin of the pulse-taking tip that other doctors had been sharing with me. What had seemed like practical knowledge to some clinicians became threatening information in a formal pedagogical setting. My teacher had felt compelled to defend the distinctiveness of the Chinese medicine body.

In transgressing the boundaries between Western medicine and Chinese medicine, I had met with the almost identical response as had my classmate the previous year. The alarm of these two teachers captures some of the generalized anxiety about inappropriately conflating the bodies of Chinese medicine and Western medicine. As students, we were frequently reminded of the potential "dangers" of trying to draw equivalences between Chinese medicine and Western medicine. Teachers would recount cases where apparent equivalences between the two medical systems had proved illusory, where a Western medicine concept or diagnosis had colored the physician's assessment and a failed treatment had only been averted by returning to a "pure" Chinese medicine interpretation of the patient's condition at the last minute.

Contrary to my teacher's concern that I did not understand the dangers of conflation, I found myself, at least during my later student years, vigorously defending the uniqueness of Chinese medicine and its understanding of the body. By my final year of medical school, I was particularly concerned about the trend toward "integrated medicine" or "integrating Chinese medicine and Western medicine" (*zhongxiyi jiehe*). This phrase had been popularized by Mao Zedong in 1950s, when he proposed recruiting doctors of Western medicine to undergo intensive Chinese medicine training. This program was technically still in operation in a small way when I was a student in the 1990s. But the meaning of the phrase had changed. There was no urgent need to recruit doctors of Western medicine into the practice of Chinese medicine. All doctors of Chinese medicine were combining the two medical systems in their work. But some doctors wanted to associate their practice explicitly with "integrated medicine," championing it as a "best of both worlds" approach. To my eyes, this slogan was a justification for doctors who preferred to draw more heavily on Western medicine than Chinese medicine in their clinical work. I thought this trend threatened to erode the practice of Chinese medicine and decided to explore it more deeply in my graduation thesis.

During our fifth and final year of medical school, my classmates and I were dispersed throughout various Chinese medicine hospitals in the city doing clinical clerkships. We were no longer just observing other doctors but working with them. In May, not long before the end of the school year, each student was required to complete a graduation thesis. Many of my classmates were frantically searching for their first job, and they were hoping to get through this assignment with a minimum of effort. Since I wasn't facing these existential concerns, I was looking forward to this project as a chance to collect my thoughts on some issues related to my ethnographic research, specifically on the challenges of "integrated medicine." I chose to write about Chinese medicine herbal therapies for chronic viral hepatitis.

There is an unusually high incidence of chronic viral hepatitis (primarily hepatitis B) in China. I had become interested in this disease because the clinical benefits of Chinese medicine therapies are widely recognized in China, even by some doctors of Western medicine, who were known to sometimes prescribe herbal remedies for their hepatitis B patients. Over the Chinese New Year holiday, I got a chance to learn more about Chinese medicine therapies for this problem. While most of my classmates were busy with family festivities, one of my teachers introduced me to Dr. Su, a clinical specialist in viral hepatitis at Dongzhimen Hospital. She agreed to let me shadow her for several weeks during the holiday and "copy her prescriptions." Over the next three weeks, I had five mornings of clinical observation with her. There was a steady stream of patients each day, and I furiously scribbled everything I saw into my notebook.

It was only after I had returned to my regular hospital clerkship and was looking back over my notes that I was struck by a certain style in Dr. Su's clinical approach to hepatitis. In particular, I noticed that her prescriptions often included herbs that were known to address Liver patterns of disharmony. But as I had observed, most patients complained of gastrointestinal symptoms— poor appetite, nausea, abdominal discomfort, loose stools, and so on—that would more often be associated with Spleen and Stomach patterns of disharmony. These symptoms could have an indirect relationship to the Liver's main properties to "store blood" (cangxue) and to "course and drain" (shuxie). But to my admittedly inexperienced eyes, I felt that most patients' presentation did not have strong evidence for patterns of Liver disharmonies. I began to wonder if Dr. Su's basis for including these herbs was the patient's Western medicine diagnosis. As I explored the literature on this topic, I noticed that many other contemporary scholars writing about hepatitis B seemed to share Dr. Su's integrationist logic: diseases of the anatomical liver required treatment of the Chinese medicine Liver. Although my time with Dr. Su was too limited to judge the efficacy of her treatments, the integrationist approach that she and many other published clinicians had adopted seemed to me to conflate the Chinese medicine body with the Western medicine body, precisely the problem that so many of my teachers had warned me about.

As my research progressed, I reviewed classical scholarship about conditions that I thought most resembled hepatitis B, a modern disease category that does not exist in classical medical texts. I believed this literature supported my view that Chinese medicine therapies would be more effective when traditional approaches were followed instead of integrationist ones. Ultimately, I argued that clinically effective treatments of chronic hepatitis needed to be based on a clear separation of the bodies of Chinese medicine and Western medicine. Treatments that addressed Liver patterns simply because of the Western medicine diagnosis of hepatitis were unlikely to have positive results. I asserted that an effective Chinese medicine treatment of chronic hepatitis should focus instead on the Spleen and Stomach. I gave three reasons for this claim. First, when considered from the perspective of pattern recognition, most chronic viral hepatitis patients suffer from gastrointestinal symptoms—the abdominal bloating and discomfort, nausea, vomiting, and irregular stools that I had observed with Dr. Su—which are most directly associated with patterns of the Spleen and Stomach. Second, when considered from the perspective of Chinese medicine nosological categories (known as *bing*, see Chapter 3), I argued that the closest approximation to chronic viral hepatitis would be "Jaundice" (*huang dan*). Chronic hepatitis patients do not usually present with jaundice—a dark yellow discoloration of the skin, the eyes, and the urine. But many patients do in the acute stage, and I argued that this diagnosis was the best way to impose some classificatory rigor on the otherwise unremarkable gastrointestinal symptoms of most chronic hepatitis patients. Furthermore, it is also important because, according to Five Phases doctrine, the yellowish color of jaundice corresponds to the Spleen (and Stomach) and not the Liver. Lastly, classical Chinese medicine scholarship on Jaundice supports this approach. I found that in most ancient references to the treatments for Jaundice, doctors almost always emphasized the role of Spleen and Stomach and rarely mentioned the Liver.

The oral defense took place about a month before graduation. The thirty-odd classmates of mine who had been training at Dongzhimen Hospital at the time crowded into a hospital classroom. The thesis committee sat toward the front of the classroom behind several long desks. One after another, they called on individual students to take a seat at a desk directly in front of them. Each student was given a few minutes to briefly summarize his or her research and then another ten minutes to respond to the committee's questions. The rest of the class watched uncomfortably, as the thesis committee was surprisingly sharp in its questioning. Many of my classmates had dashed off their essays, and the thesis committee rebuked them without mercy.

In contrast to many of my classmates, I had worked quite hard on my thesis and was perhaps overly pleased with the final product. I thought my conclusions were well supported and might possibly have some clinical significance. I also asked several friends to help me polish the final draft, so that I could be sure that my argument would not be muddled by errors of grammar and diction. But I felt my confidence ebb as I watched my classmates, one after another, wilt before the thesis committee. When my turn finally came, I stumbled through a very poor summary of my argument. One committee member, Dr. Xia, took the lead in posing most of the questions. I had been introduced to her a couple years earlier when she was a Ph.D. student, and she had agreed to let me interview her on her experience as a Chinese medicine graduate student. I remembered that her advisor was one of the most famous doctors in the hospital, a specialist in gastrointestinal disorders, and I even recalled that her Ph.D. research had been on alcohol-related liver disease. My project was about a topic she knew well. Her stern demeanor gave no hint as to whether she remembered me. "In your graduation thesis, you argued that chronic hepatitis should be diagnosed as Jaundice, correct?" "Yes," I said quietly, suddenly feeling much less certain about this claim. ". . . and therefore, therapy should center on the treatment of the Spleen and Stomach." "Yes. . . ." Her examination technique was quite simple. She turned all my claims into questions and then threw them back at me. At the end of her long list of questions, she paused for what seemed like a very long time. Then she delivered her concluding point. "Ai Like (艾理克)," she said, addressing me by my Chinese name. "The treatment of the Spleen and Stomach are important for cases of chronic viral hepatitis, but you absolutely must not ignore the Liver. Soothing the Liver, softening the Liver, supplementing the Liver, clearing the Liver, and other Liver pattern therapies are essential to the treatment of hepatitis. . . . Hepatitis is a disease of the liver. It would be dangerous not to treat the Liver."

In the last vignette, Dr. Xia seemed to be directly contradicting the lessons of the previous two. Instead of carefully defending the boundaries of the Chinese medicine body from neophytes who may not fully understand the epistemological and political stakes of doing so, Dr. Xia was embracing the opposing strategy of integrating the two medical systems and finding points of congruence in their respective "bodies." In fact, she even performed this integration through a linguistic ambiguity. When she cautioned that "hepatitis is a disease of the liver" and that "it would be dangerous not to treat the Liver," it was impossible to know with certainty to which medical system and to which organ she referred. Based on context, I have assumed the Western medicine *liver* in the first sentence and the Chinese medicine *Liver* in the second. And I have followed the convention of Western scholars of using lowercase and uppercase letters to distinguish the organs of Western medicine and Chinese medicine, respectively. But this convention reinforces the assumed divide between the two medical systems, positing two L/livers, not one. In Chinese, no such convention exists. There is only one word for this organ—*gan* (肝)—and there are no orthographic devices to distinguish its different connotations in Chinese and Western medicine. Sometimes these distinctions are readily discernible from context. At other times, the grammatical flexibility of Chinese makes it possible to slip between meanings or even imply both at once. We will see doctors grappling with and sometimes intentionally using similar semantic ambiguities in other situations (see Chapter 3).

My argument to eliminate anatomical considerations from the Chinese medicine treatment of chronic viral hepatitis was in the spirit of defending the distinctiveness of the Chinese medicine body, a calling many of my teachers had passionately instilled in me. But it was flawed from the onset because I was applying Chinese medicine therapies to a Western medicine diagnosis. I had already conflated the categories that I was seeking to purify. Dr. Xia's critique implicitly recognized this problem with her call to integrate the two medical systems. And perhaps, equally important for her response, my project dealt directly with therapeutic interventions. We were no longer engaging in an intellectual debate about the uniqueness of the Chinese medicine body—a position she might possibly defend in other circumstances—but how to design a Chinese medicine treatment for a Western medicine pathology. Her integrationist approach was no less important than the contravening trend to segregate. Just as doctors might warn their students about the dangers of conflation, doctors (sometimes the same doctor) also told stories about the risks of not combining both medical systems. These stories usually turned on the perceived diagnostic strengths of Western medicine, with cancer often playing the role of the bogeyman. "The patient has a persistent cough, but you don't recognize that it's caused by lung cancer. . . ." "You spend weeks, even months, treating a patient's chronic abdominal pain, and then you discover the patient has stomach cancer. . . ." In stories like these, the doctor of Chinese medicine is always guilty of "delaying the patient's therapy," allowing the cancer to metastasize, permitting a treatable situation to become a life-threatening one, and presumably using less efficacious Chinese medicine therapies when better Western medicine treatments would be indicated. These same doctors may readily admit that Chinese medicine therapies could be an important, perhaps even crucial part of the patient's therapy, but only after a correct Western medicine diagnosis has been made.

The conflicting admonishments captured in these vignettes highlight the challenges that contemporary doctors of Chinese medicine face when negotiating the boundaries between Western medicine and Chinese medicine. In the everyday clinical practice of Chinese medicine, contemporary doctors of Chinese medicine seem caught between the dynamics of purification and hybridization. They must navigate between two contradictory positions: either the bodies of Chinese medicine and Western medicine are radically incommensurate, or they have definite points of congruence; either they represent two distinct ontological realms, or they are related through a hybrid space of intervention. Upon first reflection, one might think that the uncertainties of this relationship would make clinical work impossible. Yet contemporary doctors are surprisingly adept at negotiating this problem. Indeed, the great rapidity with which doctors at crowded urban hospitals conduct their consultations every day suggests that this problem hardly slows them down at all.

It is my contention that this intellectual agility is based on a small "toolbox" of conceptual devices, such as the dualisms explored in this book, that help doctors negotiate this postcolonial predicament. The structure-function dualism is one such tool that guides everyday clinical practice and allows doctors to navigate two medical practices that are simultaneously incommensurable and occasionally analogous. It reifies the divide between East and West, between "Chinese medicine" and "Western medicine," and provides techniques for bridging this divide.

Relating to Anatomy

Like Nathan Sivin and Manfred Porkert, most contemporary doctors assert that the bodies of Western medicine and Chinese medicine are radically different. But the belief that Chinese medicine describes a functional body and Western medicine a structural body only emerged in the Communist period. During the Republican era, doctors claimed that the bodies of the two medical systems were roughly analogous. I want to first illustrate this transformation visually by comparing two images, the first from a textbook published in 1937 and the second, published over two decades later, from a 1959 textbook. Then I will return to a more detailed examination of this historical transition.

Beginning in 1937, new students at the China Institute of Medicine (中國 醫學院) in Shanghai, a well-known private academy of Chinese medicine, would have encountered Figure 10 in a textbook called Lecture Notes on Anatomy (解剖學講義). Like many textbooks from this era, it was a handwritten document created by the individual who would teach the course.[2] This anatomical drawing, titled "Image of the Anterior-Posterior Intersections of the Organs," appeared relatively early in the textbook, in a section called "Overview of Anatomy." It depicts a crude side view of the head and torso as an empty shell that contains nothing but two intersecting tracts, crossing

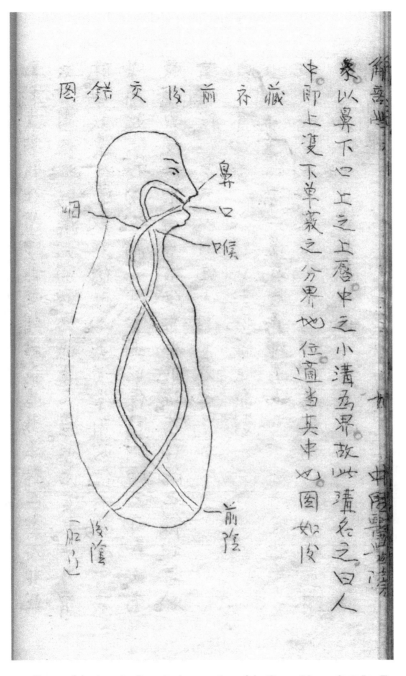

臟腑前後交錯圖

系以鼻下口上之上唇中之小溝為界故此溝名之曰人
中即上復下單裝之分界地位適當其中也圖如後

鼻
口
喉
咽
前陰
後陰
肛门

Figure 10. "Image of the Anterior-Posterior Intersections of the Organs." Image from Bao Tianbai's Lecture Notes on Anatomy (Bao Tianbai 1937).

three times at the throat, chest, and lower abdomen. In spite of the title, no organs are shown in this image. One tract begins at the mouth, becomes the pharynx (咽), and weaves toward its terminus at the "rear yin" (後陰) or anus (肛門). The other tract begins at the nose, becoming the larynx (喉), and after crossing the first tract two more times ends at the "front yin" (前陰), a shorthand for the genitals (Bao Tianbai 1937). The first tract may represent the gastrointestinal tract in a highly schematic form, but the second one does not have a single anatomical referent. Is it a mistake? Does it refer to connections and resonances beyond anatomy? Why is this seemingly crude drawing one of the first images that a student would encounter in a textbook on anatomy, a field that has been called "iconophilic," because of its long historical association with detailed, realistic drawings of the human body (Moxham and Plaisant 2014)?

It is worth reflecting on this image because it does not, and arguably could not, appear in any contemporary medical textbook in China. Neither traditional nor modern, neither Chinese nor Western, and perhaps according to the critics of the age, "neither donkey nor horse" (Lei 2014), this image probably never circulated beyond this textbook itself. Nonetheless, I believe it captures some important features of the Chinese medicine profession and its relationship to the discipline of anatomy during the Republican period. *Lecture Notes on Anatomy* is a Chinese medicine text with an expansive understanding of the field of anatomy. It borrows terms and rubrics from this modern field of medicine, but primarily to organize concepts and claims from the Chinese medicine corpus. For the author Bao Tianbai (包天白), a well-known Chinese medicine educator of this era, the writing of this textbook was an opportunity to bring together the "anatomical theories (*jiepou xueshuo*) of National medicine that have been scattered across various texts and present them in two parts, an Overview of Anatomy (解剖學總論) and Specific Anatomical Systems (解剖學各論)."[3] In other words, *Lecture Notes on Anatomy* is not a conventional biomedical anatomy textbook; rather, it is very much a Chinese medicine textbook, presenting an overview of how the physical body was depicted across various ancient Chinese medical texts.

What is striking here is that Bao Tianbai was perfectly comfortable assembling traditional statements about the body under the modern rubric of anatomy. His side view of the torso was reminiscent of classic drawings of the body found in late imperial texts. But his intertwining tracts were original. In the accompanying text, he gave only a brief explanation of the image.

The system of the five *zang* [Lungs, Heart, Spleen, Liver, and Kidneys] begins at the larynx and ends at the genitals. The system of the five *fu* [Stomach, Gallbladder, Large Intestine, Small Intestine, and Bladder][4] begins at the pharynx and ends at the anus. Their anterior and posterior positions mutually intersect. This is truly the Creator's miraculous work. Without this, we could not exist (Bao Tianbai 1937).

Bao Tianbai did not explain how mutual intersection was achieved or even what entities were coming together. For lack of a better term, I have used the word "tracts" to describe the image itself. Bao does not use this term himself, but instead discusses the systems of the five *zang* and five *fu*, two terms that reference the major organs in Chinese medicine. The pathway of the inter-twining "tracts" in the image are only vaguely suggested by verbs, such as "begins," "ends," and "intersect." Although he states that the miracle of life is represented by this drawing, he made only a few brief remarks to explain its significance.

When I first came across Bao's image and description, I was taken aback by its simplicity and crudeness, particularly since it was part of an anatomy textbook. I immediately interpreted it against the iconophilia of standard anat-omy texts, and I suspect today's textbook editors would, as well. Contempo-rary textbooks of Chinese medicine do not contain visual images of the inner structures of the body. Images of the body in classic medical texts were also uncommon. When they did appear, they tended to share some of the stylistic traits of Bao's drawing, such as the images found in the late Ming acupuncture classic, *Compendium of Acupuncture and Moxibustion* (針灸大成), published by Yang Jizhou (楊繼洲) in 1601. Like Bao's, Yang Jizhou's images are quite distinct from the European fascination with detailed, realist portrayals of hu-man anatomy.

Although more detailed than Bao's drawings, Yang's representation of the organs was also schematic. Yang captured the main organs recognized in Chi-nese medicine but omitted most other structures, such as bones, muscles, con-nective tissue, the circulatory system, and so on. He highlighted some of the relationships within the body, using tracts to connect the Heart to the Spleen, Liver, Kidneys, and the genitals. Bao Tianbai's image could be understood as a further simplification of Yang's. He uses the same side view of the torso but omits the organs and lets a simplified set of tracts stand in for them.

Despite the interesting stylistic continuity, Bao Tianbai's image was dif-ferent than Yang Jizhou's because it was clearly in dialogue with the new academic field of modern anatomy. The China Institute of Medicine, in fact, taught the basics of anatomy in a separate course that used a textbook called *Lecture Notes on Physiology and Public Health* (生理衛生講義) (Wu Keqian 1937). But Bao's relationship to anatomy was very different than today's doctors

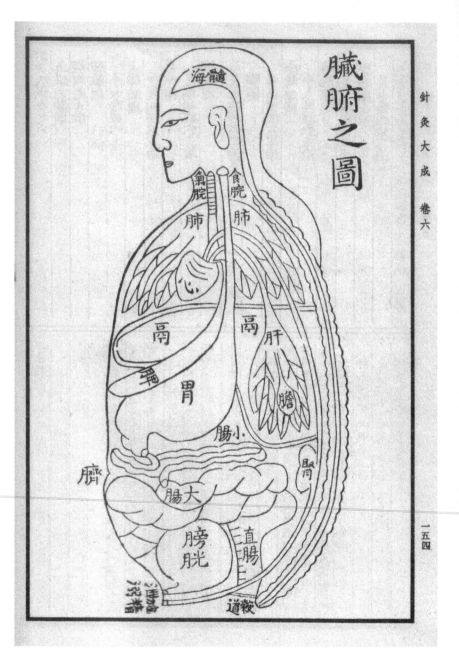

Figure 11. "Drawing of the Human Viscera," Yang Jizhou, Compendium of Acupuncture and Moxibustion, 1601. Image from a 1955 reproduction of this medical classic (Yang Jizhou 1955 [1601], 154). Many medical classics were republished in the early Communist era to help disseminate medical knowledge.

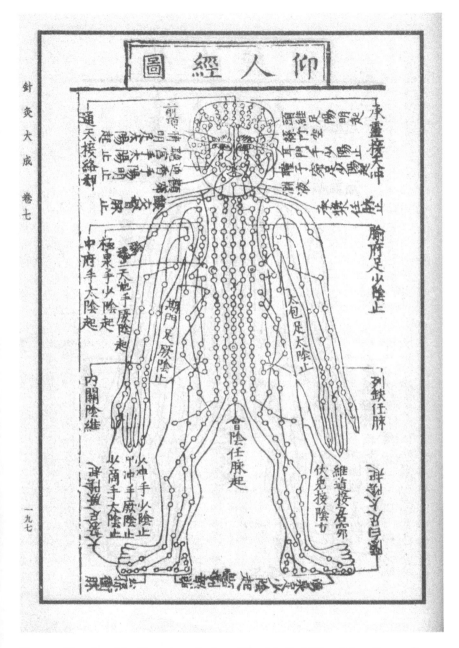

Figure 12. "Drawing of the Channels on the Front Side of the Body," Yang Jizhou, Compendium of Acupuncture and Moxibustion, 1601. Image from a 1955 reproduction of this medical classic (Yang Jizhou 1955 [1601], 197). Note the stylistic differences with the modern textbook images (see Figure 13) that were published just four years later.

for two reasons. First, Bao recognized the strengths and weaknesses in each medical system, but he did not adjudicate them according to the standards of anatomy.

> Our Chinese medicine still does not have the name of anatomy. It only has the approximate [descriptions of] the viscera and bowels, the shell of the body, the meridians, the tendons and bones, the five senses and the four limbs. Western medicine has used the power of scientific instruments to exhaustively study the form, depiction, and significance of the human body (Bao Tianbai 1937, 1–2).

If taken out of context, this passage would almost seem to echo modern critics of Chinese medicine, such as Yu Yanxiu (see Chapter 1) who rejected Chinese medicine categorically because of its inaccurate description of the body's inner structures. But in an interesting reversal, Bao Tianbai asserted that this apparent weakness was balanced by his second key point: Chinese medicine was the clinically superior form of medical practice.

> With regard to the practicalities of treatment, [Western medicine] does not have one-tenth the value [of Chinese medicine]. Although our Chinese medicine lacks the precise anatomy of Western medicine, it contains the more unique doctrines (Bao Tianbai 1937, 2).

Today, Chinese medicine is widely assumed to be the inferior form of medical practice, even by doctors and scholars of Chinese medicine. But claims about the therapeutic advantages of Chinese medicine were actually quite commonplace in the Republican period. In our discussion about acute illnesses, we have already established that there are ample reasons to accept these Republican-era claims of clinical superiority at face value. But scholars have rarely acknowledged this point. Perhaps only Bridie Andrews has gestured toward it in her studies of Republican-era medicine in China. She has argued that early adopters of Western medicine in China were attracted to the medical system for a host of reasons but not primarily its curative efficacy. She noted that Ding Fubao (1874–1952), a key figure who helped to popularize Western medicine through his voluminous writings, once stated that "Western medical arts have not yet advanced to a state of completion; some of China's drugs and prescription surpass Western ones" (Andrews 2014, 141). One of my central claims of this chapter is that to correctly interpret Republican-era medical texts, we must begin with this widely shared assumption that Chinese medicine was the clinically superior form of medicine, even if it was being attacked for its supposedly unscientific foundations. It will not be possible to understand how doctors of Chinese medicine related to the anatomical claims of Western medicine without recognizing this basic conviction.

When did these attitudes about clinical efficacy change, and was there a corresponding shift in the way doctors of Chinese medicine related to the field of anatomy? In Chapter 1, we discovered that a major shift in how doctors perceived the clinical efficacies of the two medical systems was underway in the first decade of Communist rule in the 1950s. Figure 13 suggests that doctors' relations with modern anatomy were changing at roughly the same time. This image appeared in an early textbook, *Concise Acupuncture and Moxibustion Studies* (简明针灸学), produced at the Nanjing College of Chinese Medicine and published in 1959. Here we can observe one of the twelve major meridian channels, the Hand Greater Yang Small Intestine Channel, mapped onto a realistic image of the human body. The comparison with Bao Tianbai's drawing, produced twenty-two years earlier, is instructive. Both images appear in textbooks. The first was produced by the author himself for a course he taught in a private institute. The second was created with the support of the state at the Nanjing College of Chinese Medicine, one of the most important sites for textbook production in the early PRC. Bao Tainbai's image claimed an association with modern anatomy in the titles of the textbook and the image, yet the entities had no clear correspondence to actual anatomical structures, flouting the realist traditions of accuracy and precision in anatomical drawing. The Nanjing image depicted a meridian channel, a Chinese medicine entity that is considered to have no underlying anatomical substrate (Porkert 1974; Hu Xianglong and Cheng Shennong 1997). Yet the rest of the image conforms to conventional human dimensions. The solid lines indicate the meridian pathway on the surface of the body. The dots are its associated pressure points. The broken line depicts an interior branch of the meridian, which "attaches to the heart, follows the pharynx, descends through the diaphragm, arrives at the stomach, and belongs to the small intestine" (Acupuncture and Moxibustion Teaching and Research Group of the Nanjing College of Chinese Medicine 1959). Although schematic, each of these internal structures is drawn in roughly the correct location. The pathway of the channel follows an identifiable topography of the body, and one might reasonably use the image to identify this pathway on an actual human body. The broken lines do not correspond to internal structures, like the "tracts" found in Yang Jizhou and Bao Tianbai's drawings, but merely suggest certain relationships.

This text was not the first to use realistic drawings or even photos to map the meridian channels onto an anatomically correct body. But it is one of the earliest textbooks of the Communist era, and it helped establish a trend that continues to this very day. In current textbooks, all drawings of meridian channels follow this basic style. Each channel is drawn on a young adult, male model of realistic proportions. If the inner structures of the body, such as bones, organs, and other tissues, are included, they are always sketched

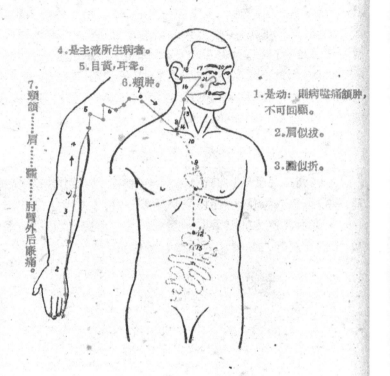

(六)手太阳小腸經脉循行与病候关系示意图

1.起于小指之端, 2.循手外侧上腕，出踝中， 3.直上循臂骨下廉，出肘内侧两骨之間， 4.上循臑外后廉， 5.出肩解， 6.繞肩胛， 7.交肩上， 8.入缺盆， 9.絡心， 10.循咽， 11.下膈， 12.抵胃， 13.屬小腸， 14.其支者，从缺盆， 15.循頸， 16.上頰， 17.至目銳眥， 18.却入耳中， 19.其支者，別頰上䪼，抵鼻， 20.至目内眥， 21.斜絡于顴。

Figure 13. "Hand Greater Yang Small Intestine Channel Pathway and Its Relationship to Its Illness Presentations." Image from 1959 textbook *Concise Acupuncture and Moxibustion Studies* (Acupuncture and Moxibustion Teaching and Research Group of the Nanjing College of Chinese Medicine 1959). Note the stylist differences with the Yang Jizhou images (see Figures 11 and 12), republished just a few years earlier.

according to their appropriate anatomical size and proportion. In short, this style of drawing superimposes the "functional body" of the meridian channel on the "structural body" of anatomy. Perhaps it is just this blending of structure and function that gives this style of drawing currency in contemporary acupuncture textbooks.[5]

One Body or Two?

With these images in mind, separated by a mere twenty-two years, we will begin a deeper exploration of the transformation captured by their stylistic differences. In contrast to the Communist era, where doctors of Chinese medicine oscillate between policing the boundaries of ontologically distinct bodies and awkwardly trying to find points of congruence, we will see that Republican-era doctors moved relatively smoothly between the bodies of Western medicine and Chinese medicine. For doctors of Chinese medicine with an interest in anatomy during this period, the bodies of Chinese medicine and Western medicine were considered roughly analogous. But doctors and scholars of this period also recognized that there were areas of significant divergence between the bodies of the two medical systems. When confronted with differences, these scholars accounted for them in two basic ways. First, they would attack Chinese medicine itself. They often argued that Chinese claims were erroneous because doctors of the late imperial period had not faithfully transmitted the correct meanings of the texts from early China. Second, they would be critical of Western medicine. When they wanted to champion the Chinese medicine perspective, they would argue that differences reflected the greater theoretical subtlety and refinement of the Chinese explanation.

In certain circumstances, doctors might resort to a third strategy, what historian Sean Hsiang-lin Lei has called the claim to incommensurability. This position was a precursor to the purifications that became commonplace in the Communist era, but it is important to recognize that this strategy emerged as a response to attacks by the biomedical critics. It was significant in the political clash between the two professions, but, given the circumscribed nature of those debates (see Chapter 1), it had minimal influence in the realm of clinical practice. As we will see, the structure-function dualism did not exist in the Republican period, even though Lei's research captures some of the discursive developments that would enable its emergence in the Communist era. To clarify the relationship between Lei's research on this topic with my own arguments about how doctors of Chinese medicine related to the field of anatomy during the Republican period, it is helpful to examine the work of the late Qing scholar and physician Tang Zonghai (唐宗海). Lei's analysis of the claim to incommensurability centers on the concept of "qi transformation" (氣化), which was developed by Tang Zonghai and later used by Republican-era doctors to assert the fundamental ontological distinctions between the bodies of Chinese medicine and Western medicine (Lei 2014). While Lei astutely tracked the evolving uses of this concept, it is important to explore other aspects of Tang Zonghai's work that were even more influential for Republican-era doctors.

Tang Zonghai was one of the first doctors of Chinese medicine to write seriously about the differences between Chinese medicine and Western medicine. In his groundbreaking work *Essential Meanings of the Medical Classics in Light of the Convergence of China and the West* (中西匯通醫經精義), published in 1892, Tang was forced to grapple with a basic epistemological challenge: what is the significance of modern anatomy for the practice of Chinese medicine? Do the different descriptions of the human body found in Chinese medicine and modern anatomy refer to one body or two?[6] Tang's answer was complicated. On the one hand, Tang was sensitive to the growing imperialist incursions of this period. As he stated in his preface, "Today all the countries of the Far West have penetrated Chinese territory. Not only are their machines dominating, but they slander the medicine of China as false" (Wang Mimi and Li Lin 1999, 3). Throughout the text, he felt compelled to defend the greatness of Chinese civilization. "The writings of the three dynasties of the Qin and Han, the *Inner Canon*, the *Classic of Difficulties*, and Zhongjing's treatises, were extremely precise and refined, far beyond the achievements of Western medicine" (Wang Mimi and Li Lin 1999, 3).

Tang's pride in Chinese civilization is balanced by his concern that this cherished heritage was in decline. "The true transmission [of Chinese medicine] gradually declined after the Jin and Tang dynasties. It has been full of errors since the Song dynasty" (Wang Mimi and Li Lin 1999, 3). As I will discuss in greater detail in Chapter 3, Tang was not alone in his belief in the late imperial decline in Chinese civilization. His views were part of the intellectual trend known as evidential scholarship that rejected neo-Confucianist thought, the philosophical movement that had dominated Chinese society since its emergence in the eleventh century during the Song dynasty (Bol 2008). From the perspective of evidential scholars, neo-Confucianism was a speculative and corrupting philosophical trend that had diverged from the original writings of Confucius and his disciples (Elman 1984). Tang's solution to the problem of neo-Confucianism and the corruption of late imperial medical writings was to correct them with insights from Western medicine. Many doctors from the Republican period who believed it was essential to reform Chinese medicine adopted precisely this same approach.

Tang was particularly interested in anatomy but also critical of its limitations. He admired European anatomical descriptions because of their precision, but he also argued that they lacked an account of qi transformation.
"Western methods . . . are very detailed about the form [of the body] but ignore its qi transformation" (Wang Mimi and Li Lin 1999, 4). Although "qi
transformation" indexed the theoretical subtlety of Chinese medicine, Tang
believed that it was anatomy that would clarify it. In the "Introductory Remarks," he notes:

> I have selected the anatomical drawings of Westerners but have not
> followed their explanations. They demonstrate that the descriptions
> of the *Inner Canon* were indeed correct. By using these drawings to
> seek the meaning of the canons, qi transformation will be even more
> evident (Wang Mimi and Li Lin 1999, 4).

In this passage, Tang Zonghai's belief in the "convergence" of the two
medicines was evident. Anatomy could illuminate qi transformation. But at
other moments, Tang seemed to waver on this point, stressing the divergence
of the two medicines.

> One must first understand Heaven and Earth, yin and yang, before
> one can know the qi transformations of the human body. Through
> dissection and examination, Western medicine has described in detail
> every layer of the human body, front and back, left and right, inside
> and outside. But it cannot separate each layer into yin and yang, and
> therefore only knows its form but not its qi. Dissection can only exam-
> ine the structures of the corpse. How could it reveal the qi transforma-
> tions of the living person (Wang Mimi and Li Lin 1999, 5)?

Did Tang Zonghai believe in one body or two? Were the distinctions between
the structures of the corpse and the qi transformation of the living body incommensurate or not? On the whole, Tang believed in the convergence of
the two medicines, but later scholars would turn to this strategy of ambiguity
when needed.

Defending the Body of Chinese Medicine

Tang Zonghai's strategy of ambiguity become important only several decades
later when the new doctor of Western medicine Yu Yunxiu launched an attack on the theory of Chinese medicine with his book *Deliberations on the
Divine Pivot and Simple Questions* (靈素商兌), published in 1916. Yu is the
same figure we encountered in Chapter 1 who led an unsuccessful legislative

proposal to ban Chinese medicine in 1929. His theoretical attack preceded his political maneuverings by more than a decade. Yu was originally trained in Chinese medicine and later learned Western medicine when he traveled to Japan in 1908. Although his book was very polemical—he claimed that Chinese medicine was responsible for the deaths of countless individuals over its 4,000-year history—it was not easily refuted because of his strong knowledge of Chinese medicine. The basis of his critique was that Chinese medicine was not grounded in a knowledge of anatomy, making its theoretical claims fallacious. It might be excusable for the ancients to claim that "Liver stores essence and doesn't drain" in light of their level of technological development, he claimed, but for contemporary doctors to adhere to these canonical views was pure dogmatism and ignorance.

Much to Yu's frustration, his challenge to traditional practitioners was ignored until the early 1920s, when it finally elicited a response. As Sean Lei has pointed out, that response, led by Yun Tieqiao (惲鐵樵) and Yu Jianquan, was to mobilize Tang Zonghai's concept of qi transformation to emphasize the differences between the bodies of the two medical systems. Building on Yu Yunxiu's claim that this strategy was "avoiding the place of confrontation," Lei has argued that Yun Tieqiao and Yu Jianquan went beyond Tang's position of ambiguity to make an ontological defense. In other words, they asserted that the two medical systems were incommensurate (Lei 2014, 82–86). In 1922, Yun Tieqiao responded to Yu Yunxiu through his book *A Record of Insights from the Canons* (群經見智錄), building on the concept of qi transformation to advance his new concept of the "four seasons" (*si shi*).

> The five organs of the *Inner Canon* are not the five organs of anatomy, but the five organs of qi transformation (Yun Tieqiao 1948, 104).

> The *Inner Canon* associates the liver with the spring, the heart with the summer, the spleen with late summer, the lungs with autumn, and the kidneys with winter. The liver gives qi to the heart, the heart gives qi to the spleen, the spleen gives qi to the lungs, the lungs give qi to the kidneys, and the kidneys give qi to the liver. Therefore, the five organs of the *Inner Canon* are not the five organs of flesh and blood, but the five organs of the four seasons (四時). Whoever doesn't understand this principle will be clutching at brambles. Not one word of the *Inner Canon* will make sense (Yun Tieqiao 1948, 43).

By insisting on the radical differences between "the five organs of the four seasons" and "the five organs of flesh and blood," Yun was indeed relying on the strategy of incommensurability. Instead of capitulating to Yu Yunxiu's insistence that Chinese medicine must be evaluated by the standards of anatomy, he tried to turn the tables on him.

> If [Yu Yunxiu] states that it is preposterous to study medicine without
> knowing anatomy, I respond in the same tone. It is preposterous to
> study medicine without knowing the principles of the four seasons,
> hot and cold, yin and yang, production and conquest (Yun Tieqiao
> 1948, 109).

Frustrated by this refusal to engage in the terms of his debate, Yu Yunxiu called Yun's strategy "avoiding the place of confrontation." While Lei is not incorrect in his analysis of this particular debate, we need to be cautious about extending his claim that the bodies of Western medicine and Chinese were henceforth viewed as ontologically distinct. On the contrary, Yun Tieqiao and many of his like-minded reformist colleagues more commonly insisted on the fundamental *commensurability* of the two bodies, as we will see in the surprising story of the nervous system.

Locating the Nerves in the Chinese Medicine Body

Despite Yun Tieqiao's renowned defense of Chinese medicine based on the principles of the four seasons, he was deeply interested in anatomy and Western medicine more generally. Moreover, the overall trajectory of his engagement with Western medicine followed the strategy of convergence first laid out by Tang Zonghai. We can explore the implications of this trend by looking at how he and other reformist doctors, inspired by biomedical discourses on the nervous system, developed new treatments for emotional disorders. The innovations of this period have had a significant effect on contemporary practice, even though most doctors are unaware of their unusual origins (Karchmer 2013).

The key development that emerged out of Republican-era innovations in the treatment of emotional disorders was a focus on the Liver and its associated patterns of disharmony. Classically, the emotions are associated with all the viscera or five *zang*: joy correlates to the Heart, anger with the Liver, pensiveness with the Spleen, sadness with the Lungs, and fear with the Kidneys (Wu Dunxu, Liu Yanchi, and Li Dexin 1995, 130). Contemporary doctors, however, take a more expansive view of the role of the Liver in regulating the emotions. The Liver's capacity to "course and drain" (*shuxie*) qi is considered essential to one's emotion life in general. When the Liver is constrained and qi does not flow freely, emotional volatility ensues (Wu Dunxu, Liu Yanchi, and Li Dexin 1995, 68–69).

The Republican-era interest in treating emotional disorders through the Liver were spurred by the disease of neurasthenia, a new concept to Chinese society in the early twentieth century. Neurasthenia, which literally means "weakness of the nerves," became a fashionable term in the late nineteenth century for describing the physical and emotional exhaustion thought to be caused by modern lifestyles. When the concept arrived in early twentieth-century China, it found a receptive audience. It seemed particularly fitting for the semi-colonial Chinese urbanites, where the feeble, sickly Chinese individual was considered to be at the root of national weakness (Shapiro 1998, 2003). For Chinese medicine, neurasthenia was not just a trendy new disease concept but also a vehicle for thinking about the nervous system, which was an aspect of anatomy that was still being intensely investigated at the turn of the twentieth century.[7] There is no entity in Chinese medicine that directly corresponds to the nervous system of Western medicine. As Hugh Shapiro has pointed out, Chinese medicine physicians had previously encountered anatomical descriptions of the nervous system and its centrality to cognition and volition. But these physiological and philosophical claims had limited utility in the pragmatic world of clinical practice. With the arrival of neurasthenia, doctors of Chinese medicine now had an entry for thinking about the role of the nerves in treating emotional disorders (Shapiro 2003).

Spurred by the encounter with neurasthenia, reformist doctors of Chinese medicine began to make a surprising claim: the biomedical concept of the nerves was roughly analogous to the Chinese medicine description of the Liver. Therefore, neurasthenia could be treated by addressing Liver-related pathologies. This claim is surprising because no doctor of Chinese medicine today would make this assertion. It would be dismissed as "contrived" (*qian-qiang fuhui*), the sort of novice mistake that might merit a serious reprimand from one's teacher. But the doctors making this claim in the Republican period were hardly novices. They were excellent clinicians, great scholars, and careful students of Western medicine. For example, Zhang Cigong (章次公), a highly respected clinician from the Republican period, referred to this principle in his clinical cases. Commenting on the insomnia of a patient named Mr. Liang, Zhang explained the relationship of the Liver to the nerves: "The ancients would consider this a case of Liver deficiency because the Liver stores the ethereal soul (*hun*). Most herbs that tonify the Liver have the function of strengthening the nerves" (Zhu Liangchun 1980, 229). In another case, he treated Mr. Zhou's neurasthenia with a prescription in which seven out of eight total herbs in the prescription directly or indirectly treat the Liver. He commented, "This formula is like a Chinese medicine tranquilizer, and it is appropriate for insomnia due to neurasthenia" (Zhu Liangchun 1980, 231).

Zhang Cigong's claim that the Liver was roughly analogous to the nervous system and could therefore guide the treatment of emotional disorders was a widely shared viewpoint among his reformist colleagues. Although Yun Tie-qiao had seemingly "avoided the place of confrontation" in his debate with Yu Yunxiu in 1922, he made a similar argument in *Exploring the Subtleties of the Pulse* (脈學發微), one of the textbooks for his correspondence school, published a few years later in 1926. In the following passage, he argued that a wiry pulse (*xian mai*), the classic pulse associated with Liver pathologies, indicated emotional imbalances resulting from the actions of the nervous system.

> Why is the pulse of the Liver wiry? Wiry indicates tension in the nerves of the arterial walls. Liver disease in the *Inner Canon* actually refers to brain disease. The classics usually associate anger with the Liver, which is why the Liver is the General, but in fact [the emotions of] the Liver include melancholy, hatred, neuroticism, and all seven emotions (*qiqing*). Its diseases are integrally related to the brain and therefore are neurogenic (Yun Tieqiao 2008, 48).

> All diseases and symptoms that are related to the nerves should be discussed in terms of the Liver. Our generation cannot afford not to know this fact (Yun Tieqiao 2008, 24).

Another famous Republican-era physician, Zhu Weiju (祝味菊), known for his virtuoso clinical skills, also shared this understanding of the nervous system. Zhu Weiju had a strong background in Western medicine, having spent two years studying it at the Sichuan Military Medicine Academy and another year studying medicine in Japan. In his 1931 book *Elaborations on Pathology* (病理發揮), he argued that both Heart qi and Liver qi conditions in Chinese medicine referred to nervous system pathologies.

> The more the world's level of civilization progresses, the more knowledge advances, the more functional nervous disorders spread. . . . The ancients were not good at anatomy and did not know what the nerves were. They speculated about the pathology of functional nervous disorders based on the symptoms, sometimes even attributing particular presentations to the various organs. . . . References to all Heart qi and Liver qi diseases in the old medical texts correspond to what we today call nervous diseases. The correspondence is, in fact, quite good most of the time, just the names are different. Heart qi refers to functions of the voluntary nervous system; Liver qi refers to the functions of the autonomic nervous system. The ancient term "qi" encompasses all the functions of the nervous system (Zhu Weiju 2005, 14).

Although we can see Zhu Weiju invoking the language of structure and function in this passage, his larger interest is not to separate the two bodies of Western medicine and Chinese medicine but to demonstrate their congruences by relating Heart qi and Liver qi to the nervous system. As these three passages suggest, there was relative unanimity among these reformist voices: the Chinese medicine Liver was roughly analogous to the biomedical nervous system. Therefore, the emotional disorders of the day, such as neurasthenia, could be treated by therapies that addressed Liver pathologies. Although the historical origins of these innovative new treatments have been forgotten, in part because contemporary textbooks of Chinese medicine carefully eschew most references to Western medicine, this therapeutic approach is widely used by practitioners today (Y. Zhang 2007; Karchmer 2013). Soon another feature of this story may be forgotten. Neurasthenia was a disease category that was already falling out of favor in the West just as it was becoming popular in China, and it was eventually abandoned as a biomedical diagnosis (Kleinman 1986, 21). The term has remained popular in China, although it is gradually being displaced by other psychiatric diseases and their accompanying pharmaceutical treatments since the 1990s.

Geographic Imaginaries and the Body

It would be misleading to suggest that Zhang Cigong, Yun Tieqiao, Zhu Weiju, and other reformist doctors of the Republican period represented or somehow spoke for the vast number and incredible diversity of Chinese doctors that were practicing in the Republican period. There were elite doctors and scholars, working primarily in Shanghai during this time, but they were influential writers and educators who shaped medical discourse. Their interest in anatomy built upon and continued the trend toward "convergence" launched by Tang Zonghai's *Essential Meanings*. As Bao Tianbai, Deng Tietao (see Chapter 1), and Lu Yuanlei (see Chapter 3) would attest, their confidence to borrow from the modern claims of anatomy almost certainly related to their prowess as clinicians and their confidence in the clinical advantages of their medical practice over Western medicine.

By the late 1950s, however, there was a shift in how doctors of Chinese medicine wrote about anatomy. Scholars turned away from the pursuit of congruences with Western medicine. With the rapid growth of the Western medicine profession in the early Communist period, it became essential to emphasize the distinctive features of Chinese medicine, not the "convergences" with Western medicine. The ontological divide, first suggested in Yu Yanxiu's debate with Yun Tieqiao and Yu Jianquan, re-emerged and began to be codified in new textbooks. But this new focus on the uniqueness of the Chinese medicine body was also an exercise in negotiating the problem of double truths. Distinctive features of the Chinese medicine body had to appear epistemologically reasonable and at least have the aura of scientific plausibility. Doctors turned to the discourse of structure and function, which became the primary means for purifying the distinctions between the bodies of Chinese medicine and Western medicine. This new divide was already prominently featured in the first state-produced Chinese medicine textbook, *Overview of Chinese Medicine* (中医学概论), published in 1958. It is perhaps not insignificant that this textbook was written specifically for doctors of Western medicine who were enrolled in the new "integrated medicine" programs to study Chinese medicine. The concepts of structure and function become indispensable tools for translating and explaining difficult classical terms, such as "viscera manifestation" (*zangxiang*; 藏象).

The concept of viscera manifestation is essential to understanding the properties of the organs, as understood in Chinese medicine. To better understand the challenge confronting the editors of *Overview* and other textbooks, I will give a brief example of how the term viscera manifestation is described classically in the *Inner Canon* and then compare its presentation in *Overview*. In the chapter "On the Six Calendrical Units and Viscera Manifestation" (六節藏象論), the Yellow Emperor questions his minister, Qi Bo, about the meaning of this term.

> The Yellow Emperor asks: what does viscera manifestation (*zangxiang*) mean?
> Qi Bo responds: The Heart is the *root* of life, the place of the Spirit (*shen*). It *manifests* in the face and is *expressed* in the blood vessels. It *belongs* to the greater yang within yang and *opens* to the qi of Summer. The Lungs are the *root* of breath (*qi*), the place of the Corporeal Spirit (*po*). They *manifest* in the hair and are *expressed* in the skin. They *belong* to the greater yin within yang and *open* to the qi of Fall. The Kidneys are the *root* of. . . . The Liver is the *root* of. . . . The Spleen, Stomach, Large Intestine, Small Intestine, Triple Burner, and Bladdeer are the *root* of. . . . (Nanjing College of Chinese Medicine 1992 [1959], 81) (author's emphasis).

Qi Bo responds to the Yellow Emperor by discussing each major organ and its relationships within the body. Each organ is described in the same way: it "roots" an essential property of the body, stores a form of "spirit," "manifests" on the exterior of the body, is "expressed" in a related tissue, "belongs" to a system of yin-yang relationships, and "opens" to the seasons. The famous Ming dynasty commentator Zhang Jingyue (張景岳) used the multiple meanings of the ancient term *zang*, which means "organ," to "store," and to "hide," to explain the web of relationships that link the organs to the body and cosmos. "Zangxiang means stores (藏) in the interior, but manifests (象) on the exterior" (Li Zhiyong 1999, 36).

In *Overview of Chinese Medicine*, these properties and relationships are carefully teased out and presented in language that is more digestible for its modern readership. "Viscera manifestation" serves as the title of the chapter, but it is not explained as a relationship of interior to exterior; rather, the editors turned to the concepts of structure and function to lay out its distinctions from the anatomical body.

> In summary, the Chinese medicine understanding of the organs is that on the one hand, they refer in part to the substantive organs (*shizhi zangqi*). But more importantly, it refers to all the manifestations of the functional activities and pathological changes of the organs. All these manifestations do not completely represent the activities and effects of the substantive organs. Rather they indicate the activities and effects of a certain system (this system is not the modern anatomical concept of system). For example, the *Inner Canon* "On Needling Prohibitions" states: "The Liver produces on the left, the Lungs store on the right." "On Regulating the Meridians" also says: "The Heart stores spirit." These claims are completely unrelated to their anatomical references. But in terms of physiological function, pathological changes, as well as therapeutic efficacy, the theory of the *Inner Canon* is entirely accurate (Nanjing Zhongyi Xueyuan 1958, 40–41).

The stylistic contrast between this passage and the writings of the Republican scholars previously discussed is striking. Instead of a confident assertion of congruences between the Chinese medicine body and Western anatomy, we have an anxious defense of the Chinese medicine claims about the body that are "entirely accurate," even though they are "completely unrelated to their anatomical references." Moreover, the discussion of difference has shifted from Chinese medicine concepts such as qi transformation and the four seasons to the scientistic concepts of structure and function. The audience is no longer a Chinese medicine community seeking to find congruence between the two medical systems but doctors of Western medicine and other modern readers who are puzzling out the differences between the bodies of the two medical systems.

Doctors of Western medicine were not the only ones struggling to grasp the meaning of "visceral manifestation." Undergraduate students at the new state-run colleges of Chinese medicine, having just completed a standard high school education, also found themselves on unfamiliar terrain. When "viscera manifestation" was explained in the first edition of the national textbooks, published in 1960, the editors also distinguished between the "physiological function" of the Chinese medicine organs and the contrasting physiology associated with the anatomical organs.

> The origin of our nation's anatomy was early. In the *Inner Canon*,
> there are records of much anatomical knowledge. But it is important
> to point out that the understanding of physiological function of the
> organs in the *Inner Canon* is not based on modern anatomy (Beijing
> College of Chinese Medicine Inner Canon Department [Beijing
> Zhongyi Xueyuan Jiaoyanzu 1960, 66]).

In subsequent editions of the national textbooks, the concept of visceral manifestation elicited similar comparisons. The 1984 publication of *Basic Theory of Chinese Medicine*, from the highly regarded fifth edition of the national textbooks, described visceral manifestation and the relationship between the two bodies even more robustly in terms of the structure-function dualism.

> Although the names of the organs—Heart, Lungs, Spleen, Liver, and
> Kidneys—in visceral manifestation are the same as modern human
> anatomy, the physiological and pathological meanings are completely
> different. The physiological function of an organ in Chinese medicine
> visceral manifestation might encompass the physiological function of
> several organs in modern anatomy. Conversely, the physiological func-
> tion of an organ in modern anatomy also might be distributed among
> the physiological functions of several organs in visceral manifestation.
> This is because the organs of visceral manifestation are not simply an
> anatomical concept. More importantly, they summarize the physio-
> logical and pathological concept of a particular human system (Yin
> Huihe and Zhang Bo'ne 1984, 29).

In this passage, we find the structure-function dualism described almost exactly as I encountered it as a student: radical divides and awkward points of congruence, presented in a symmetrical fashion that thinly masks the power inequalities between the two medical systems. The two incommensurate bodies of Western medicine and Chinese medicine are "completely different," but they also interpenetrate in complicated ways. The organ of one system can be "encompassed" or "distributed" amongst several organs of the other. In the late nineteenth century, Tang Zonghai celebrated the convergence of East and West and noted points of theoretical divergences between Western and Chinese medicine. He and many of the Republican-era scholars that followed in his wake acknowledged the important insights of Western medicine but were secure in the belief that Chinese medicine was the clinically superior form of medicine. A century later, biomedicine was recognized as the superior form of medicine and the unquestioned epistemological authority on the nature of the body. It was no longer possible to assert that the two medical systems had one shared body. Instead, doctors and scholars insisted on an ontological divide, based on the concepts of structure and function, between the bodies of East and West. Against this dynamic of purification, they would find points of hybridization, limited areas of congruence that might have clinical significance.

Strengths and Weaknesses

One of the most important consequences of the structure-function dichotomy is that it generates a comparative matrix through which one can assess the clinical strengths and weaknesses of each medical system. Just as the acute-chronic dualism began limiting the clinical scope of Chinese medicine in the late 1950s and early 1960s, the structure-function dualism also reshaped clinical practice in a similar way.[8] In my observations, this dualism has often operated as a purifying technology that reinforces the supposed limits of Chinese medicine. Yet what counts as a structural pathology and a functional one is not absolute and may depend on the interpretations of the doctor trying to determine how to make a treatment intervention. Typically, many obvious physical lesions to the body are considered "structural" and beyond the reach of Chinese medicine. Conversely, the absence of an identifiable lesion will enable doctors to identify the condition as "functional" and perhaps amenable to Chinese medicine therapies. I encountered a typical example of this kind of clinical decisionmaking several years ago when visiting with a former classmate who works as an acupuncturist at major hospital in Beijing. She was having significant neck pain that day. I offered to give her an acupuncture treatment and explained to her that it was something I treated frequently in my clinic in the U.S. She waved her hand and declined the offer. "I've already had an X-ray, and I have lost the physiological curve to my cervical spine. I don't think it would help. Acupuncture is not effective at treating structural pathologies." On another occasion, I remember asking a former clinical teacher from Dongzhimen Hospital for some advice about a new patient of mine who was struggling with some complicated digestive issues. Despite seeing several biomedical specialists, the patient had not received a confirmed biomedical diagnosis. I wondered what the prospects would be for a Chinese medicine treatment. My teacher listened carefully as I recounted the patient's medical history and symptoms. Then she said, "It sounds like a 'functional' condition to me. Give it a try. Functional conditions usually respond well to Chinese medicine therapies."

While the structure-function dualism frequently limits the arenas in which Chinese medicine is considered useful, it can also lead to interesting clinical hybridities. These innovations may vary according to a doctor's specific interpretation of the points of congruences between the bodies of Western and Chinese medicine. Dr. Xia's treatment for chronic hepatitis B discussed at the beginning of the chapter represents such an intervention. She used the slippage between the anatomical liver and Chinese medicine Liver to guide her treatment strategies. Cancer therapies are a popular example of similar hybrid innovations. In the early 2000s, I had the opportunity to shadow Dr. Wang Pei (王沛), one of the leading Chinese medicine oncologists at Dongzhimen Hospital. Like most specialists in this field, he thoroughly embraced Western medicine techniques such as surgery, chemotherapy, and radiation to deal with mass of the cancer itself. His Chinese herbal treatments also attempted to treat the cancer cells, the pathological structures, as the root of the patient's illness. But just as importantly, they were designed to correct the "functional" impairments of the disease, the patient's experienced discomforts, including the side effects from the biomedical interventions.

Despite the ways in which the structure-function dualism can limit clinical practice, we should not underestimate the ability of virtuoso doctors to mobilize it to their clinical advantage. I got to witness this kind of innovative hybridity most extensively at Guang'anmen Hospital in Beijing, where I copied prescriptions with Dr. Han Fei (韩斐) over many years. Dr. Han has developed a national reputation for her unique treatments of Tourette's syndrome. Although there is no obvious structural lesion for this difficult-to-treat condition, Dr. Han has mobilized the structure-function dualism to help guide her therapies. Many Chinese medicine pediatricians consider the tics—the physical jerks and vocalizations—of this troublesome condition to be caused by Liver wind. Dr. Han rejects this approach to Tourette's syndrome, even though it would seem to be well grounded in the basic theory of Chinese medicine. A famous passage from the *Inner Canon* states that "all wind with shaking and dizziness is ascribed to the Liver" (*zhu feng diao xuan, jie shuyu gan*). But treating Tourette's syndrome through the Liver leads to poor clinical results, Dr. Han asserts, because she considers it to be "above all a psychiatric condition." The closest approximation to the mind and consciousness in Chinese medicine is the concept of Heart Spirit. Based on this congruence, Dr. Han's formulas always contain at least five or six herbs to treat the Heart.

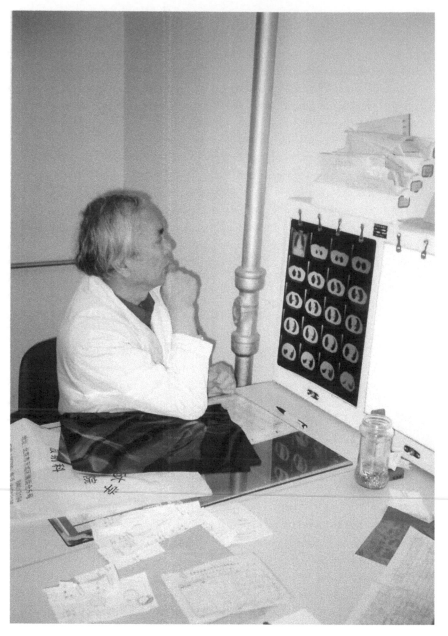

Figure 14. Wang Pei examining the CT scan of one of his cancer patients at Dongzhimen Hospital, 2002.

Over the years, I have watched her successfully treat hundreds of children with Tourette's, gradually bringing their tics, anxieties, and emotional dysregulation under control, through her unique hybrid approach to this condition.

As the previous examples suggest, the degree to which the structure-function dualism constrains the work of Chinese medicine doctors is ultimately determined by the skill of the practitioner. This lesson was delivered most emphatically to me during an interview with the famous physician Jiao Shude (焦树德) in the spring of 1999. I was joined by two local collaborators, Guo Hua, a graduate student in the Department of Inner Canon Studies, and Lai Lili, my research assistant. The three of us had been conducting a series of interviews about the key clinical methodology in Chinese medicine, known as "pattern discrimination and treatment determination" (*bianzheng lunzhi*; 辨证论治) (see Chapter 4). We were overjoyed when Jiao Shude agreed to be interviewed. He was considered to be one of the best Chinese medicine doctors in the whole country. At the request of Jiao Shude, the interview was transformed into something of a small colloquium. He invited one of his former students, Nie Huimin (聂惠民), the chair of the Cold Damage Teaching and Research Group at the Beijing University of Chinese Medicine and a highly respected scholar in her own right. In turn, I invited my academic advisor, Judith Farquhar, a medical anthropologist and leading scholar on Chinese medicine, and Wang Jun, one of my graduate school classmates, who also did research on Chinese medicine. Both just happened to be in Beijing at this time. Nie Huimin arranged for us to meet in a small office at the university, close to the Sino-Japanese Hospital where Jiao Shude worked.

One of the things that distinguished Jiao Shude from other contemporary doctors of Chinese medicine doctors was his unusual medical training. Born in 1922, he had studied Chinese medicine in the classic apprenticeship style during the Republican era. In 1949, he attended a medical school for biomedicine and received a formal degree in this field. Then in 1955, he joined the first class of the program to train young doctors of Western medicine in Chinese medicine, the "integrated medicine" program discussed earlier. Because of the strong support from the CCP, some of the most famous doctors of Chinese medicine from all over China were brought to Beijing to teach in this program. Having just completed his Western medicine training, Jiao Shude was able to join the first class of the integrated medicine program, held at the newly founded China Academy of Chinese Medicine (中国中医研究院). Despite his formal training in biomedicine and his involvement in the high-profile integrated medicine program, he saw himself as a traditionalist, defending the clinical merits of Chinese medicine.

Jiao Shude was famous for his clinical virtuosity, and some of the most scintillating moments of the interview were the cases that he recounted to us. He clearly took great pleasure in telling these stories, describing his treatments in great detail, as if he were proving the efficacy of Chinese medicine to us with each case. The most memorable case from that afternoon included an interesting reference to the structure-function dualism. The events took place in the late 1960s during the height of the Cultural Revolution. Jiao Shude had been sent to the Peking Union Hospital, China's most prestigious hospital of Western medicine, to teach "integrated medicine." During his stay there, a CCP branch secretary personally sought him out on behalf of a patient with an unusual case of bleeding gums that had not responded to any other therapies. He managed to stop the bleeding with just a couple doses of herbs. The party secretary was so impressed that she asked if he might be able to help her husband.

Jiao Shude recalled, "Later she said to me that she had another patient and asked if I could help. This patient turned out to be her husband. . . . I asked what kind of illness it was. She said it had to do with the kidneys. The nerves to the urethra had been severed accidentally during an operation. Once severed, they could not be reattached, and from this point on, he had been incontinent. . . . He had to put thick pads of cotton in his pants, because the urine would just leak out. When the cotton became soaked, he would go to the bathroom and change it. Back then there weren't any "Pampers," just cotton, which he would continually change. This was an agonizing experience for the husband. How could it be treated it, I wondered? The nerve had been severed. The wife had seen me treat the patient with the bleeding gums and knew that Chinese medicine had its unique strengths. When she asked me if I could treat her husband's illness, I said I could try. Maybe it would get better; maybe it wouldn't, because this was a structural lesion (*qizhixing bingbian*), a severed nerve. To my surprise, he drank about ten doses and got better. Not just better, but good enough to act as a representative at the World Health Organization, living abroad for four years with his wife. He was like a normal person, urinating when he wanted to."

At the conclusion of this brief anecdote, Jiao Shude immediately launched into another. His bushy white eyebrows danced over his eyes as he spoke. I glanced up at the others and noticed looks of astonishment on their faces. We were all trained in Chinese medicine to one degree or another. We were all aware that "structural pathologies" were considered beyond the reach of Chinese medicine, and a severed nerve was beyond the reach of any type of medicine. Was it possible that Jiao Shude had embellished this anecdote to impress us? With so many well-documented cases of successful treatments, he had little to gain by doing so. But he had hardly paused to let us appreciate the remarkable claim he had just made. Finally overcome by curiosity, Professor Nie Huimin interrupted. Stepping out of her role as interviewee and back into her former relationship of student to Jiao Shude, she turned and questioned him.

Nie Huimin: "Old Jiao, . . . just now you didn't mention a prescription or a pattern."

Jiao Shude: "I just supplemented the Kidneys. Nothing special!" He raised his voice, as if annoyed by the question. "Don't think that to cure an illness, you need some special medicine. You don't. I just used Rhizoma dioscoreae (*Shan Yao*), Fructus corni (*Shan Zhu Yu*), Radix rehmanniae (*Shou Di Huang*), Rhizoma alismatis (*Ze Xie*), Scleortium poriae cocos (*Fu Ling*), Cortex moutan radicis (*Mu Dan Pi*), and things like Ootheca Mantidis (*Hai Piao Xiao*), and Restrict the Fountain Pill (*Suo Quan Wan*). Just the typical stuff [for supplementing the Kidneys and retaining urine]. If you identify a pattern correctly, you can have miraculous effects. If you don't, then you can take two hundred doses, and nothing will happen."

In this account, Jiao Shude acknowledged his own doubts about treating a condition that was supposedly caused by a structural lesion. But he resolved it in a manner that was stunningly straightforward from the perspective of Chinese medicine. The first six herbs in his list make up a famous, widely used formula, Six-Ingredient Rehmannia Pill (*Liuwei Dihuang Wan*), that all students of Chinese medicine learn by heart. This formula is famous for supplementing the Kidneys, which are known to "rule water" (*zhu shui*), managing the body's distribution and elimination of liquids. In Jiao Shude's analysis, the "root" of this patient's incontinence was a deficiency of the Kidneys. To enhace the effects of this formula, Jiao Shude also added several common herbs to address the "branch," the symptom of leaking urine. Ootheca Mantidis and the three herbs found in the Restrict the Fountain Pill (*Wu Yao, Yi Zhi Ren*, and *Shan Yao*) all served this complementing role by "restricting urine and stopping leakage" (*suoniao zhiyi*). His lesson for us was that correct methodology, properly using "pattern discrimination and treatment determination," rather than secret formulas and exotic medicinals, was all that one needed to treat even the most intractable conditions. In other words, pattern discrimination and treatment determination, when done well, can overcome the structure-function dichotomy. This methodology is so important to contemporary practice that it will be one of the central themes of the remainder of this book. I will argue that this methodology emerged out of a third dualism, the disease-pattern dualism, that shares the same social and political conditions as the acute-chronic and structure-function dualisms. In the hands of a virtuoso clinician like Jiao Shude, it may yield dramatic results. But for the less experienced physicians, this methodology can remain entangled in the power inequalities of postcolonial China.

3

Frail Bodies and the Problem of Diagnosis

In 1929, the Chinese medicine scholar and prolific writer Lu Yuanlei (陸淵雷) captured one of the perplexing qualities of clinical practice in Chinese medicine, a feature of Chinese medicine that could only be confounding when compared to Western medicine, in an article entitled, "Chinese Medicine Cannot Identify Disease (*shi bing*; 識病) But Can Treat Disease (*zhi bing*; 治病)." Lu Yuanlei clearly intended this title to be provocative. But why? Was he criticizing Chinese medicine for its failures of diagnosis? Was he attacking Western medicine for its limitations in treating disease? This intriguing article, together with other writings by Lu Yuanlei and like-minded scholars of this period, was part of a new discourse on Chinese medicine, a style of scholarship that was shaped by a confluence of trends that defined this semi-colonial period of Chinese history. In fact, Lu was criticizing both the Chinese and Western medicine professions, but even more importantly he was also proposing a revaluation of two key terms in his title—*bing* (病) and *zheng* (證). These two terms, usually translated as "disease" and "pattern" today, constitute the most important and complicated of the three dualisms addressed in this book. In this chapter, we will trace the tentative beginnings of this modern dualism in the early and mid-twentieth century. In the remainder of the book, we will follow its emergence and significance for contemporary medical practice.

To appreciate the significance of Lu's essay, it is helpful to first consider how a present-day practitioner would interpret the riddle of Lu Yuanlei's title. How can one treat that which one cannot identify? For today's physician of Chinese medicine, the answer is straightforward: "pattern discrimination and treatment determination" (*bianzheng lunzhi*; 辨证论治). Today's doctor would agree with Lu Yuanlei that Chinese medicine is not sufficient for "identifying disease" because it uses an alternative diagnostic category: the concept of pattern (*zheng*). On the surface, there would seem to be nothing surprisingly or unfamiliar with Lu Yuanlei's title. Yet as soon as we explore this text a little deeper, we will find that our semantic sureties begin to slip away. Lu Yuanlei was not talking about *bianzheng lunzhi* because that term had not yet been invented. Even more importantly, Lu Yuanlei's use of *bing* and *zheng* turn out to be quite different than the way contemporary doctors use them.

To understand why, let's look more closely at these two terms. We begin with *bing*. In contemporary medical practice, *bing* has two meanings. The first is the biomedical concept of "disease." This connotation has a relatively short history in China that can be traced back to nineteenth- and twentieth-century translation efforts in Japan and China to standardize biomedicine terminology (Luesink 2017). The second refers to the much older, indigenous use of the term as a Chinese medicine nosological category. I use "disease" to refer to the former and leave "*bing*" untranslated for the latter. Disease and *bing* have important convergences and divergences. Sometimes a *bing* will closely resemble a biomedical disease. For example, Stomach Pain (胃痛) can be regarded as a relatively close equivalent of gastritis or peptic ulcer in Western medicine. In other cases, a Chinese medicine *bing* may seem like an amalgam of distinct and unrelated biomedical entities. For example, Foot Qi (腳氣) is thought to describe both coronary heart disease and beri beri. As Hilary Smith has shown in her excellent study of the condition, classical usages of this *bing* also closely resembled the disease of gout, and contemporary colloquial usage most often refers to athlete's foot (Smith 2017). Today's doctors insist that an accurate biomedical diagnosis is essential to acquiring a reliable understanding of the patient's condition and prognosis. At the same time, they would also agree with Lu Yuanlei that Chinese medicine can treat, at least in many instances, the very diseases that it fails to describe accurately. The key to this clinical possibility is the concept of "pattern" *zheng*, as described in the methodology of *bianzheng lunzhi*. Doctors can achieve clinically efficacious results by correctly identifying and treating the "pattern" of a patient's illness,

Today's practitioner knows this answer to Lu Yuanlei's question because it is inscribed in the national textbooks. He or she would understand Lu Yuanlei's second key term of *zheng* through the lens of national textbooks, which are organized around the methodology of *bianzheng lunzhi*. But in Lu Yuanlei's essay, there is no reference to *bianzheng lunzhi*. As Volker Schied has argued, this term did not exist until after 1949 (Scheid 2002). Although he could not have known it at the time, Lu's essay (and the work of many others) helped lay the groundwork for the emergence of this methodology a few decades later. He accomplished this task by urging his readers to reengage with one of the great medical texts of early China, the *Treatise on Cold Damage* (*Shanghan Lun*; 傷寒論). But he asked his readers to shift their attention away from the concept of *bing*, a term that was used widely in the text, toward *zheng*—a term used far more sparingly (Mayanagi Makoto 2013).

> Zhang Zhongjing could identify disease (*shibing*) and also treat it. He was, of course, a master of medicine and not a technician. But his method of treating disease (*bing*) only requires the *identification of presentations* (*shizheng*) not disease (*bing*). It turns out that *identifying presentations* (*shizheng*) is easy but *identifying disease* (*shibing*) is difficult. Chinese medicine only seeks to satisfy the need to treat disease (*bing*) but doesn't pay much attention to the difficult and useless methods of *identifying disease* (*shibing*) (Lu Yuanlei 2010b, 1,448). (author's emphasis)

The newness of Lu Yuanlei's argument is evident from the language of this passage: "only" *zheng* is needed to treat *bing*; it "turns out" that *zheng* is much easier to identify than *bing*. Much of this essay and many of Lu Yuanlei's writings on the *Treatise* are devoted to rethinking the meanings of *bing* and *zheng*, arguing that a correct understanding of *zheng* enables the clinician to sidestep the problem of disease diagnosis, which only quasi-mythical sages like Zhang Zhongjing or modern physicians empowered with scientific knowledge could do.

To help clarify Lu's use of *bing* and *zheng*, I have translated *shibing* and *shizheng*, the key terms in the title of his essay, as "identify disease" and "identify presentation," respectively. These translations may surprise some readers. With regard to the first expression, Lu makes clear in the essay that he wants to assert an equivalence between *bing* and "disease." Although I will generally leave *bing* untranslated whenever I refer to the Chinese medicine usage of this concept, I have translated the term as "disease" here because Lu Yuanlei and other reformist doctors of this period rejected an indigenous notion of *bing* that was distinct from the concept of disease. For the second term, I have intentionally chosen "presentation" instead of the today's usual gloss of "pattern" to clearly indicate that Lu Yuanlei was not referring to the methodology of *bianzheng lunzhi*. I believe "presentation" is an excellent term to capture both the late imperial connotations of *zheng* and Lu's own use of the term.

Although these questions of translation may seem like an obscure point of academic debate, I believe essential issues in the history of medicine in twentieth-century China turn on the correct understanding of these terms. A good example can be found in Sean Lei's *Neither Donkey nor Horse*. In this otherwise excellent history of the medicine in Republican China, Lei mistakenly read the clinical writings of this period through the lens of "pattern" and the modern connotations of *zheng*. He acknowledged that the phrase *bian-zheng lunzhi* was not used in this period but argued that the "conceptual content and linguistic fragments were already present and had been correlated with each other" (Lei 2014, 188). As a result, he called this period the "pre-history of pattern differentiation and treatment determination" and argued that this emergent methodology was responding to various challenges posed by the arrival of biomedicine in China (Lei 2014, 190–92). In this chapter, I make a very different claim. The innovators of the Republican period had no conception of *bianzheng lunzhi* and in fact hoped to promote a very different clinical methodology. Although the encounter with biomedicine did indeed spur some of the innovations of this period, its role was far more complex than the impact-response model suggested by Lei. Reformers like Lu Yuanlei were not threatened by biomedicine. In fact, they often were inspired by biomedicine as they responded to other crises that I describe in this chapter. Lei's misinterpretation with regard to the term *zheng* is understandable. Indeed, it could not be more widely shared. Most doctors and scholars of Chinese medicine are unaware of the linguistic shifts I will discuss in this chapter and almost universally read classical texts through the modern connotations of *zheng*. For this reason, I will argue in Chapter 4 that the emergence of "pattern discrimination and treatment determination" (*bianzheng lunzhi*) in the Communist period is best understood as a paradigm shift or epistemic break that has thoroughly transformed our perceptions of late imperial and Republican styles of clinical practice.

My understanding of *zheng* is more closely aligned with the work of Volker Scheid, who has argued for multiple translations of *zheng* to track each major historical period and its corresponding epistemic shifts in medical theory and practice (Scheid 2014). For the purposes of this chapter, however, I differ with Scheid's suggested translations and prefer the single term "presentation" as a gloss for both late imperial and Republican-era usage. This choice has two advantages. First, it emphasizes the continuities between the late imperial and Republican period. Although Lu Yuanlei was not alone in calling for a new understanding of the term, these innovations were tentative, exploratory, and not radically different from late imperial usage. Moreover, they had only limited impact on the general habits of clinical practice. Second, *zheng* only became a key diagnostic term for the majority of practitioners in the Communist era. By emphasizing the continuities between the late imperial and Republican periods with the translation of "presentation," the shift to a new gloss of "pattern" for the Communist era helps to highlight the far more radical shift in connotation that happens in this period.

Lu Yuanlei's essay is a reminder of the challenge of understanding pre-modern Chinese medicine texts, particularly if readers assume the continuity of terms, concepts, and principles over even relatively short historical time spans. In this chapter, I argue that two concepts, *bing* and *zheng*, which are essential to clinical practice today, have profoundly different connotations and uses in the early twentieth century. I show, moreover, that a confluence of social, political, and intellectual forces set in motion a revaluation of *bing* and *zheng* and laid the groundwork for more radical shifts in meaning during the Communist era. It is important to recognize that the current paradigm of clinical practice, based on the methodology of *bianzheng lunzhi*, was not the inevitable outcome of Republican-era innovations. Indeed, I show that Lu Yuanlei and his colleagues seem to be imagining a very different form of clinical practice that had the *Treatise of Cold Damage* as its center. Although their vision of reform was ultimately never realized, or only in a fragmented form, their efforts were extremely important because they had the effect of altering the historical relationship of *bing* and *zheng*, diminishing the former term and elevating the latter. In so doing, they created the intellectual possibilities for new theoretical formations to emerge. To understand this process, it is essential to explore the broader context of medical discourse in the Republican period. We will begin with an important but nearly forgotten feature of this historical period: the intense debates that swirled between adherents to the *Treatise on Cold Damage* and its associated clinical approaches and those who followed a competing current of practice, the Warm Disorders school.

The Problem of Frail Bodies

Lu Yuanlei's discussion of *bing* and *zheng* was part of a larger discussion in the Republican period about the proper interpretation of the *Treatise on Cold Damage*. Over the next three sections of this chapter, I will explore some of the key dimensions of the debates about the *Treatise* before examining how these debates influenced the concepts of *bing* and *zheng*. It's particularly important to begin with the *Treatise* because historical accounts of medicine in the Republican period have tended to present the conflict between the Western medicine and Chinese medicine professions as the central dynamic, the driving force for reforms in traditional medical practice. As we discussed in Chapter 1, this assumption has probably emerged out of scholarship that documents the growing power of the Western medicine profession in China at this period and its intensifying connections with the Chinese state, particularly following the establishment of the Nationalist government in 1928 (Croizier 1968; Andrews 2014; Lei 2014). But if we turn away from the master narrative of the state and move toward the most pressing clinical issues of this period, it becomes clear that the rise of the Western medicine profession was a relatively minor concern for most doctors. We have already explored how Yun Tieqiao responded to the attacks of Yu Yanxiu in Chapter 2. But he and other reformist doctors were far more concerned with two other issues: the apparent weakness of Chinese bodies and the late imperial decline in medicine. These two concerns were closely tied to each other, and their urgency was intensified by the colonial context in which these doctors were working. I begin with the problem of frail bodies.

During the Republican era, European and Japanese colonial encroachments were spurring rapid social and political changes, and medical reform became a pressing issue for many leading physicians in China's urban centers. But the urgency and direction of reform varied to a large extent on how one viewed the Chinese body and its vulnerabilities. Politics and medicine, revolution for the nation and reform in medical practice, were intimately linked. One aspect of the fear of weak Chinese bodies can be traced to the famous colonial epithet that China was the "sick man of Asia," an expression that first appeared in the English-language newspaper *North China Daily News* (字林西報) in 1896. This phrase was a derivative of a similar epithet for the Ottoman Empire known as the "sick man of Europe." In the context of social Darwinism and fears of racial extinction, leading Chinese intellectuals and political figures latched onto this phrase and seemed to readily accept that physical inadequacies were a compelling explanation for political weakness. For example, Mao Zedong's first publication in 1917, "A Study on Physical Education," his only known publication that predates his encounter with Marxism, endorsed exercise as a means of transforming society. Challenging the religious and philosophic proclivities toward the stillness of meditation and the social preference for flowing gowns not suited for vigorous activity, Mao exhorted his readers to embrace the slogan "Civilize the spirit by making savage the body" (Mao Zedong 1917). Chiang Kai-shek, as president of the Republic of China, lamented the inadequacies of the Chinese physique in his address to the Fourth National Games in 1930.

> The Chinese nation's status in the world, its international ranking, is not even third class. This is our Chinese nation's greatest shame. And the reason is that our national physique is weak, causing people of other nations not to take us seriously (Morris 2004, 100).

It may have been this equation between the individual and national body that later inspired Mao Zedong to demonstrate his fitness to lead by swimming the

Yangtze River, most notably at the age of seventy-three, on the eve of launching the Cultural Revolution.

The ambitious reform-oriented doctors of the Republican period also believed themselves to be besieged by a culture of weakness and an embrace of physical frailty. Diseases of depletion seemed to be rampant, perhaps confirming the colonial mindset that was already pervasive among China's political elite. Old diseases such as spermatorrhea—the leaking of sperm thought to be caused by depleted male bodies—became ubiquitous in the mainstream press; new ones such as neurasthenia, literally "weakness of the nerves," were embraced by medical professionals, becoming a mainstay of neuropsychiatry for decades in China long after this diagnosis had fallen out of favor in the West (Kleinman 1986; Lee 1999; Shapiro 1998, 2003). Other activists perceived this same disconcerting problem of physical frailty and proposed their own solutions—social, political, and otherwise—to reinvigorate weak constitutions. The famous Daoist innovator Chen Yingning (陳攖甯), for example, advocated a form of Daoist practice, the Immortals Learning (仙學), that he developed in response to his own struggles with consumption. Stressing activism, practice, autonomy, innovation, Chen promoted the Immortals Learning techniques of self-cultivation to create a robust body strong enough to repel foreign influences (X. Liu 2009).

Although there was colonial overtones to these concerns about frail Chinese bodies, debates about physical weakness had its roots in late imperial medical discourse. As Marta Hanson has shown, southern constitutions had long been considered delicate compared to those of robust northerners (Hanson 1998, 2011). They could only withstand treatment with gentle herbs. Volker Scheid's authoritative study of doctors from the Jiangnan city of Menghe, home to one of best-known medical lineages of the nineteenth and twentieth centuries, illustrates this broad regional concern with fragile southern bodies. Fei Boxiong (費伯雄), the most iconic figure of the Menghe tradition, famous for making two trips to the Daoguang imperial court to successfully treat the emperor and the empress, was celebrated for "using gentle therapies to achieve big results."

> Even during his lifetime, Fei Boxiong was renowned for his gentle approach to treatment. . . . [One gazetteer] of 1888 noted, "In treating [medical] disorders, [Fei Boxiong] did not like to use fierce and harsh prescriptions. He [held instead that] the right [way was for them] to be governed [by the principles of] harmonization and gentleness." . . . He did not invent this method, however, but merely followed a style of prescribing that had become popular throughout the Jiangnan area

during the Qing. Its mode of drug usage responded to, and in turn amplified, long-established local beliefs that attributed to Jiangnan southerners a more delicate constitution than to the robust northern Chinese. Jiangnan people thus had become increasingly suspicious of taking drugs like Ephedrae herba [*Ma Huang*], Aconiti radix lateralis praeparata [*Fu Zi*], or Rhei radix et rhizoma [*Da Huang*] that were associated with potent effects, fearing that these might kill rather than cure them (Scheid 2007, 162–63).

Fei Boxiong's approach was not only suited to southern sensibilities; it may also have been even more perfectly tailored to his many wealthy, upper-class clientele who considered themselves to be more refined than the average southerner. Scheid argues that their complaints, conditions such as "exhaustion (*xu lao*)" or "damage from the seven emotions (*qi shang*)" may have had psycho-emotional etiologies and would have been particularly amenable to Fei's principles of "harmonization and gentleness."

The discourse on delicate southern constitutions was significant far beyond the clinical styles of Fei Boxiong and other members of what later became known as the Menghe lineage. It also shaped the emergence of the Warm Disorders current in the late imperial period, a system of clinical practice that was very popular throughout Jiangnan and other areas of southern China. The Warm Disorders current evolved rapidly during the Qing era, and by the nineteenth century it was considered to be a distinct medical school with its own unique system of diagnosis and formulary, one that competed with the long-standing Cold Damage tradition (Hanson 2011).

By the early twentieth century, the once-celebrated sophistication of a doctor like Fei Boxiong and the widespread practices of the Warm Disorders current had become a source of alarm for Republican-era medical reformers. They bristled at this apparent embrace of weakness and mild-acting formulas, particularly as found in the Warm Disorders current, and resented that the belief in southern fragility undermined the authority of Zhang Zhongjing's *Treatise*. The following passage by Yao Shichen (姚世琛) captures the frustration of a Cold Damage advocate. In the preface to *Records of Experiments with Canonical Formulas*, the influential Republican-era book by Cao Yingfu (曹穎甫) on clinical applications of the *Treatise*, Yao Shichen directs his vitriol at the Warm Disorders innovators and their pampered patients.

By the time the history of medicine got to the Qing dynasty, ancient formulas had already been gradually overturned and the "Light and Nimble School" had emerged. Developing the theory that "warm pathogens enter from above, first violating the lungs, then adversely

transmitting to the pericardium," Mr. Ye Tianshi (葉天士) became
known for his "light touch," as can be fully seen in his *Guide to Clinical Practice*.

Then Mr. Wu Jutong (吳鞠通) appeared. Because of his devotion to Ye, he brushed aside the "Six Jing Theory" of the sage Zhang
Zhongjing, cleverly promoted his "Triple Burner treatment," and
produced *Systematic Differentiation of Warm Disorders* (溫病條辨).
Subsequently, China from Jiangsu, Zhejiang, Anhui, and Fujian to
the border provinces, one after another began to use these formulas,
teacher transmitting to discipline, father instructing son, until a world
of "mint and burdock seed" had been created!

But are these the crimes of Ye and Wu alone? . . . Because Mr. Ye
lived in the dynamic city of Suzhou, and Mr. Wu hung his shingle in
the south-central city of Huaiyin, the patients they saw were princes,
aristocrats, and wealthy businessmen. These people enjoyed high position and lived in comfort, indulging their appetites and lusts. Their
discomforts were slight, nothing more than an occasional cold or mild
exhaustion. Thus, ephedra and cinnamon twigs were not needed
to dispel Cold and Wind. . . . As a result, the sage's superb text was
mocked to the point that no one dared to mention it (Cao Yingfu 2004
[1936], 17–18).

Although tension between Cold Damage and Warm Disorders proponents
had been simmering for a long time, the former celebrating Zhang Zhongjing as the one true sage of medicine, the latter proclaiming Ye Tianshi as a
second sage, Yao's diatribe against the "world of 'mint and burdock seed'"
seems to have a new urgency to it, as if to say, in these troubled times, weak
bodies and weak medicine can only perpetuate national weakness. Although
Yao Shichen's critique does not explicitly refer to the geopolitical context of
his times, another famous voice for reform in this era did. Lu Yuanlei was dismayed by the great popularity of the Warm Disorders approach. For him, the
future of Chinese medicine lay in the return to the *Treatise*. Writing in 1929, as
the political confrontation with Western medicine was coming to a head, Lu
Yuanlei reminded his readers of the importance of the *Treatise* in the struggle
with this new competitor.

I often hear of doctors of Western medicine attacking Chinese medicine, but I have been unwilling to acknowledge their insolent assaults,
believing them too vulgar to debate. I have usually mocked them
with a few ludicrous words, not wanting to waste a day on these types,
nor was I eager to protect the rice bowls of today's so-called doctors

of Chinese medicine. The reason Chinese medicine is superior to Western medicine is its treatments, and in treatment there is nothing greater than [Zhang] Zhongjing. . . . Today's so-called doctors of Chinese medicine all follow Ye [Tianshi], Wu [Jutong], and Wang [Shixiong]. They don't read Zhongjing's book; they don't use Zhongjing's methods. This is heresy and not the great lineage of Chinese medicine (Lu Yuanlei 2008a, 82).

Like Yao Shichen, Lu expressed his frustration that his contemporaries no longer follow the methods that Zhang Zhongjing lays out in the *Treatise* but instead trust the diagnoses and treatments of the Warm Disorders innovators such as Ye Tianshi, Wu Jutong, and Wang Shixiong. Thus in 1929, the year of Yu Yanxiu's abolition proposal, Lu Yuanlei was reminding his readers that the real danger to the profession came from within, not from the new profession of Western medicine. Moreover, when we connect this claim to the article with which we opened the chapter, we can see that Lu thought correct interpretation of the *Treatise* required a correct understanding of *bing* and *zheng*. We will return to this point later in the chapter.

In today's world of Chinese medicine, these sorts of polemical attacks on the Warm Disorders current or any other major aspect of Chinese medicine theory and practice are unimaginable. Both the Cold Damage and Warm Disorders currents are considered respectable fields of study and important clinical methodologies. The impassioned debates of the Republican period remind us of the colonial anxieties that stirred them. To understand the motivations of these writers, we need to first explore why they found the mild therapies of the Warm Disorders so threatening.

The Perils of Mildness

Both the Cold Damage and Warm Disorder camps were fearful of the other's treatments. They regularly accused their adversaries of nothing less than murder. But they perceived very different kinds of danger in their opponent's therapies. For the Warm Disorders advocates, the problem with Cold Damage herbs and formulas was that they were too powerful for frail southern bodies. Many Jiangnan physicians viewed "Ephedra and Cinnamon twigs like they were snakes and scorpions" (*magui ru shexie*) as the popular expression went (Zhu Weiju 2005, 52). In contrast, the Cold Damage advocates saw Warm Disorders treatments as pernicious not because they were poisonous, but because they frequently exacerbated the illness process, driving it deeper into the body. In a passage from *Collection of Insights from Discussions of Medicine in the Reading Room,* Zhang Shanlei (張山雷) provides a typical example of this counterintuitive claim.

> When the warm heat theory of Ye Xiangyan [Tianshi] became popu-
> lar, there was the possibility that some of the inspirations of these later
> scholars could modestly augment that which was missing in Zhang
> Zhongjing's *Treatise.* But who could have imagined that Old Ye [Tian-
> shi], the first to propose this theory, and [Wu] Jutong, the first to write a
> treatise about it, would both shun Zhang Zhongjing's established prin-
> ciples, erroneously creating new formulas, using cloying herbs that trap
> the pathogen, causing innumerable harms without a single benefit?
> Everyone has followed in this path without reflection, adopting habits
> that completely mislead the people, devoting one's entire life [to this
> mistaken approach] without ever awakening (Zhang Shouyi 2008, 78).

How is it possible that the cooling herbs of the Warm Disorders current could be both gentle and dangerous? The opposing argument against the warming herbs of the Cold Damage current was straightforward: strong herbs were toxic and would overwhelm delicate bodies. For the Cold Damage advocates, the dangers of cooling herbs were more pernicious. Although supposedly "mild," they were also "cloying" and could therefore "trap the pathogen." Rather than curing disease, they would hasten its natural progression. Zhu Weiju (祝味菊), a highly respected clinician from this period, argued that the Warm Disorders therapies masked their dangers behind familiar clinical presentations, creating the impression that the patient's worsening condition was caused by the natural progression of the disease rather than the physician's own error. He gave a detailed accounting of this process.

> In the sixteenth year of the Republic [1927], I came to Shanghai to
> escape political turmoil. I often heard that people's constitutions
> were different due to the environment here. When traveling to a new
> country, one must ask about the customs, so I didn't dare to impetu-
> ously hang up my shingle. I kept a low profile in Shanghai for a year,
> lingering around the clinics of famous physicians and the preparation
> counters of the pharmacies. Sure enough, the illnesses were the same
> as Three Xiang [Hunan] but the treatments were very different. . . .
> Why were the symptoms the same, but the treatments different? Could
> it really be due to the environment? I decided to humbly study with a
> famous physician, a Mr. Zhu [no relation]. After three months, I was
> in awe of his ingenuity and incredible skill at predicting the course of
> a disease. The illnesses usually went from mild to serious, ending in

death, the doctor predicting every step in the process but unable to prevent the fatality. The doctor would take every appropriate action—from releasing the Exterior with pungency and coolness and driving out dampness with sweetness and blandness, to transmitting heat through the Qi sector, to clearing the Ying sector and dispersing the Blood sector; or from dispersing dampness and turbidity, to nourishing yin and clearing heat, to cleansing phlegm and opening the orifices, to settling the Liver and extinguishing wind—but could not halt this progression. To my disbelief, I quietly realized that famous doctors became famous for predicting the course of an illness, not from stopping it and saving a life. Alas! What is the point of being a famous doctor if you know the progression of an illness but you cannot do anything about it! And the patients, believing the disease to be beyond a cure, not faulting the murderous actions of the medicine, die without a regret. . . . Although I had a desire to reform medicine, how could a solitary tree stand when heretical ideas are flowing all about? . . . Who would be the companion of the one sober man in a crowd of drunks? (Zhu Weiju 2005, 63)

In this passage, "the heretical ideas" and "the crowd of drunks" refer to Warm Disorders theories and the adherents to this current. Zhu's long list of therapies, the doctors' "appropriate actions," is the standard progression of treatment strategies within the Warm Disorders current. Zhu's critique clearly resonates with his fellow reform-oriented colleagues: Warm Disorders therapies are deceptively dangerous. But he also draws our attention to another concern. Warm Disorders therapies are a threat because they are based on a principle of regionalism: in different locales, the same set of symptoms may be treated differently. Zhu and his fellow reformers not only favored strong therapies, but they also sought a universal form of medical practice, true for all time and places. If Chinese medicine were to compete with Western medicine in an increasingly global world, it must also aspire to a universal understanding of the body and treatment regimens that applied to all. Only the *Treatise*, in their opinion, could provide the edifice for such a complete medical system. As we will see, it would turn out that many Japanese enthusiasts of the *Treatise* would share, and even seek to disseminate, just such a vision of the *Treatise*.

The Problem of Orthodoxy

Reading these attacks, one might reasonably ask, if Warm Disorders therapies were so dangerous, how did they ever become so popular? The answer from major figures of the Warm Disorders movement was straightforward: the inadequacies of the Cold Damage therapies necessitated these innovations. Wu Youke (吳又可) (1582–1652), the late Ming physician who is generally considered the first scholar of the Warm Disorders current, made this point emphatically. In his *Treatise on Febrile Epidemics* (瘟疫論), he argued that febrile epidemics (*wenyi*), a concept that later merges with Warm Disorders (*Wen Bing*), were actually far more prevalent than Cold Damage (Hanson 2011, 95). Wu Youke's critique of the Cold Damage tradition was only slowly taken up, his therapeutic innovations generally considered too piecemeal to constitute an alternative tradition. The next major innovator in the Warm Disorders current, the famous Qing dynasty physician Ye Tianshi (1667–1746), was actually a careful reader of Ke Qin (柯琴), one of the great Qing scholars of the *Treatise on Cold Damage* (Scheid 2014). An eclectic practitioner and virtuoso clinician, Ye Tianshi also read Wu Youke's treatise and adopted some of his ideas (Hanson 2011, 116). In his brief but seminal essay the *Treatise on Warmth and Heat* (溫熱論), published posthumously in 1777 by his students, it is unlikely that Ye Tianshi imagined himself founding a new current of medical practice. As Marta Hanson has shown, it was only subsequent scholarship, such as *Systematic Differentiation of Warm Disorders* (溫病條辨) published by Wu Jutong (吳鞠通) in 1813, *Warp and Woof of Warmth and Heat* (溫熱經緯), published by Wang Shixiong (王士雄) in 1852, and an emerging Jiangnan regionalism that allowed Warm Disorders therapies to become a medical current that stood in opposition to Cold Damage (Hanson 1998).

Ironically, if there were one point on which Republican-era Cold Damage advocates could agree with their Warm Disorders adversaries, it would have been on the historical failures of the Cold Damage tradition. But this alignment was driven by different concerns. Warm Disorders scholars felt that the Cold Damage current was an important but limited tradition. Warm Disorders scholarship helped to address its inadequacies. Adherents to the Cold Damage current, however, perceived a more pervasive concern. Late imperial medicine was in decline, plagued by errors of transmission and philosophical speculation. The Warm Disorders current was emblematic of this deviation from the true heritage of early China. Where one's allegiances fell, whether one was receptive to new innovations or saw these same innovations as evidence of decay, depended on one's affinity for the late imperial philosophical trend known as "evidential scholarship" (*kaozhengxue*).

Evidential scholarship developed out of seemingly minor developments in the field of philology in the late Ming, but eventually became one of the most important intellectual trends of the late imperial period. It grew in popularity because it raised doubts about the authenticity of texts that were foundational to neo-Confucianism, the dominant philosophical trend since roughly the eleventh century. Confucianism—based loosely on the philosophical principles of the ancient philosopher Confucius—has been associated with Chinese dynastic rule since the Han empire (206 B.C.E.–220 C.E.). But it underwent some major revisions during the Song (960–1279), when literati attempted to reassert the universal validity of Confucianism in a world that seemed vastly different than the one Confucius had known some 1,500 years prior (Mote 1999, 149). The founders of neo-Confucianism had to respond not only to the naturalization of Buddhism in China, a once-alien religious system, and the rise of Daoism and Chinese folk religion, but also to a fracturing political landscape as various peoples and states once thought to be peripheral to Chinese civilization grew in power and influence (Mote 1999; Bol 2008). Although the great empires of the past, the Han and the Tang, seemed unattainable in the more complex world of the eleventh century, Song intellectuals believed that Confucianism could provide a universal cultural and moral grounding (Bol 2008, 14). Neo-Confucian thought gradually grew in popularity and eventually received official state support, most notably during the Ming dynasty (1368–1644). But following the Manchu conquest of China in the seventeenth century, many Chinese literati began to question the certainties of neo-Confucian thought. The shock of "barbarian" rule under the new Qing dynasty (1646–1911) cast neo-Confucian orthodoxies in a new light. From the perspective of the careful textual study and critical thinking that became the defining feature of evidential scholarship, neo-Confucianism seemed too speculative and solipsistic, too focused on the cultivation of moral perfection, too enamored of complex cosmological systems of thought to permit pragmatic action, such as resisting the Manchus. The popularity of evidential scholarship grew considerably during the Qing (Elman 1984). It also inspired late Qing revolutionaries such as Zhang Taiyan (章太炎), who viewed the Manchus as colonizers and the main obstacle to recovering the glory of the Confucian traditions of early China.

Skepticism was inherent to the project of evidential scholarship, and this attitude penetrated into the medical world. Just as evidential scholars raised doubts about the authenticity, and hence the value, of nearly all neo-Confucian writings, doctors of the same ilk questioned the merits of nearly all medical texts written since the Song. For example, the "great masters" of the post-Song period came under critical scrutiny. In the Ming, Zhang Zhongjing was considered to be one great doctor among four, the progenitor of one important branch of medicine that was complemented by the three great Jin and Yuan innovators: Liu Hejian (劉河間), Li Dongyuan (李東垣), and Zhu Danxi (朱丹溪). During the Qing, evidential scholarship elevated

Zhang Zhongjing to the status of "great sage of medicine," the progenitor of all that was great in China's medical traditions. Xu Dachun (徐大椿) (1693–1771), a rough contemporary of Ye Tianshi, exemplified the influence of this movement in medical discourse. In *Treatise on the Origin and Development of Medicine* (醫學源流論), he rejected the Ming dynasty celebration of the four masters in emphatic terms.

> The way of medicine has long been obscured. The Ming people spoke of four great masters: Zhang Zhongjing, Liu Hejian, Li Dongyuan, Zhu Danxi, who were considered the ancient forefathers of medicine. This was truly ignorant nonsense. Zhang Zhongjing is the sage that compiled [the wisdom of] antiquity, just as Confucius is the forefather of Confucianism. The knowledge of Liu Hejian and Li Dongyuan is but one aspect [of medicine]. Zhu Danxi merely deliberated on the claims of various masters, selecting and discarding to provide a convenient approach for the novice. These are the so-called famous physicians? The three masters don't amount to one ten thousandth of Zhang Zhongjing; how ludicrous to lump them all together (Xu Lingtai 2008 [1757]).

The apotheosis of Zhang Zhongjing began to reach dizzying heights in the Republican period as reformers sought a new path forward out of China's colonial situation. The work of the brilliant Zhang Taiyan offers a great example of this trend. In the aftermath of the 1911 Revolution, as the country fractured into competing regional warlord cliques and colonial spheres of influence, Zhang devoted his evidential scholarship skills to the study of medicine, becoming a mentor to many of the reformist doctors of the Republican period. Zhang Taiyan considered the *Treatise on Cold Damage* to be China's greatest medical text and the basis for a flourishing medical tradition that could withstand the challenge of Western medicine. "The only reason that Chinese medicine is superior to Western medicine is the *Treatise on Cold Damage*" (Zhang Taiyan 2009, 111) But he was also dismayed by the scholarship on the *Treatise*, which he expressed in a preface to Lu Yuanlei's opus, *A Modern Interpretation of the Treatise on Cold Damage*.

> Since the Jin, there have been many commentators on the *Treatise on Cold Damage*. They can be divided into three groups: the ugly like Tao Hua, the reckless like Shu Zhao, and the heterodox like Huang Yuanyu. . . . Cheng Wuji used ancient canons to discourse systematically [on the *Treatise*] but he did not understand Zhongjing's intent. Fang Youzhi and Yu Chang rearranged the original text and cleverly

defended their uses [of the *Treatise*] and occasionally explained their forefather's views but often went too far. Zhang Zhicong and Chen Nianzu borrowed the doctrine of five evolutive phases and six climatic factors, mistakenly applying the Suilu Chapter [of the *Inner Canon*] and making an efficacious text into mystical blather. Who has been able to avoid these three errors and brilliantly stand on his own, establishing and explicating the great principles? There is no one greater than Master Ke, from Zhejiang. Who has been able to analyze clearly and insightfully? There is no one greater than Master You from Suzhou. Alas! After more than one hundred commentators, there are no more than two that can stand on their own. What a tragedy! (Lu Yuanlei 2008b [1931], 1)

The techniques of evidential scholarship were essential for Zhang Taiyan and his colleagues in recovering (what they considered to be) the original meaning of the *Treatise*. This commitment to evidential scholarship further predisposed these Republican reformers to oppose the Warm Disorders current, which fit perfectly into their narrative of the late imperial decline. As Zhang Taiyan bluntly remarked, "The superficial writings of Ye Tianshi and Wu Jutong are not worthy of respect" (Zhang Taiyan 2009, 222). But it was easier to dismiss the scholarly trend than the clinical issues that supposedly gave rise to it. As a result, Republican reformers had to demonstrate that Cold Damage approaches could handle the sorts of problems that most Jiangnan doctors believed best suited to the Warm Disorders approach. For example, Zhang Taiyan tackled this problem in an essay entitled, "Yangming Disorders Are Disorders of Warmth and Heat." Against the claims of the Warm Disorders school, he argued that the *Treatise* already had clear explications on what constituted disorders of warmth and heat. Moreover, the *Treatise* also clearly articulated the dangers of sweating therapies for these conditions, a treatment principle that the Warm Disorders school believed to be unique to their tradition. Lastly, Zhang Taiyan points out that Warm Disorders advocates had failed to recognize that Zhang Zhongjing's formula Five Poria Powder (*Wu Ling San*) is actually a key formula for the treatment of warmth and heat conditions (Zhang Taiyan 2009, 10–16).

Yun Tieqiao, one of the leading scholars and clinicians of the Republican period (see Chapter 2), adapted a similar strategy. In 1925, Yun Tieqiao opened a Chinese medicine correspondence school, using a series of textbooks that he wrote himself. One textbook, *Clarifying the Principles of Warm Disorders* (溫病明理), was written explicitly to address confusions that he believed were caused by the Warm Disorders current. Like Zhang Taiyan, with whom he had a very close relationship, he dismissed Warm Disorders scholarship.

> My humble ambition is to help Chinese medicine flourish, and there-
> fore I cannot avoid correcting false theories. . . . The books of Wang
> Mengying, Wu Jutong, Ye Tianshi are filled with flaws and errors. If
> I were to correct each one, the stack of papers would be as high as
> me . . . (Yun Tieqiao 2008, 122).

Yun Tieqiao also argued that treatments for Warm Disorders are already present in Zhang Zhongjing's work. He directed his students to passages from Zhang Zhongjing's other text, *Essentials of the Golden Casket* (金匱要略), where the second chapter contained therapies for dampness (*shi*; 濕) and heatstroke (*ye*; 暍), conditions that he considered to be true Warm Disorders (Yun Tieqiao 2008). Perhaps more importantly, he believed that only a small number of diseases fell into the Warm Disorders rubric. If his contemporaries would stop misdiagnosing so many conditions as Warm Disorders, they would soon recognize that Zhang Zhongjing's work already contained the treatments they needed, and, moreover, the dangerous formulas of the Warm Disorders current could be avoided (Yun Tieqiao 2007 [1924]).

The Diagnosis Problem

These intellectual trends—the concern about frail bodies and the debates about the value of late imperial medical scholarship—are essential to understanding how leading Chinese medicine reformers were beginning to reinterpret the meanings of *bing* and *zheng* during the Republican period. To further explore the shifting connotations of these concepts, I want to now turn to a very public and impassioned debate about the nature of Chinese medicine diagnosis. It was well documented in medical journals of this period, but scholars have often misinterpreted its significance. At the beginning of this chapter, we encountered Lu Yuanlei's claim that Chinese medicine was ill equipped to "identify disease." These claims, made in 1929, were influential in the development of a 1933 policy proposal made by the government-sanctioned Institute of National Medicine (國醫館) to "unify disease names" (*tongyi bingming*). I have used the term "disease" as a gloss for *bing* here because the proposal explicitly stated that the disease names of Western medicine should be used as the basis for reforming the *bing* names of Chinese medicine. This proposal elicited a great deal of debate and a wide range of responses. The proposal was rewritten to address the many critiques, but controversy continued, and it was ultimately shelved, as the institute turned to other issues. The written responses this proposal engendered, many of them published in the Chinese medicine journals of this period, are an excellent resource for tracing the early twentieth-century shifts in the meanings of *bing*.

The Institute of National Medicine was a new government organization that emerged out of the 1929 bill to abolish Chinese medicine. This bill was proposed by Yu Yunxiu, a member of the Central Board of Health, just a few months after the KMT had established the new Nationalist government in Nanjing. Sean Lei has shown that, although the bill failed to become law, it sparked an unprecedented mobilization of the Chinese medicine community and actually led to important political gains for the Chinese medicine profession, as it learned to cultivate allies within the government (Lei 2014). The establishment of the Institute of National Medicine in 1931 was one such political victory. But this achievement was partial, like many others under the Nationalist regime. Proponents of Chinese medicine imagined an institute with true political power to "reform national medicine, to study national drugs, and manage the affairs of national medicine," but opponents maneuvered to make sure that the institute never had any true administrative functions and was nothing more than an "academic association" (Deng Tietao 1999, 309).

Reflecting the original administrative goals of its supporters, the Institute of National Medicine consisted of a network of regional bodies that all reported to a central institute in Nanjing. Despite the limited powers of the institute, the leaders pursued their agenda vigorously. Deng Tietao has identified three major undertakings of the institute: first, the promulgation of "The Institute of National Medicine Outline of Academic Standards for Sorting Out National Medicine"; second, the proposal "to unify disease names"; and lastly, the support and ultimate success in passing "Regulations for Chinese Medicine" in 1936 to confer legal status on Chinese medicine doctors. The first two projects were tackled in rapid succession in 1933 and clearly demonstrated the reformist orientation of the leadership at the Institute of National Medicine.

One defining element of the reformist platform was a strong embrace of modern science and Western medicine. This stance was clearly visible in the first undertaking of the institute, the Outline of Academic Standards for Sorting Out National Medicine. This document was originally drafted by Lu Yuanlei, revised by Guo Shoutian, and approved on May 1, 1933, by the Standing Council of the Institute (Deng Tietao 1999, 298). In the opening line of the outline, the authors state their allegiance to the institute's charter to use "scientific methods to gradually sort out" national medicine and drugs. For example, Article II of Part I calls for "demonstrations with modern theory" when "treatments have true efficacy but lack a clear theoretical explanation" (Deng Tietao 1999, 299). Critics charged that this approach was "too Westernized" or too hybrid (literally, "neither old nor new, neither East nor West") (Deng Tietao 1999, 300). A close look at the outline itself reveals that its basic claims were anchored in two key perspectives of the reformist camp that we have already explored: first, Chinese medicine had been in decline since the late imperial period, and second, "scientific methods" were needed to rectify these errors of transmission.

The proposal to "unify disease names" was motivated by a similar desire to use elements of Western medicine to improve Chinese medicine. Less than two months after the approval of the Outline for Academic Standards, the Reform Committee of the Institute, under the leadership of Shi Jinmo, developed the "Central Institute of National Medicine Proposal by the Reform Committee for the Unification of Disease Names" and sent it and related documents to all branch offices. The proposal outlined a procedure for branch offices to review the names of all *bing* in Chinese medicine and determine their equivalent disease categories in Western medicine. Consistent with the principles delineated in the outline, the reform committee offered the following justification.

> Why rely on Western medicine disease names? The Institute of National Medicine has declared that it will use scientific methods. The disease names of National medicine have never been scientific. To bring them in line with scientific methods is hardly the sort of project that a small number of reform committee members can do in a short period of time. Even if we could, [we are faced with the problem] that there is only one truth for all phenomena. Western medicine disease names have a scientific foundation. If new disease names must be created, they cannot differ from Western medicine. If they differ from Western medicine, then they cannot be scientific (Zhao Hongjun 1982, 236).

Based on statements such as this, contemporary scholars have often misunderstood the proposal to unify disease names as a well-intentioned but misguided act of radicalism. For example, both Zhao Hongjun and Deng Tietao criticized the reform committee for insisting that there is "only one truth for all phenomena" and thereby assuming a single standard by which to judge what Zhao calls "two different systems of knowledge." Moreover, both historians expressed surprise that disease/*bing* was the committee's starting point for reforming Chinese medicine. Chinese medicine "discriminates patterns," not diseases, both scholars have argued, and this project therefore risked "forsak-

ing pattern discrimination and treatment determination *bianzheng lunzhi"*
(Deng Tietao 1999, 99–100; Zhao Hongjun 1982, 240–41).

These assessments, shared by two respected historians of this period, are
a reminder of the difficulty of the historian's task. Because the contemporary
practice of Chinese medicine is dominated by the methodology of *bianzheng
lunzhi*, both scholars mistakenly read this Republican-era debate through the
modern connotations of *bing* and *zheng*. But this hermeneutic act is only
possible if the Orientalist geographies of the body (Chapter 2), and other ontological divides between the two medical systems were already in place. It
assumes that doctors of this period understood Western and Chinese medicine
to represent "two different systems of knowledge." However, if we recall that
reformist doctors in the Republican era considered the bodies of the two medical systems to be "roughly analogous," then we should not be surprised that
these individuals also insisted they share a single diagnostic category. Just as
Zhu Weiju and the Cold Damage advocates disparaged the apparent regionalism of the Warm Disorders current, the Reform Committee was motivated by
a similar concern, hence the need to assert that there is only "one truth for all
phenomena." In their judgment, an alternative set of Chinese *bing* concepts
would imply a regionalism that rejected the principles of science.

The reform committee's proposal to "unify disease names" was debated in a
special issue of the journal *The Annals of the Medical World* (醫界春秋). What
is significant for the story of *bing* and *zheng* is not the merits of this proposal
but how the various commentaries reveal that vastly different understanding
of these terms in the Republican period. With regard to the term *bing*, we can
see that all commentators gave far greater importance to this term than either
the historians Deng Tietao and Zhao Hongjun did or contemporary doctors
would. For example, critics of the proposal argued vigorously that the concept of *bing* was essential to the practice of Chinese medicine. Conservative
critics issued dire warnings that implementation of the proposal would lead
to nothing less than a collapse of the theoretical edifice of Chinese medicine.
For example, Xia Yingtang stated:

[When I state that] national medicine disease names cannot be
unified, this is not to say that there isn't important work to be done in
reforming them. But the purpose should be to seek the unification of
the national medicine community not unification with Western medicine. . . . If we follow Western medicine in adopting disease names,
then we must also follow Western medicine in adopting its theory. If
national medicine disease names perish, then national medicine must
inevitably also perish (Zhao Hongjun 1982, 238).

Members of the Shanghai branch office of the Institute of National Medicine resigned in protest over the proposal. Leading figures of that office, including well-known physicians such as Qin Bowei, Yan Cangshan, Zhang Xianchen, Wu Keqian, and Sheng Xinru, collectively authored a response that asked the following rhetorical questions.

> (1) If we rely on Western medicine disease names to unify national medicine *bing* names, are we fully prepared [for the challenge] of relating treatment principle to drugs? (2) If we rely on Western medicine disease names to unify national medicine *bing* names, can we really avoid discrepancies between the [Chinese medicine] diagnosis and Western medicine diagnosis? (3) Do sponsors of this proposal and the Reform Committee really understand Chinese medicine in any depth? (4) In the future, will the Academic Reform Committee of the Central Institute of National Medicine continue these freeloading practices (Deng Tietao and Cheng Zhifan 2000, 193)?

The apocalyptic claims of Xia Yingtang and the repudiation of the Shanghai branch office are striking reminders about the centrality of *bing* to Republican-era doctors. Even though they vehemently opposed the reform committee proposal, they concurred about the importance of *bing* to clinical practice.

Given the deep divisions between Cold Damage and Warm Disorders advocates, between progressives and conservatives, it is perhaps not so surprising that the proposal met with such strong opposition. But even doctors within the reformist camp such as Yun Tieqiao were critical of the unification proposal. In his response, Yun articulated a more nuanced understanding of the nature of science. While he accepted the reform committee's assertion that there could only be one truth, he argued that the different methods for approaching this truth were of equal value.

> My humble opinion is that science is progressive. What was right yesterday is wrong today. We cannot say that today's science is the truth. This is clearly demonstrated by the fact that Western medicine has numerous discourses that do not correspond to reality. This is my first point. Ultimately, there is only one truth in the world. But with regard to the methods of studying this truth, there are many paths that lead to the same end. There is not just one method. . . . Western science is not the only path of scholarship. Eastern medicine has its perspective. This is my second point. The adoption of Western [medicine disease] names will destroy Chinese [medicine] theory and make names and facts incompatible. If Chinese [medicine] theory is destroyed, then

> Chinese learning will be bankrupt. . . . The honorable Institute's
> decision to rectify names is one method. But when determining
> names, attention must be directed at one's own theory, because theory
> is primary and names are secondary. To be only concerned with names
> is like having guests without a host (Deng Tietao and Cheng Zhifan
> 2000, 192).

There is much in this fascinating passage that merits close attention, such as
Yun Tieqiao's play on Confucian principles of hosting and the rectification of
names, his sensitivity to the historicity of science, and his critical perspective
on the epistemological claims of Western medicine. Yun straddled the uni-
versalist position of the reform committee ("there is only one truth") and a
modest pluralism ("Western science is not the only path of scholarship"). But
he ultimately aligned more closely with the conservative critics on this issue:
Chinese medicine *bing* categories are an integral part of its theoretical edifice.

These dire warnings were not the only reasons for the failure of the proposal. The reform committee had requested a written response from all
branch offices in a mere ten days, vastly underestimating the difficulty of the
task, as even Lu Yuanlei complained (Deng Tietao and Cheng Zhifan 2000,
193). Moreover, the reform committee announced that all practitioners would
be required to follow the finalized list in their practice or face heavy fines and
possibly a prohibition from practicing medicine. It is not clear how the institute would have monitored or enforced such standards. Despite the collapse
of this proposal, it is significant for our story for two reasons. First, the inten-
sity of debate, both for and against the proposal, was evidence of the significance of *bing* as a diagnostic concept for Republican-era doctors. It is almost
unimaginable that contemporary practitioners would make such a vigorous
defense of this concept today. As we shall see, it is the concept of *zheng* that is
indispensable to today's doctors. Second, in the response of Yun Tieqiao, we
see a premonition of what I call the strategy of "double truths." Adversaries on
both sides of the "unification of disease names" debate implicitly recognized
the epistemological vulnerability of the Chinese medicine concept of *bing* vis-
à-vis the Western medicine concept of disease. Advocates for the unification of
disease names wanted to deal with this inherent weakness by eliminating any
deviation from the scientific standards of Western medicine. Yun Tieqiao, on
the other hand, called on his readers to broaden the definition of science, to
recognize that there are "many paths that lead to the same end [of truth]." As
we will see, Yun's approach ultimately won the day, but the epistemological
authority of *bing* was greatly weakened in the process. The more important
solution to the problem of disease names was the eventual emergence of the

new diagnostic concept of *zheng*, which has no immediate parallel in Western medicine.

Redefining *Zheng*

At the opening of this chapter, we discussed how Lu Yuanlei believed that Chinese medicine could treat disease without being able to "identify disease." This claim was further articulated in a series of essays published in *Medicine of China Monthly* (中國醫學月刊) in January 1929, where he explained that *zheng* should be the focus of therapeutic interventions. For example, in one essay he wrote, "Chinese Herbs and Formulary Have a Special Effect on *Zheng* and No Special Effect on *Bing*" (Lu Yuanlei 2010a, 1,439). This series of essays, together with writings by other reformist doctors, calls on readers to understand *bing* and *zheng* in new ways. We can best appreciate the novelty of these claims when we compare them to more conventional perspectives of the era, such as the one captured in Xie Guan's (謝觀) *Comprehensive Dictionary of Chinese Medicine*, the first dictionary of Chinese medicine, published in 1921. The following passage is from the dictionary's definition of *zheng*, but it is also a remarkably clear statement of the relationship of *bing* to *zheng* at this unique historical conjuncture.

> *Zheng* (證): the external expression of an internal disorder (*bing-zhuang*), like the verification of an object. . . . For example, Liver *bing* [is manifested] by poor vision; Kidney *bing* by poor hearing; Lung *bing* by poor olfaction; Heart *bing* by a rigid tongue; Spleen *bing* by diminished sense of taste. The Liver, Kidneys, Lungs, Heart, and Spleen are located in the interior of the body and are hard to see, but the changes of the five sense organs can be observed. They testify to the affliction of the internal organs and guide therapy. Likewise, the Greater Yang Meridian travels between the skin and muscle and is hard to see. But a headache, a stiff and painful neck, and a fear of cold can testify to a *bing* of the Greater Yang Meridian and guide therapy. . . . Later generations replaced this character with [a different] *zheng* (症), egregiously departing from the original meaning of the term (Xie Guan 1994 [1921]).

In this passage, *bing* and *zheng* exist in a relationship of mutual implication. Xie Guan's *bing*, which can be associated with organs and meridians alike, is clearly not the biomedical concept of disease but rather a general term for an internal pathology. *Zheng* is its "external expression," the observable manifestation of an internal pathology, its "presentation." I choose this latter gloss to emphasize this inside-outside relationship, that *bing* and *zheng* are two aspects of a single phenomenon. Thus, Xie Guan explains this relationship by reference to widely known correspondences of the body. The Liver "opens at the orifice of the eye" (*kaiqiao yu mu*); therefore, a Liver *bing* is expressed, becomes "evident," or "presents" in the *zheng* of poor vision. As we will see, this use of *zheng* is distinct from Lu Yuanlei's connotation and even more radically different than the modern textbook definition.

Xie Guan's definition of *zheng* (and *bing*) is not an idiosyncrasy of the dictionary. It is not only consistent with many other works from this period, but I believe it is the key to correctly reading much late imperial medical writing. For example, the well-known Republican-era physician Wu Keqian (吳克潛) wrote in a passage on the pulse exam in 1933, "*Bing* is concealed in the interior, *zheng* is expressed on the exterior" (*bing cang yu nei, zheng jian hu wai*; 病藏於內, 證見乎外) (Wu Keqian 1933, 211). Likewise, He Liancheng (何廉臣) used *zheng* in a kindred sense in his popular collection of case records, *Classified Cases of Efficacious Treatments by Famous Doctors of the Nation*, published in 1927. He Liancheng arranged each case according to the following categories: *bing* name, cause, "presentation" (*zhenghou*; 證候), diagnosis (*zhenduan*; 診斷), treatment principle, prescription, and outcome. In He Lianchen's usage, *zhenghou* (this term is synonymous with *zheng*) was simply a list of the patient's signs and symptoms. It clearly lacked the modern meaning of "pattern," which is written as a pithy four- or eight-character summary of the illness process. The closest one gets to a description of a contemporary "pattern" of disharmony is in the "diagnosis" section, which included a description of the patient's pulse, tongue, and underlying cause of the patient's illness (He Lianchen 2003 [1927]).

When we turn to Lu Yuanlei's writing on *zheng* in 1929, we capture a glimpse of an emerging epistemic shift. In his essay "Chinese Herbs and Formulary Have Special Effect on *Zheng* and No Special Effect on *Bing*," Lu Yuanlei asked directly, "What is *zheng*?" His answer echoed Xie Guan's definition of "presentation," but he does not want to suggest it is merely the expression of an internal pathology. *Zheng* has other qualities, and for this reason I leave it untranslated in this passage.

> What is *zheng*? *Zheng* is *zhenghou*, and also the standard for using
> medicine. All the terms from the *Treatise on Cold Damage* and *Essentials of the Golden Casket* are *zhenghou*, such as fever, chills, stiffness
> in the neck and back, fullness in the chest and flanks, irritability, thirst,
> palpitations of the heart, palpitations below the umbilicus, fullness
> below the heart that is soft to the touch, sweating, absence of sweating,

hard stools, flatulence, diarrhea with undigested food, etc. These are *zhenghou* and they can't be simply understood by just looking at a text. A famous teacher must explain them, or one must read [about them in] excellent commentaries (Lu Yuanlei 2010a, 1,439).

To the reader unfamiliar with Zhang Zhongjing's texts, the long list of clinical terms in this passage might seem to be a mundane, even random list of symptoms. But in the very next paragraph, Lu argues that they are far more.

Zhenghou (證候) is not the same as the concept of "symptoms" *zhengzhuang* (症狀) found in Western medicine texts. Symptoms only describe the abnormal state of the patient but have nothing to do with diagnosis and treatment. The *zhenghou* of Zhongjing's work are the criteria for how to use medicine (Lu Yuanlei 2010a, 1,439).

Lu's careful parsing of *zhenghou* (presentation) from *zhengzhuang* (symptoms) needs to be understood in its historical context. Contemporary doctors of Chinese medicine see these terms as distinct and unrelated. But up until the 1920s, the initial character for each word—證 and 症—were often used interchangeably (Mayanagi Makoto 2013). Xie Guan complained about this phenomenon in the dictionary definition discussed earlier when he wrote, "Later generations replaced this character with [a different] *zheng* (症), egregiously departing from the original meaning of the term." In Lu's essay, "symptom" was described as a simple marker of ill health with little diagnostic value, while *zhenghou* pointed to deeper illness mechanisms. Why was this seemingly minor distinction so important to Lu Yuanlei and his reformist colleagues? What was the significance to the practice of Chinese medicine as a whole? In order to explore these questions, we must turn to Japanese scholarship on the *Treatise on Cold Damage* and its influence on reform-minded Chinese scholars of this period.

Clinical Experiments in Diagnosis

Japanese scholarship on traditional medicine was relatively unknown in China until the mid 1920s. But as Japanese medical texts began to disseminate more widely, they became part of the dialogue about reform. Many reformist doctors, who were already keenly interested in the *Treatise on Cold Damage*, also became interested in Japanese scholarship on Zhang Zhongjing during this period. For example, Lu Yuanlei was so impressed by the originality of this scholarship that in his two major works on Zhang Zhongjing, *A Modern Interpretation of the Treatise on Cold Damage* (傷寒論今釋) and *A Modern*

Interpretation of the Essentials of the Golden Casket (金匱要略今釋), he cited Japanese scholarship 674 times and 629 times, respectively (Lu Yuanlei 2008 [1931], 3). I've explored how Japanese scholarship influenced Chinese writings on the *Treatise* in greater detail elsewhere (Karchmer 2015a). Here I want to focus specifically on the role it played in new interpretations of *zheng*. At just the moment that doctors were debating the centrality of *bing* to the diagnostic processes of Chinese medicine, Japanese scholarship was suggesting that *zheng* should be the focus instead. As these academic inquiries preceded in the 1930s, it became essential to define both terms against similar concepts in biomedicine. The older interior-exterior, pathology-presentation relationship of *bing* to *zheng* captured in Xie Guan's definition began to shift. Several decades later, in the Communist period, that relationship would be fundamentally reworked in ways that could not have been anticipated in the 1930s.

How did the colonial context, the problem of frail bodies, and the debates between Cold Damage and Warm Disorders advocates drive innovative new approaches to clinical diagnosis in Chinese medicine? One of the clearest examples of how experimental thinking about the concept of *zheng* was affecting clinical practice can be found in the case records from the Suzhou Hospital of National Medicine (蘇州國醫醫院). Established in 1939, this hospital was a unique medical institution. First, it was an attempt to bring institutional administration to the practice of Chinese medicine when the great majority of doctors worked in private clinics at the time (Leung 2017). Second, the hospital was established at a politically unstable moment, not long after the Japanese occupation of Suzhou. The hospital was founded with the official approval of the Reform Government of the Republic of China (中華民国維新政府) (March 3, 1938–March 20, 1940), the Japanese puppet government in control of Jiangsu, Zhejiang, Anhui Provinces. Third, the hospital explicitly wanted to put into practice many of the reformist principles discussed earlier, focusing on the use of Cold Damage formulas in their treatments. Lastly, the founding doctors of the Suzhou College of National Medicine (蘇州國醫學校) were enthusiastic readers of Japanese scholarship on the *Treatise* and were in regular communication with leading Kampo physicians in Japan prior to the outbreak of war.[1]

Although it might be tempting to think that this hospital was an imperialist project orchestrated by Kampo phsyicians in Japan, there is little evidence to support such a claim. Kampo medicine had been in decline in Japan since 1875, when the Meiji government began to aggressively promote modernization in Japan, passing laws to promote the rapid development of Western medicine and simultaneously using policy to hinder the practice of Kampo medicine. In the early twentieth century, a small group of Japanese doctors began a movement to revive Kampo medicine. These physicians, many of whom were first trained as doctors of Western medicine, had later become enthusiastic followers of the Ancient Formulas School (古方派) of Japanese Kampo medicine. The Ancient Formulas School was a current of traditional Japanese medicine that was inspired by the famous eighteenth-century physician Yoshimasu Tōdō (吉益東洞). His scholarship was focused almost exclusively on the work of Zhang Zhongjing, to the point of dismissing almost all other facets of ancient Chinese medical writings. Early twentieth-century physicians such as Wada Keijurō (和田啟十郎) were inspired by the apparent empiricism and clinical efficacy of the Ancient Formulas School and championed it over other Japanese schools of traditional medicine. As the Japanese empire expanded into East Asia, other doctors seeking to revive Kampo medicine began to hope that Japan's imperialist aspirations might work to their benefit. They anticipated that the large numbers of traditional doctors in the conquered areas would be attracted to their unique style of traditional medicine, which they called "Eastern medicine," thereby making their work relevant to Japanese authorities. In reality, these hopes for a circuitous revival of Kampo medicine via Japan expansion into East Asia never received serious attention from Japanese authorities, who remained focused on disseminating biomedicine in Japan's new colonial possessions (M. S. Liu 2009). Kampo physicians in Japan remained a powerless group, unable to establish even their own hospital in Japan (Yakazu 1988).

Nonetheless, the intellectual affiliation between the founding doctors of the Suzhou Hospital of National Medicine and the Japanese revivalist doctors was clearly signaled in the opening issue of the hospital's journal, *Journal of the Suzhou Hospital of National Medicine* (蘇州國醫醫院院刊). One of the leaders of the twentieth-century movement to revive Kampo medicine, Yumoto Kyūshin (湯本求真) (1876–1941), was asked to write the preface to the journal.

> Eastern Civilization excels at the metaphysical; Western Civilization excels at the physical. How can medicine be any different? Eastern medicine (*dongyang yixue*; 東洋醫學) is synthetic, inductive, and best at internal medicine. Western medicine (*xiyang yixue*; 西洋醫學) is analytic, deductive, and superior at surgery. If the two could be forged into one, then they would make an incomparable new medicine for the world. . . . The first step is to revive and develop the withering and ailing Eastern medicine. . . . Today my comrade, Dr.

Tang Shenfang . . . has given medicine something truly valuable in the launching of the *Journal of the Suzhou Hospital of National Medicine* (Yumoto Kyūshin 1939).

In this fascinating passage, we can glimpse the fragile state of traditional medicine in Japan "withering and ailing." Yumoto is clearly expressing his hope that a "comrade"—Tang Shenfang (唐慎坊), director of the hospital—in one of the conquered areas would contribute to the revival of traditional medicine. Because the writings of Yumoto Kyūshin were influential in China, it is perhaps most important to notice that he framed the relationship between traditional East Asian medicine and biomedicine through purified, Orientalist tropes: Eastern civilization and Western civilization, Eastern medicine and Western medicine. Perhaps not unlike some of the military leaders of Japan, Yumoto Kyūshin was envisioning the two types of medical practice through the lens of two competing civilizations. In the hospital journal, there is little to suggest that Chinese doctors had any serious interest in the Japanese political projects such as the East Asian Co-Prosperity Sphere. But these Orientalist tropes are significant because eventually Chinese doctors would abandon their commitment to congruence and begin to view the two medical systems through a similar purifying lens.

Yumoto Kyūshin was also quite likely the inspiration for Lu Yuanlei's distinction between *zheng* as presentation and symptom. Yumoto's most important text was *Sino-Japanese Medicine* (皇漢醫學), published in 1927 and translated into Chinese in 1928, shortly before Lu Yuanlei's aforementioned essay. Yumoto's ontological distinction between the medicines of East and West shaped his interpretation of the concept of *zheng*, which is known as *shō* in Japanese. In the following passage, he insisted on distinguishing between the two characters of *shō/zheng* (證) and *shō/zheng* (症) (the two characters are homonyms in both Japanese and Chinese), which had previously been used interchangeably in the medical writings of China and Japan. I have used the glosses of presentation and symptom accordingly in my translation and italicized these terms for clarity.

The *symptomatic* therapy (對症療法) of Western medicine and the "adjust the therapy to the *presentation*" (隨證治之) approach of Kampo medicine look similar but are different. The former focuses on the patient's uncertain self-reported symptoms (自覺症狀) and seeks to repress them. This approach is called treating the branch in Kampo medicine and is completely different than the "adjust the therapy to the *presentation*" approach. Kampo medicine combines the self-reported *symptoms* with the observed *symptoms* (他覺症狀) to discover and treat the confirmed and unchanging *symptoms* (症狀). For Kampo medicine, treating the *presentation* (證) is a causal therapy (原因療法) and a treatment of special efficacy (特効劑) (Yumoto Kyūshin 1983 [1927], 60).[2]

Yumoto's views are significant because they would have been read by elite, urban practitioners in China. Borrowing a famous phrase from the *Treatise*, "adjust the therapy to the presentation," Yumoto attributed a new meaning to *shō/zheng* (證) by opposing it to symptomatic therapy. In the process, he argued that Western medicine only treats the "branch," while Kampo medicine addresses the root cause.

In order to understand how Yumoto's semantic distinction, reinforced with new orthographic conventions, could indicate a fundamental difference between root and branch, we can look ahead a few years to the work of one of his most important students, Ōtsuka Keisetsu (木塚敬節). The doctors of the Suzhou Hospital of National Medicine were in close communication with Ōtsuka and other Japanese scholars during the mid 1930s. Before the founding of the hospital, many of these doctors had been involved with the Suzhou College of National Medicine, which was established in 1933 with Tang Shenfang as president (Deng Tietao 1999, 203). The college published its own journal, *Suzhou Journal of National Medicine*, and often featured works by Japanese scholars in translation. For example, the journal published the new book by Ōtsuka Keisetsu, *Key to Classifying and Discriminating Clinical Presentations in Kampo Medicine* (類證鑒別漢醫要訣), serially across its 1934 volumes. In this work, originally published in Japanese in 1932, we can see that Ōtsuka, like his teacher, was also keenly interested in the concept of *shō/zheng* and insisted on the distinction between the two characters *shō/zheng* (證) and *shō/zheng* (症).

> *Presentation* (*shō/zheng*; 證) means evidence, verification, confirmation. It also means proof. It is completely different than *symptoms* (*shō/zheng*; 症). . . . If you are examining a patient with pneumonia, who has fever, chills, floating and tight pulse, absence of sweating, and panting, then this is called the Ephedra Decoction *presentation* (*shō/zheng*; 證). If the patient only has a fever or wheezing, then this is a *symptom* not a presentation (Ōtsuka 1934). (author's emphasis)

This passage was significant for its clinical implications. Ōtsuka was showing that a specific cluster of symptoms indicated treatment with a specific formula. Scholars familiar with the *Treatise* will recognize that this cluster—fever, chills, floating and tight pulse, absence of sweating, and panting—was derived directly from a passage discussing the use of Ephedra Decoction (*Ma Huang Tang*). This approach to diagnosis and treatment, known in Japan as "match the formula to the presentation" (*fangzheng xiangdui*), was an invention of the Ancient Formula School. This methodology rejected all theories of pathology, claiming they were speculative and unreliable. Instead, it advocated for a close reading of the *Treatise*, as Ōtsuka suggested, where specific descriptions of an illness presentation are the only guide for the use of a particular formula. In other words, there was no need to determine an underlying *bing*. Only the presentation (*shō/zheng*; 證) was needed for diagnosis and treatment.

When we compare Ōtsuka description to Xie Guan's definition, we can recognize three important distinctions. First, the new character, *shō/zheng* (症), is no longer a poor substitute character for the original term, *shō/zheng* (證). The newer term has been reserved exclusively for Western medicine, the older exclusively for traditional Kampo (or Chinese medicine). Second, Ōtsuka has *narrowed* the meaning of the original term *shō/zheng* (證). It still referred to an external "presentation," but the underlying *bing* or internal pathology was no longer a concern. Instead, the presentation has been reframed through the clusters or groupings of symptoms as found in Zhang Zhongjing's classic texts. This more limited connotation was also referred to as the "formula presentation" (*fangzheng*) (方證). Third, Ōtsuka, building on the work of his teacher Yumoto Kyūshin, was driving a conceptual wedge between the two medical systems. Whereas *zheng*—regardless of the character—was used loosely by Republican-era doctors to refer to a clinical presentation, Ōtsuka was suggesting a more radical divide between traditional Chinese/Kampo medicine and biomedicine. As we will see in Chapter 4, the nature of that divide would continue to evolve substantially in the Communist era.

It is precisely this new approach to diagnosis and treatment, inspired by both Japanese and Chinese scholars, that was central to the mission of the doctors at Suzhou Hospital of National Medicine. The hospital was dedicated to using the classic formulas of Zhang Zhongjing, and, according to the statistical analysis presented in the journal, the doctors did so in 75 percent of their treatments. The clinical methodology promoted for this purpose in the journal was called "presentation diagnosis" (*zhenghou zhenduan*; 證候診斷). Using the two-character compound *zhenghou* to refer to the term presentation, the editors of the hospital's journal highlighted the importance of this diagnostic practice in a box insert.

Our Goals
     To study practical medicine and treatment techniques, to focus on presentation diagnosis (證候診斷) and the uses of formulas and drugs,

to absolutely refuse to do speculative research and empty theorization. Although our national medicine has accumulated thousands of
years of history and can truly cure illnesses, it still can't take its place
among the sciences of the world, because it has been influenced by
mysticism. We should clarify our goals, not cling to the empty words of
Five Phases and qi transformation and select the best from the ancient
books.—The Editors (Suzhou Hospital of National Medicine 1939,
Treatment Cases 24).

In this passage, we can see how the editors have inserted "presentation diagnosis" into the debates between Cold Damage and Warm Disorders advocates.
This methodology was positioned as a counterbalance to the negative influences of neo-Confucianism, here marked by derogatory expressions, such as
"speculative research," "empty theorization," "mysticism," "empty words," and
so on.

In the many clinical cases recorded in the journal, we can observe doctors
trying to put this principle into action. Ye Juquan (葉橘泉), perhaps the most
famous doctor at this hospital, explicitly used the term "presentation diagnosis" and emphasized the critical importance of the concept of "presentation" several times in his cases. For example, in the case of Chen Zhenhua, a
twenty-three-year-old male sick with typhoid fever, he wrote, "Treatment with
Chinese herbs takes the presentation (證候) as its object" (Suzhou Hospital
of National Medicine 1939, Treatment Cases 13). Ye invoked the expression
"presentation diagnosis" another three times in his cases. Each time, the expression appears parenthetically to explain how he reached a particular "diagnosis" (診斷). Two of these diagnoses referenced concepts from the *Treatise*
("Cold Damage Greater Yin Disease" [傷寒太陰病] and Cold Damage Yang
Brightness Presentation [傷寒陽明症]) and one referenced a *bing* from the
Essentials of the Golden Casket (金匱要略) called Phlegm-rheum (痰飲).

Ye Juquan indicated that he was privileging the presentation over other
diagnostic approaches in one case with a reference to Yoshimasu Tōdō, the
eighth-century progenitor of the Ancient Formulas School. The patient,
Zhang Yuyi, suffered from "a cough with blood, nocturnal emissions, dis-
tention in the left flank, twitching when sleeping on the left side, fever in
the afternoon, red face, strong heart palpitations." He also noted the patient
claimed to have tested negative for tuberculosis elsewhere. Ye Juquan made
the following diagnosis: "neurasthenia, flu-like symptoms, coughing up blood,
and the presentation of Buplureum Dragon Bones and Oyster Shell Decoction" (Suzhou Hospital of National Medicine 1939, Treatment Cases 3). In
the treatment section of this case, he explained:

According to the method of Zhang Zhongjing, one doesn't ask the cause of the illness. [Rather] one uses the method that corresponds to the presentation. This is the treatment philosophy espoused most forcefully by the Japanese doctor, Mr. Tōdō. As a result, I administered the Buplureum Dragon Bones and Oyster Shell Decoction and after seven to eight doses the patient was cured (Suzhou Hospital of National Medicine 1939, Treatment Cases 3).

Ye Juquan did not base his treatment on a biomedical diagnosis of neurasthenia, possible tuberculosis, or some other respiratory condition, but focused on the totality of the presentation, which aside from the patient's cough, most closely matched the presentation associated with "Buplureum plus Dragon Bones and Oyster Shell Decoction," a classic formula from the *Treatise*. In other words, he was matching the patient's presentation to a formula.

Returning to the case of Chen Zhenhua, we observe Ye Juquan using a similar approach in a case of typhoid fever, complicated by intestinal bleeding. Instead of one treatment for one disease—as one might expect with biomedicine—he used a series of different formulas (all from the *Treatise* except one) to negotiate the perils of this complicated condition and guide the patient back to health. As he summed up, he alternately used "Unripe Bitter Orange Decoction to Drain the Epigastrium (*Zhi Shi Xie Xin Tang*), Major Bupleurum Decoction (*Da Chai Hu Tang*), Reach the Source Drink (*Da Yuan Yin*), Regulate the Stomach and Order the Qi Decoction (*Tiao Wei Cheng Qi Tang*), Pulsatilla Decoction (Bai Tou Weng Tang), Polyporus Decoction (*Zhu Ling San*), Five Ingredient Formula with Poria (*Wu Ling San*), and Ginseng, Aconite, Astragalus, Atractolydes, and other herbs (*Shen Fu Qi Zhu deng*), using [each formula] according to the presentation (*duizheng shizhi*; 對症施治)" (Suzhou Hospital of National Medicine 1939).[3]

The hospital never published another journal issue and eventually closed in 1941. The single journal issue has provided a fascinating glimpse of an emergent style of medical practice based on Zhang Zhongjing's classic texts and the new concept of "presentation diagnosis." Unfortunately, the devastation of war cut short the exchange between Japanese and Chinese doctors, and the influence of Japanese scholarship in China declined precipitously in its aftermath.

The experimental nature of the medical writings of the Republican period set the stage for even more radical changes with the establishment of the People's Republic of China in 1949. But these changes were not, in most cases, the continuation or the coming to fruition of ideas proposed by Republican-era doctors. For example, the intense animosity between the Cold Damage and Warm Disorders advocates faded rather quickly under the Communists. Likewise, Japanese-style diagnosis and treatment based on the "formula presentation" was not widely embraced. Instead, a new approach, "pattern discrimination and treatment determination (*bianzheng lunzhi*; 辨證論治)," became established as the leading clinical methodology. This new expression was indeed centered on the concept of *zheng*, but its meaning was open to competing interpretations. Writing in the *Journal of Chinese Medicine* in 1958, Ye Juquan argued that *bianzheng lunzhi* should follow the principles of "presentation diagnosis" that he had practiced almost twenty years earlier in Suzhou. "So-called *bianzheng lunzhi* does not mean just anything. . . . [We must] determine which formulas match which presentations" (Ye Juquan 2014 [1958], 1). But other views prevailed, and the connotations of the term *zheng* continued to evolve. In Chapter 4, we will explore how the Republican-era concepts of *bing* and *zheng* become transformed through the processes of purification and hybridization into our third and most important dualism of disease and pattern.

4

New Textbooks, New Medicine

Shortly after finishing my medical school degree at the Beijing University of Chinese Medicine in June of 2000, I returned to the University of North Carolina (UNC) at Chapel Hill to complete my graduate degree in Anthropology. Over the next two years, when my schedule permitted, I audited some of the courses offered at the University of North Carolina Medical School. The contrast with my medical school experience in Beijing was striking. Lectures at UNC were presented in an auditorium-style lecture hall, well suited for the PowerPoint presentations that almost all lecturers used. Courses were taught collectively; each lecture was presented by a different professor speaking about his or her specialization. I was impressed both by the breadth of these lectures, which covered a range of materials well beyond my Western medicine courses in Beijing, and by the ability of each professor to distill each lecture down to a few key ideas. Before each class, students would receive a printed handout of the upcoming PowerPoint slides. To my surprise, it seemed that most students did not take notes other than making a few jottings in the margins of their PowerPoint handouts. Whenever I glanced about the hall during a lecture, I noticed students relaxing in their cushioned chairs, putting their feet up, sipping a drink, munching on a bagel, talking in quiet tones with a neighbor. With the lights dimmed, the projector whirring, I often felt as if I had come to watch a movie. I quickly learned that the casual atmosphere was deceptive. Whenever a professor posed a question to the class, I was always impressed that students would volunteer a quick, well-considered answer.

These cursory glimpses into the training at an American medical school made my experiences at the Beijing University of Chinese Medicine feel more austere and old-fashioned, as if a remnant of a bygone era. In Beijing, our classrooms were spartan. There were no computers and no PowerPoint presentations. (The revolution of cell phones, computers, and internet would come to China in the early 2000s.) We sat on wooden chairs behind long wooden tables, all of which were bolted to a cement floor. During the winter, we almost always kept our jackets on during class, because cold air often poured through a couple of broken windows. Even when the windows were intact, they were poor defenses against the chilly weather outside, and everyone preferred to stay bundled up. Professors lectured throughout the class period. Some wrote on the blackboard, but not all. They rarely paused to question students directly or encourage class discussion. Students, on the other hand, were much busier than their UNC counterparts. We assiduously took notes on everything that the professor said and wrote on the blackboard. Even the students sitting in the back rows looked quite busy.

Classroom protocol was important, and lapses in propriety would often be interpreted as an affront to the professor. Eating food in class was unthinkable. With our immovable desks and chairs, it was physically impossible to do anything more than slump forward when exhausted. Putting one's feet up would have been seen as disrespectful. Students always arrived before the professor. When the professor walked in, the student designated "class leader" (*banzhang*), a position of prestige, would bellow, "Attention," and everyone would stand in unison. With a nod of acknowledgment from the professor, we would sit down, and the lecture would begin promptly. There were some dimensions of classroom etiquette that, much to my dismay, I only learned about much later. For example, I often chewed gum to help me stay alert throughout our long days of classes, usually six to eight fifty-minute periods per day. Shortly before graduation, one of my classmates reminded me that I used to chew gum in class. I was surprised that she had even noticed and even more that she still remembered. Shaking her head, she told me, "No Chinese student would have been allowed to chew gum like you in class. Our teachers were very tolerant with you, probably because you were an American."

Perhaps the most notable difference between UNC Medical School and Beijing University of Chinese Medicine was the structure of the class lecture. Although I only attended a limited number of lectures at UNC, I was impressed that each lecture was unique to the invited professor. Each professor focused on summarizing his or her field of expertise, articulating fundamental principles, but leaving specific details to the textbooks, which students were expected to learn on their own. At the Beijing University of Chinese Medicine, the organization of the lecturers was driven by the textbooks. It was only the best professors, usually the most experienced clinicians, who felt like they could lecture on topics not found in the textbooks. I will never forget my course on the *Treatise on Cold Damage* taught by Pei Yongqing. He rarely spent time discussing specific content from the textbook; instead, he illustrated key points with thrilling stories from his own clinical cases. But most professors were much more conservative. One of the main reasons was that our tests, which were always given in the same format—sixty points worth of multiple-choice questions and forty points worth of short essay questions—were based entirely on the textbooks. Since test scores alone determined students' grades, most teachers felt that they had an obligation to teach the textbook.

I had never had a college-level educational experience that was so reliant on textbooks. And the more I studied them, the more they became peculiar objects for me. They were unlike the heavy, highly illustrated, expensive textbooks that I had grown up with. Our Chinese medicine textbooks were slender and delicate. They were printed cheaply on thin paper with soft paper covers that would easily fray or tear. They rarely contained images. The few textbooks that did, such as anatomy, included only simple ink sketches. The price tag was modest.[1] I frequently marveled at the bare-bones style of these textbooks. Who could have guessed that these unpretentious books were invaluable resources, our essential guides for learning both Chinese medicine and Western medicine? We read them closely, studied them intensively. Becoming a doctor meant mastering them.

During my second and third year of classes, I began to reflect more critically on the textbooks. Universities and colleges of Chinese medicine around the country were in the process of transitioning from the fifth edition of the national textbooks to the sixth edition. In nearly every course, but especially the Chinese medicine courses, our teachers complained about the new edition of textbooks. Up to that point, I had not given much thought to the content of the textbooks. I had innocently assumed that we were learning the basics, the standards, the kind of content that specialists would all agree upon. But the complaints about the sixth edition stirred me out of my uncritical inertia. As I began to inquire about the problems of this latest edition, all my tidy assumptions about the knowledge and standards captured in the textbooks slowly began to unravel. Most professors considered the fifth edition to be the best of all the editions and truest to the traditional principles of Chinese medicine. But others insisted that textbooks must reflect the latest, up-to-date knowledge of the field. Like Western medicine textbooks, they argued, Chinese medicine textbooks should be updated every decade or so. I decided to research this topic in earnest and was able to interview almost two dozen scholars who worked as editors on various editions of the national textbooks—in particular, many who contributed to the Chinese Internal Medicine (中医内科) textbook, the most important course for our clinical training. Eventually I would discover that the development of the national textbooks, these humble-looking guides to contemporary clinical practice, was deeply intertwined with profound changes in the theory and practice of Chinese medicine. These changes culminated in the emergence of the clinical methodology of "pattern discrimination and treatment determination" (*bianzheng lunzhi*) (辨证论治), which the fifth and sixth editions of the national textbooks explicitly claim as one of the key characteristics of Chinese medicine. This chapter explores how the textbooks became the driving force behind the subsequent evolution of Republican-era concepts of *bing* and *zheng*. As these terms developed new connotations, particularly as *zheng* lost the meaning of "presentation" and became the diagnostic concept of "pattern," the third dualism in the postcolonial transformation of Chinese medicine took shape. The new disease-pattern dualism made possible the emergence of *bianzheng lunzhi* and the new institutionalized practice of Chinese medicine.

Two Histories of *Bianzheng Lunzhi*

"Pattern discrimination and treatment determination" (*bianzheng lunzhi*) is unquestionably the "essence" of Chinese medicine today. It is the concept around which the national textbooks are designed. In my experience, nearly all doctors of Chinese medicine agree upon the singular importance of *bianzheng lunzhi* to Chinese medicine. The *Basic Theory of Chinese Medicine* textbook states unequivocally that *bianzheng lunzhi*, together with the principle of "holism" (*zhengtiguan*), are the two "basic characteristics" of Chinese medicine (Wu Dunxu, Liu Yanchi, and Li Dexin 1995, 4–8). I have observed countless doctors reminding their students—and me—of its importance. "You must *bianzheng lunzhi*," doctors insist. Good clinical results can only be achieved by following this methodology. Likewise, poor outcomes are inevitable when one fails to do a proper pattern discrimination. The famous gynecologist Xiao Chengzong (肖承宗), whom I had the pleasure of interviewing, came up with a clever way to explain its importance: "Without *bianzheng lunzhi*, Chinese medicine doctors would be nothing more than barefoot doctors; Chinese medicine formulas would be nothing more than folk prescriptions (*pianfang*)."[2] In other words, without *bianzheng lunzhi*, doctors would have nothing but one-size-fits-all treatments. They would not know how to tailor their treatments to the specific conditions of individual patients. Instead of theoretical sophistication and nuanced therapies, doctors would practice medicine by the numbers.

In the eyes of most practitioners, *bianzheng lunzhi* is a timeless concept. But it presents a conundrum to historians and potentially a political minefield to those who question its antiquity. Outside of China, some scholars have argued that *bianzheng lunzhi* is a creation of the Communist period (Scheid 2002, 6–7; Scheid and Karchmer 2016; Karchmer 2010). But within China, such a claim can be politically charged. In 1999, when I was still a student at the Beijing University of Chinese Medicine, Wang Yuchaun (王玉川), a retired professor at the university and highly respected scholar, published a controversial article that challenged both the antiquity and uniqueness of *bianzheng lunzhi* to Chinese medicine. Wang Yuchuan was born in 1923, trained during the Republican era, and became of one of the founding members of the Inner Canon Teaching and Research Group at the Beijing University of Chinese Medicine. He was an important figure in edit-ing the early editions of the *Inner Canon* textbook in the late 1950s and early 1960s. In this article, he noted that the phrase *bianzheng lunzhi* cannot be found in Xie Guan's 1921 *Comprehensive Dictionary of Chinese Medicine*. Likewise, "eight principles pattern discrimination" (*bagang bianzheng*), one of the key techniques in pattern discrimination, he told his readers, was a phrase coined by Zhu Weiju in 1950, not in the distant past.[3] Perhaps most importantly, as one of the individuals that participated in the textbook writing process of the 1950s, Wang Yuchuan credited the scholars who contributed to writing of the national textbooks for systematizing *bianzheng lunzhi*.

> It was after the establishment of New China [in 1949] that the various styles and content of the methodology of pattern discrimination and treatment determination were synthesized and written into the Chi-nese medicine textbooks. A large group of Chinese medicine educators and researchers (including Yin Huihe, Wang Mianzhi, Wang Youren, specialists at the China Academy of Chinese Medicine, as well as the author himself) worked under the auspices of the Party's Chinese med-icine policy to make this contribution (Wang Yuchuan 1999).

Wang Yuchuan went even further in this article to suggest that *bianzheng lunzhi* was not unique to Chinese medicine. "Is not the differential diagnosis and the selection of therapies according to the specific circumstances of each patient in Western medicine . . . just another form of *bianzheng lunzhi*?" he asked (Wang Yuchuan 1999).

I happened to notice this article shortly after it was published and was curious to discuss it with my classmates and teachers. But my acquaintances seemed to wave me off. Several dismissed it as the eccentric ramblings of a well-known curmudgeon. One individual even suggested that Wang had lost some of his prestigious positions at several national medicine associations as a result of this article. If there were such political reverberations, they were short-lived, because in 2009 he was named as one of thirty "Great Masters of National Medicine" (*guoyi dashi*), the first ever state-level honor conferred on doctors of Chinese medicine since the founding of the People's Republic. Nonetheless, the political sensitivities around the significance and uniqueness of *bianzheng lunzhi* at the time made such a story plausible.

For the historians, the challenge posed by *bianzheng lunzhi* is that it should derive its authority from the classics. But as Wang Yuchuan claimed, this four-character term cannot be found in any of the ancient canons or even in late imperial and Republican-era medical texts. This contradiction was readily apparent in the commemorative history *Scientific and Technological Achievements of Chinese Medicine in the Forty Years since the Founding of the Nation*, published in 1989, one of the few texts to attempt a history of this supposedly unchanging principle. The following passages gives an example of this tension.

The editors acknowledged that, when measured against the great time spans of Chinese medicine, the term *bianzheng lunzhi* was a recent invention. Depending on one's hermeneutic proclivities, they suggested it was either about two hundred years old or four hundred and fifty years old.

> The term *bianzheng lunzhi* first appears in Zhang Xugu's (張虛谷) *Medical Awakening* (一門棒喝) [c. 1829]. The term *bianzheng shizhi* first appears in Zhou Zhigan's (周之干) *Posthumous Writings of Shenzhai* (慎齋遺書) [c. 1586] . . . (State Administration of Traditional Chinese Medicine and Hu Ximing 1989, 70).

Part of the reasons for this ambiguous origin story is that during the early years of the People's Republic, these two expressions, *bianzheng lunzhi* and *bianzheng shizhi*, were used interchangeably—the former emphasized the "determination" (*lun*) of treatment and the latter referred to "application" (*shi*) of treatment—until the latter term dropped out of favor.

I have intentionally not translated passages from *Medical Awakening* and *Posthumous Writings of Shenzhai* that would seem to support these claims. As the reader might have already surmised based on the discussion of *bing* and *zheng* in Chapter 3, these expressions could not have the same connotation as today's "pattern discrimination and treatment determination." The editors of *Scientific and Technological Achievements of Chinese Medicine, 1949–1989* seemed to recognize this tenuous genealogy and made no attempt to provide textual evidence for their claims. This apparent omission may be because they gave greater emphasis to another history of *bianzheng lunzhi*, in which they specifically acknowledged the contribution of three modern scholars, Zhu

Yan (朱颜), Ren Yingqiu (任应秋), and Qin Bowei (秦伯未), to development of the methodology.

> In the 1950s, Mr. Zhu, Mr. Ren, and Mr. Qin decisively put forward the concept of *bianzheng lunzhi*. Subsequently, the Chinese medicine community launched a broad exploration into the system of diagnosis and treatment in Chinese medicine and its distinguishing features. They argued that Zhang Zhongjing brought together the experience of the ancients and laid the foundations of the theory of *bianzheng lunzhi*. As later generations of physicians carried it forward, they made it more systematic, until it became the distinguishing feature of Chinese medicine clinical practice (State Administration of Traditional Chinese Medicine and Hu Ximing 1989, 70).

After briefly making visible the scholarly labor of systematizing *bianzheng lunzhi*, the editors quickly covered their tracks. They pushed the origins of *bianzheng lunzhi* as far back into Chinese antiquity as possible, citing the scholarship of Yue Meizhong (岳美中), another revered figure of the mid-twentieth century.

> But the *bianzheng lunzhi* system emerged long before the Ming and Qing dynasties. As Yue Meizhong and others have noted: the basics of *bianzheng lunzhi* theory were laid down in the *Yellow Emperor's Inner Canon*, and the system of *bianzheng lunzhi* was established [in the *Treatise on Cold Damage* and *Essentials of the Golden Casket*] by Zhang Zhongjing. From the Jin and Tang dynasties until the middle of the Northern Song, the organ systems and the meridians were the heart of *bianzheng lunzhi*. In the Song, Jin, and Yuan dynasties, physicians both improved the pattern recognition of Zhang Zhongjing's three yin three yang doctrine and developed their own insights based on personal experience. During the Ming and Qing dynasties, doctors not only recognized yin and yang, interior and exterior, hot and cold, depletion and repletion patterns, but also established the Wei Qi Ying Xue patterns of the Warm Disorders school. With the founding of the People's Republic, *bianzheng lunzhi* was definitively recognized as the distinguishing feature of Chinese medicine clinical practice and has been the subject of research and systemization (State Administration of Traditional Chinese Medicine and Hu Ximing 1989, 70).

Thus, the editors resolved the historical conundrum posed by *bianzheng lunzhi* by weaving the objective newness of the term into an evolutionary narrative of its development through every major period in the history of Chinese medicine, beginning with the *Yellow Emperor's Inner Canon* (ca. 100 B.C.E.) and continuing through the works of Zhang Zhongjing (220 C.E.), the four masters of the Jin and Yuan dynasties (1115–1368 C.E.), and the Warm Disorders innovators of the Ming and Qing.

Working between *Scientific and Technological Achievements of Chinese Medicine, 1949–1989* and Wang Yuchuan's article, it is possible to identify two (or more) histories of *bianzheng lunzhi*, one that is less than seventy years old and one that is more than 2,000 years old. Few contemporary doctors espouse the former, but the historical evidence does not support the latter. The term *bianzheng lunzhi* did not exist in the Republican period, but after the aforementioned articles by Zhu Yan, Ren Yingqiu, and Qin Bowei in 1954, 1955, and 1957, respectively, there was an explosion of literature on this topic that continues to this day (Zhu Yan 1954; Ren Yingqiu 1955; Qin Bowei 1957). When I had the opportunity to interview senior physicians about the history of *bianzheng lunzhi*, I almost always got the same response. Doctors like Zhang Jingren (张镜人) and Deng Tietao more or less reiterated the dual historical claims of Wang Yuchuan and *Scientific and Technological Achievements of Chinese Medicine, 1949–1989*. The term *bianzheng lunzhi* did not exist in the Republican period, they concurred, but the spirit of the concept has always been part of Chinese medicine.[4] The national textbooks will be the key to understanding this apparent paradox, but first we need to understand how the textbooks became so central to the teaching of Chinese medicine.

Learning through Apprenticeships

Apprenticeships were the primary form for transmitting medical knowledge in premodern China, and this trend continued into the Republican period, despite the development of many private schools during this period (Deng Tietao and Cheng Zhifan 2000, 198). Deng Tietao and Cheng Zhifan have argued that even with the advent of these new medical schools, most new doctors were trained through apprenticeships, including two-thirds of the leading doctors profiled in the *Encyclopedia of Medicine in China* (中国医学百科全书) (Deng Tietao and Cheng Zhifan 2000, 198). Moreover, my interviews with doctors who attended some of these schools indicated that the clinical training within these school programs often involved an apprentice-style relationship to an established physician, arranged either through the school or the student's personal family networks.[5] With the establishment of state-run colleges of Chinese medicine and their affiliated hospitals of Chinese medicine in the late 1950s, a new institutionalized model of education became the dominant mode of transmitting knowledge in the world of Chinese medicine.

What were the effects of this new form of education, and how did it alter the practice of Chinese medicine? To answer these questions, we need to first explore the nature of apprenticeship training more broadly.

Anthropologists have studied apprenticeship styles of learning across a wide range of societies for a diverse number of specialized crafts. Drawing on their insights, we can more readily appreciate how the institutionalization of Chinese medicine education profoundly reshaped the profession. There are four key elements to apprenticeships in general that have particular relevance for Chinese medicine. First, apprenticeships are inherently risky ventures from the perspective of the master. The master's reputation and the quality of his or her work are at stake. A bad apprentice can affect the quality of the master's product or otherwise reflect poorly on the master. Conversely, a successful apprentice might become a future competitor for the master. As a result, masters tend to select disciples with care (Lancy 2012). One unique feature for the Chinese medicine apprenticeships compared to craft specializations in other societies is the centrality of texts and the apprentice's degree of literacy. Unlike pottery, stonework, weaving, blacksmithing, carving, and the transmission of other skilled crafts in nonliterate societies, learning medicine in China could be dependent on the mastery of textual knowledge, at least in its elite forms. Yang Nianqun's research on Li Zeqing (1914–97), a well-known physician from Hubei Province, helps capture this aspect of medical apprenticeship in China.

> According to his recollections, when Li Zeqing sought out Chen Wenqing to become his apprentice . . . , Chen Wenqing was unconcerned about his [peasant] attire. He simply picked up a copy of Wang Ang's *Essentials of Materia Medica* (本草備藥) and asked him to take it home and punctuate it. Like classical Chinese texts in general, classical herbal texts did not have modern punctuation. To be able to correctly punctuate the sentences of a classical herbal text was a measure of one's ability to read and understand classical Chinese. With his foundation from ten years of old-style private education, Li Zeqing completed the punctuation for *Essentials of Materia Medica*. When Chen Wenqing saw it, he said, "This child can be taught. This child can enter the way of medicine," indicating that he had passed the test, so to speak, to become an apprentice (Yang Nianqun 2005, 245).

In the elite, literary tradition of medicine, the apprentice was expected to be proficient in classical Chinese, the difficult written language of ancient China, in order to read and master certain classic medical texts. Once the master and the family of the disciple had come to terms, the apprenticeship was ritually formalized and confirmed with a payment to the doctor, perhaps in the form of rice. Over several years, usually between three to five years, the disciple was expected to gradually master the skills needed to open his own clinical practice.

Second, because of the inherent risk in apprenticeships, the master reluctantly passes on his or her knowledge, and then only when the disciple has demonstrated sufficient loyalty. Often devotion to the master was demonstrated through the completion of innumerable menial tasks. The historian Yang Nianqun has captured some of the work typical of a premodern medical apprentice in China.

> During the apprenticeship, the master would provide board and give a yearly allowance of roughly three strings (one string contained 100 copper coins). The apprentice's workload was varied and heavy. In addition to washing, cutting, collecting, and drying herbs, the apprentice had to do a large number of chores, such as opening and closing the clinic, fetching water, sweeping the floor, sharpening knives, meal preparation, providing a basin of water for the master to wash his face or feet, and removing ash from the stove. In the evening, the apprentice would roll a "paper coal" (making a thin, long roll from rough straw or bamboo paper to be used as a lighter for smoking tobacco) and extract the cores of Ophiopogonis tubers (*maidong*) (pulling it with his teeth or a tool). Each evening, he would make a small pile of cores (Yang Nianqun 2005, 245).

David Lancy has surveyed the anthropological literature on apprenticeships and found countless examples of disciples performing similar menial work (Lancy 2012). In the early stages of the apprenticeship, the master certainly benefits from the labor of the apprentice. But he also uses this period to determine whether the apprentice is worthy of further instruction. As David Lancy points outs:

> At first, the apprentice learns by observing the work of those more expert but is mostly occupied with menial chores such as fetching and cleaning up or simple, repetitive tasks such as bobbin winding or bringing clay, water, or wood to the master. The apprentice demonstrates through hard work and diligence, over a sometimes lengthy period, his or her worthiness for instruction. . . . "Before the neophyte [Mande blacksmith] can master techniques and form, he has to master pain. He begins at the bellows, where he spends many hours each day" (Lancy 2012).

The worthiness of the disciple and therefore the willingness of the master to teach him is only firmly established through this initial period of hard work.

Among elite practitioners of medicine, there was an additional requirement of attracting a literate discipline, as Li Zeqing's case so clearly reminds us. The reason for this requirement is that the early stages of medical apprenticeship also involved large amounts of rote memorization. The centrality of memorization helps illustrate a third key difference with modern education systems, which is that the master, unlike today's professor, only provided minimal instruction. Lancy has argued that apprenticeships proceed through laddered or staged degrees of difficulty, putting the burden on the apprentice to learn through careful observation (Lancy 2012). Although this combination of extracting menial labor, requiring rote memorization, and providing only minimal instruction would seem to run counter to contemporary principles of pedagogy, there is good evidence that it could work quite well for training Chinese medicine doctors. For example, we have a famous account of the merits of apprenticeship in a letter that has colloquially come to be known as "The Petition of the Five Elders" (五老上书) (the actual title was "Some Opinions on Reforming the Instructional Plan for Colleges of Chinese Medicine" (对修订中医学院教学计划的几点意见). The letter was written by five professors on the eve of the graduation of the first class of students at Beijing College of Chinese Medicine and delivered to the Ministry of Health on July 16, 1962. It was a plea for government action to address the serious challenges confronting the new colleges of Chinese medicine. The authors believed that, despite six years of education, most of the graduating students had not been adequately trained in Chinese medicine. To sharpen their point, the authors compared the new colleges with the apprenticeship-style training that they personally experienced in the Republican era.

According to our understanding of apprenticeship training, the first requirement of a doctor is to select a student with good reading skills. After the master-disciple relationship is ritually consecrated (*baishi*), the student spends the first two years reciting aloud texts, such as the *Inner Canon* (usually selections), *Treatise on Cold Damage, Essentials of the Golden Casket, Pulse Verses* (脉訣), as well as *Drug Property Verses* (藥性賦), *Formulas in Rhyme* (湯頭歌), and other works. While the student learns these texts so thoroughly that he even memorizes some of the commentaries, he also copies prescriptions (*chaofang*) with the master. Beginning in the third year, the teacher explicates key passages and indicates other required reading. The student both studies intensively and assists the teacher in his clinical work, usually spending half the day in the clinic, half the day reading. The master will allow the student to conclude his studies (*chushi*) with the completion of five years of training, but only if he believes the student has the ability to open a clinic. If the student has not studied well, he might be required to stay longer. Students from the few families with good financial resources that don't need to open a clinic immediately will also follow (*canshi*) another famous doctor. When following another doctor, the period of study would not be too long, from 3 to 5 months, enough to grasp the teacher's unique experience. . . . This was a good model of Chinese medicine apprenticeship training, which produced high quality, successful doctors (Ren Yingqiu 1984, 4).

This description of elite medical apprenticeship training, perhaps idealized for the purposes of the petition, resonates with many of the general features of apprenticeship described by Lancy and other anthropologists. It can also help highlight the distinctions between medical apprenticeships and the school-based medical training that ultimately replaced it in the Communist era. For example, the authors stressed the importance of "reciting aloud" and "memorizing" canonical texts, such as the *Inner Canon* and Zhang Zhongjing's *Treatise on Cold Damage* and *Essentials of the Golden Casket*, as well as the more technical texts on drug properties, formulas, and the pulse exam. Ren Yingqiu, one of the signatories to this letter, was known to continue this habit of recitation even as a professor at the Beijing College of Chinese Medicine. Wang Juyi, the well-known acupuncturist from Beijing whom we encountered at the beginning of Chapter 1, remembered with admiration that Ren Yingqiu would get up every morning, around 4–5 A.M., to recite passages from the canons. Wang Juyi happened to live in the room next to Ren Yingqiu in the early years of the college when professors and students shared a single building and heard these recitations through the thin wall separating them.[6] Although there is much to memorize in contemporary curriculums, the national textbooks are not written for that purpose, unlike many classical texts, which were written in verse precisely to facilitate memorization. I knew of a few classmates who would recite aloud some of the canons on their own, but it was not considered part of our training.

This passage also points to perhaps an even more significant difference with contemporary medical school programs. In premodern apprenticeships, mastering the canons was not separate from observing clinical work. Even as the disciple was memorizing texts, probably with minimal guidance from his master, he was also "copying prescriptions." In other words, he was carefully observing how the principles, concepts, drugs, and formulas that he encountered in his readings were being put to use by his teacher. This point contrasts sharply with today's training. We spent the first two and a half years of medical school studying the basics of Chinese and Western medicine, with no formal exposure to clinical practice. It was only in the second semester of the third year that we began to have short periods of clinical observations at various affiliated hospitals. In the fourth year of medical school, our days were split between clinical training in the morning and classroom instruction in the afternoon. The fifth and final year of medical school was devoted entirely to clinical training. One important consequence of this delayed exposure to clinical practice was that most students, including me, were unsure how to relate the basic concepts and terms of Chinese medicine to actual clinical situations. In fact, most students found it much easier to recognize Western medicine textbook descriptions in clinical practice. When I had the opportunity to interview Zhu Liangchun, the famous clinician from Nantong, about his training during the Republican period, I asked if he also struggled to learn the basics of Chinese medicine like today's students. He replied, "Not at all. We were copying our teacher's prescriptions for the beginning of our apprenticeship. We quickly saw what all these ideas meant in practice."[7]

The key texts mentioned in the "Petition of the Five Elders" also merit further exploration because ultimately these classic texts have all been replaced by textbooks. There were important distinctions between these texts that shaped how they and other premodern medical writings were later incorporated into the national textbooks. The early medical training of the well-known physician Jiao Shude, the doctor we encountered at the end of Chapter 2, can help us appreciate some of these distinctions. When I interviewed Jiao Shude in 1999, he emphasized that the encounter with the classic medical texts would be more varied than suggested by the passage from the "Petition of the Five Elders." He insisted that there were two types of classic texts.

> There are two ways to study Chinese medicine: one goes from the most superficial to the most profound, the other begins with the study of the canons and slowly proceeds to clinical practice. In the Chinese countryside, in the old society, life was hard. Some people saw medicine as a career and a way to put food on the table. What would this type of person do? They would study a little medicine, hang up a shingle, and make a living. There was another type of person, who wasn't poor, had plenty to eat and drink, and lived a comfortable life. This person was interested in scholarship. . . . Which path one took also depended on one's teacher. Some teachers would have their students first learn *Drug Property Verses*, then *Formulas in Rhyme*, and *Binhu's*

Pulses (瀕湖脈學). In this way, the student could begin to see patients under the tutelage of the teacher. This is the method of starting
with the superficial and moving to the profound; first learn the most
concrete and then slowly improve through practice. Other [teachers
would have their students] first memorize [the canons, such as] the
Yellow Emperor's Inner Canon, [*Treatise on Cold Damage Disorders*],
and the *Essentials of the Golden Casket*. Whether you understood it or
not, you had to memorize it. When you had memorized it, the teacher
would explain it to you, and then take you to see patients. . . . Then
you would study the four masters of the Jin and Yuan dynasties, and
the other famous physicians of different eras. . . . I took the latter route,
first studying the canons, then the classics from the Tang and Song
dynasties, the Four Masters [of the Jin and Yuan dynasties], and the
[major works of the] Ming and Qing dynasties.[8]

Jiao Shude's account emphasized a division between more technical works,
such as *Drug Property Verses*, *Formulas in Rhyme*, and *Binhu's Pulses*, and theoretical ones, such as *Yellow Emperor's Inner Canon*, *Treatise on Cold Damage
Disorders*, and *Essentials of the Golden Casket*. Through the former group,
an apprentice would learn the basics of a clinical exam, which emphasized
pulses above all else, and the essentials of herbal therapy, the properties of materia medica, and the most commonly used formulas. The latter group, however, focused on philosophical foundations, such as yin and yang and the five
phases; theoretical foundations, such as viscera manifestation and treatment
principles; and the clinical formulas and methodologies of Zhang Zhongjing.
As we will see, it is this latter cluster that gradually became deemphasized in
the new college curriculums structured around the national textbooks.

The accounts of medical apprenticeship provided by the "Five Elders"
and Jiao Shude remind us how successful this methodology could be. But
they do not fully explain why new colleges of Chinese medicine of the early
Communist era were failing in their educational mission. In my interviews
with textbook editors, particularly ones involved in the early editions, I was
struck by their accounts of the challenge of transitioning between these two
distinct forms of pedagogy. Many interviewees commented to me that the
most esteemed doctors of the Republican era often turned out to be dismal
college professors.[9] I was initially bewildered by these comments, but Lancy's
scholarship on apprenticeships reminds us that formal classroom instruction
has little to do with apprenticeship training. He has argued that knowledge
transmission in an apprenticeship is far closer to the informal methods of craft
learning than modern school pedagogy.

Craft mastery includes, as we've seen: a play stage, observation of an expert at work and imitation by the novice; a laddered or staged sequence of sub-tasks; a great deal of trial and error; the demonstration of diligence and motivation on the novice's part, to attract the attention of the expert; and little or no verbal instruction or even structured demonstration by the expert. This suite of characteristics can be found in the informal transmission of crafts as well as the formal apprenticeship (Lancy 2015, 290).

Early school administrators were aware of the challenges of training teachers skilled in classroom instruction. In the 1950s, the Jiangsu School for Advanced Studies in Chinese Medicine (江苏省中医进修学校) developed perhaps the most influential teacher training program for colleges of Chinese medicine. Meng Jingchun, a graduate of this program who became one of the founding professors at the Nanjing College of Chinese Medicine, recalled to me in an interview that professors from Nanjing Normal University were brought in to help teach the basics of classroom pedagogy. He remembered being instructed on how to use a blackboard and how to organize lectures according to "key points (*zhongdian*)," "difficult points (*nandian*)," and likely "areas of confusion (*yidian*)." I personally witnessed that this same style of organizing lectures was still in place nearly forty years later.

Lancy's work also alerts us to a fourth difference between medical apprenticeships and medical schools, one that may help illuminate the struggles of the Chinese medicine profession in the early Communist era. Lancy has argued that the sociological dimensions of apprenticeship were also essential to motivating the novice to endure the rigors of this training method. The disciple is doubly bound to the apprenticeship by the investments of both parents and master. The parents typically formalize the apprenticeship through fees or gifts with the expectation that this training will allow the child to enter an "exalted profession," often distinguished by various forms of social, political, or religious prestige. The master also invests in the relationship but reluctantly, gradually, and only if the disciple continues to demonstrate loyalty. His most valuable knowledge is only divulged at the end, if at all.

One of the most interesting aspects of apprenticeship is the understanding that the master's expertise is at least partly due to his or her knowledge of secrets or lore and that this information is not willingly passed on to apprentices. The African blacksmith, in particular, is invested with special knowledge and may be empowered to perform certain rituals. . . . None of this lore is freely given to the apprentice and a truly worthy apprentice is expected to "steal" as much of these more subtle aspects of the craft as he can winkle out (Lancy 2015, 290).

Chinese medicine apprenticeships were also driven by these complex sociological tendencies, and the issue of secret knowledge was one that disturbed government officials. In the early years of the People's Republic, the Communist Party tried to combat these tendencies by urging doctors to "make public" (*xian fang*) their most valuable prescriptions.

Forging Consensus

Regardless of the merits of premodern medical apprenticeships, social and political circumstances would ultimately make the establishment of colleges of Chinese medicine the primary means of educating new doctors in the Communist era. Reform efforts in the late imperial and Republican periods had laid the foundation for these Communist-era developments. By the late nineteenth century, noted political thinker Zheng Guanying (1842–1922) had called attention to the importance of educational reform. He wrote in 1892 that "schools are the source of talented people; talented people are the source of national strength. The strength of the Far West lies in superior learning" (See Li Jingwei and Yan Liang 1990, 8). Zhou Xueqiao, the editor of the early Chinese medicine journal *Medical News* (醫學報), was an early proponent of schools for the teaching of Chinese medicine. In 1906, he wrote, "There is nothing more important than schools to the reform of medicine today" (Deng Tietao and Cheng Zhifan 2000, 157). This interest in developing schools ultimately spread to the world of Chinese medicine and led to the foundation of many small private schools during the Republican period. But both the Beiyang government (established after the Revolution of 1911) and the Nationalist government (established in 1928) refused to incorporate schools of Chinese medicine into their national education systems. Threatened by this official hostility to the profession, leading educators within the Chinese medicine profession actively discussed how to remedy this situation. For example, at one major convention in 1929, the participants urged the development of "unified curricular textbooks" (Deng Tietao and Cheng Zhifan 2000, 213). But this task proved too difficult for these contentious times. In April 1933, the Institute of National Medicine proposed guidelines for a standardized curriculum, but they did not actually address the question of actual course content (Deng Tietao and Cheng Zhifan 2000, 219–20).[10]

Ultimately, it was the new political circumstances of the Communist era that made possible, if not outright compelled, the Chinese medicine profession to achieve the consensus on teaching standards that had been so elusive in the Republican period. Medical policy in the early 1950s was driven by the Ministry of Health, which was staffed almost exclusively by biomedical specialists openly hostile to the profession of Chinese medicine. The most important figure in shaping policy in these early years was He Cheng (贺诚), a biomedical physician who played a leading role in healthcare planning for the Red Army. He eventually became deputy director of the Ministry of Health after 1949, where he helped institute a series of policies aimed at reforming Chinese medicine. New opportunities to learn Chinese medicine—whether through apprenticeships or the few schools that survived into the post-war period—became increasingly limited. Although apprenticeships continued in the early Communist era and even garnered some legal support in 1956 (Taylor 2004, 101), they were plagued by problems. In 1962, Lu Bingkui noted that very few apprentices were learning the craft well. He stated that many were struggling to make ends meet, often lacked the needed command of classical Chinese, and were too busy with other work requirements to properly study (Cui Yueli 1993, 99). Other policies of the early 1950s actively undermined the profession. New licensing exams in 1952 that contained significant Western medicine content led to a failure rate as high as 90 percent in some areas and significantly winnowed the field (Taylor 2004, 39–40). At the same time, reform efforts were focused on retraining practicing doctors by encouraging them to enroll in "advanced studies" schools (with twelve-month curriculums) and courses (with three- to six-month curriculums). Most of these programs were designed to give doctors training in Western medicine, not in enhancing their Chinese medicine practice (Taylor 2004, 38–39; Croizier 1968, 161–62).

In 1954 and 1955, there was an important shift in medical policy toward Chinese medicine that was to have long-lasting impact on the future of the Chinese medicine profession. Denouncing the patent bias of the Ministry of Health toward Chinese medicine, the party launched a series of policy decisions that were to officially incorporate Chinese medicine into the new state-run healthcare systems. This shift was signaled with an attack on the former director of public health in the Northeast Military District Wang Bin (王斌), who had famously stated in a 1950 publication that Chinese medicine was a "feudal medicine" (*fengjian yi*) that was destined to disappear in the Communist era just like other aspects of feudal society. Although this viewpoint had been common within the party before 1949 and seemed to be grounded in standard Marxist base-superstructure logic, it was officially deemed bourgeois in 1955. Chinese medicine was reclassified as a product of the struggles of Chinese people, a "legacy of the motherland" (Croizier 1968,

170–72). These attacks then opened the way for criticism of He Cheng and his leadership of the Ministry of Health, because he had elevated Wang Bin to the position of vice minister within the ministry. He Cheng was denounced in the *People's Daily* and stripped of his leadership positions in 1955. Evidence of his mistaken policies included the fact that he had invited Yu Yunxiu to be a representative of Chinese medicine in the First National Health Conference in 1950, even as Yu continued to advocate for the abolition of Chinese medicine (Ren Xiaofeng 1955). Most scholars have interpreted this important event as a battle of red versus expert, with the party asserting its control over scientific and technical work (Croizier 1968; Lampton 1977, 45–66). For the Chinese medicine profession, the implications of this event were profound, enabling the profession to become part of the national healthcare infrastructure after decades of exclusion during the Republican period.[11]

Following the policy shift and the corresponding removal of party leaders thought to be at odds with this new direction, institution building for the Chinese medicine profession began in earnest. These efforts proceeded along two tracks. The first focused on promoting the new program of integrated medicine (*zhongxiyi jiehe*), in which doctors of Western medicine received systematic training in Chinese medicine. It was launched with considerable publicity in 1955 and based at the recently established China Academy of Chinese Medicine (中国中医研究院), which was to become the leading national research institute for Chinese Medicine. Seventy-six students took part. They were taught by some of the most renowned doctors of Chinese medicine in the country and graduated two and a half years later in 1958. Mao Zedong read the Ministry of Health's report on the first graduating class and enthusiastically endorsed it in his famous commentary of October 11, 1958, where he declared Chinese medicine to be a "great treasure house" (Taylor 2004, 120–24). The *People's Daily* soon urged the "vigorous development" of these programs, which party leaders believed would lead to the dialectical creation of a "new medicine" (*xinyi*) that combined the best of Chinese medicine and Western medicine (Cai Jingfeng, Li Qinghua, and Zhang Binghuan 2000, 426). Although these programs ultimately trained far fewer doctors than the colleges of Chinese medicine, "integrated medicine" became very influential, particularly during the Cultural Revolution, because of Mao Zedong's support for the program.

The second track, which was ultimately far more important for the Chinese medicine profession, focused on establishing the colleges of Chinese medicine and their affiliated hospitals. The first four colleges of Chinese medicine—located in Beijing, Shanghai, Guangzhou, and Chengdu—were established in 1956. They did not receive nearly as much publicity as the establishment of the China Academy of Chinese Medicine had the previous year, in part because the launch of these colleges did not go smoothly, particularly in Beijing (Taylor 2004, 105). Nonetheless, another sixteen colleges were built between 1958 and 1960, often on the site of former advanced studies schools (Taylor 2004, 125). By 1965, there were twenty-two colleges of Chinese medicine (Cai Jingfeng, Li Qinghua, and Zhang Binghuan 2000, 282). Beginning in 1956, there was a push to establish hospitals of Chinese medicine in many cities. Although these hospitals were established to provide Chinese medicine services and provide training for medical students, they were never purely Chinese medicine institutions. As we will see in Chapter 5, there was and continues to be a significant role for Western medicine in these hospitals.

The fortuitous shift in the CCP policy in 1955 not only led to the creation of the new institutions of contemporary Chinese medicine but pushed doctors to come to a consensus on what should and should not count as standard practice. The encounter with a centralized, robust, and potentially hostile state ultimately made it possible to bridge the divides within the profession that have been insurmountable in the Republican era. Leading scholars and officials began to urge unity during the 1950s. For example, in 1955, Deng Tietao, a young doctor at the time, published an article in the *Journal of Chinese Medicine*, arguing that the Cold Damage and Warm Disorders currents were complementary, not oppositional, schools of practice. He downplayed earlier conflicts between the two camps as the byproduct of the stifling effects of "feudalism, imperialism, and bureaucratic capitalism." He argued that "from a developmental perspective, the Warm Disorders current is a progressive development based on the foundations of the Cold Damage current. . . . The theories and methods of Cold Damage and Warm Disorders are both part of the precious heritage of our country's medicine" (Deng Tietao 1995, 87–93). These sentiments were echoed in an article for the same journal, published by Lu Bingkui in 1957. Already the most influential Chinese medicine doctor within the party apparatus at this time, he scolded his colleagues for their factionalism and a partial understanding of Chinese medicine theory. He reminded his readers that all late imperial medical writings were "developments based on the theoretical system of the *Inner Canon*" and that therefore "scholarly factions could not exist." He urged doctors to "to review their lessons . . . and come to a complete understanding of Chinese medicine scholarship" (Cui Yueli 1993, 94–96).

According to *The Scientific and Technological Achievements of Chinese Medicine in the Forty Years since the Founding of the Nation*, debates between these two camps continued into the 1960s but were ultimately settled by a movement to "unite Warm and Cold" (State Administration of Traditional

Chinese Medicine and Hu Ximing 1989, 105). In his 1983 publication *On the Unification of Warm and Cold*, the scholar Wan Yousheng (万友生) argued that most doctors were open to both approaches. He proposed that "the Eight Principles (*bagang*) can unify the Six Jing (*liujing*) of Cold Damage with the Triple Burner (*sanjiao*) and Four Levels (*sifen*) of the Warm Disorders" (Wan Yousheng 1988 [1983], 2).

Writing Textbooks

With these institutional developments, textbook writing became a priority. This important undertaking, as we will see, compelled scholars to not only resolve former differences but also focus on defining the central characteristics of Chinese medicine. Through the textbook editing process, *bianzheng lunzhi* would emerge as a concept and methodology that could provide a new level of coherence to the textbooks. In turn, the textbooks would popularize this term and make it indispensable to the contemporary practice of Chinese medicine.

It was not clear that *bianzheng lunzhi* would become so central to the national textbooks at the start of the editing process. But the challenging conditions under which the textbooks were produced no doubt contributed to this development. The emerging power inequalities between the Chinese and Western medicine professions had already become clear by the late 1950s (see Chapters 1 and 2). We can find another reminder of the precarity of the new Chinese medicine institutions in a letter written in 1962 by Lu Bingkui to Premier Zhou Enlai. Between 1958 and 1960, China was confronted by a devastating famine and near economic collapse because of the disastrous policies of the Great Leap Forward. Severe budgetary restrictions were being imposed in the wake of this failed policy, and there was a strong push within the central government to close many of the new colleges of Chinese medicine. Lu Bingkui impressed upon the premier the devastating impact such a decision would have on the Chinese medicine profession. He also reminded him just how small the new colleges were, each admitting classes of forty to fifty students, and therefore how small their impact on the national budget was. Altogether these new colleges were enrolling a total of roughly 1,000 students each year, less than one-tenth of the new enrollments in colleges of Western medicine (Cui Yueli 1993, 97). Perhaps because of Lu Bingkui's intercession, no colleges of Chinese medicine were shuttered at this time. Nonetheless, this letter reminds us of the significant disparity in professional manpower that was emerging in the early 1960s.

Prior to the production of the first edition of the national textbooks in 1960, scholars were trying to forge consensus and articulate standards by developing textbooks for specific institutions in the later 1950s.[12] The most important center for textbook writing during in the early Communist period was the Nanjing College of Chinese Medicine, which had emerged out of the Jiangsu Chinese Medicine School for Advanced Studies. In 1958, it published the first comprehensive, nationally recognized textbook on Chinese medicine, *Overview of Chinese Medicine* (中医学概论). It was a collective effort with well over a dozen contributors, managed by the Vice Minister of Health, Gou Zihua (郭子化).[13] In the preface, the editors state that they were entrusted with this project by the Ministry of Health to produce a "relatively complete overview" of Chinese medicine that could be "used for courses of Chinese medicine in colleges of Western medicine, for review by less advanced doctors of Chinese medicine or to show young enthusiasts for Chinese medicine the correct path forward" (Nanjing Zhongyi Xueyuan 1958, 1).

Building on this experience, the Ministry of Health began making careful preparations for producing a comprehensive set of national textbooks in 1958. This work led to the publication of the first edition of the national textbooks in 1960, followed quickly by a revised and expanded second edition of national textbooks in 1964. Kim Taylor has done an excellent job describing the political work that enabled the production of these two editions of the national textbooks, noting that the Ministry of Health considered this project to be an "extremely delicate issue," requiring thorough and systematic planning (Cui Yueli 1993, 127). Taylor has also argued that the national textbooks represented an unprecedented standardization of Chinese medicine, which clearly could not have been achieved, at least so efficiently, without strong leadership from Communist Party officials (Taylor 2004, 127–35). While I concur with her emphasis on the role of the state, I believe that the textbooks represent far more than a standardization. I consider them to be quintessential postcolonial innovations. They established the institutional foundations for Chinese medicine, allowed the profession to survive within a national healthcare system dominated by biomedicine, and set the course for the nature of clinical practice in the decades that followed.

The officials and participants in the textbook editing process were well aware of the challenges they faced. According to Lu Bingkui, the goal of the first edition of the national textbooks was to produce a comprehensive set of textbooks that "represented the theoretical system of Chinese medicine." It was to be "simple yet complete," establishing a "unified blueprint" for future efforts (Cui Yueli 1993, 107). The Nanjing College of Chinese Medicine played a leading role in these efforts, working together with the other four main colleges (Beijing, Shanghai, Guangzhou, and Chengdu). Together, they produced eighteen textbooks in total (Cui Yueli 1993, 127; Taylor 2004,

130). The experimental status of these textbooks was recognized in the series title itself, which labeled them "Provisional Textbooks for Colleges of Chinese Medicine" (中医学院试用教材).

Although the second edition of the national textbooks was produced just four years later, it has been celebrated as a major improvement over the first and continues to be highly regarded, perhaps only surpassed by the fifth edition, published twenty years later in the mid-1980s (Cui Yueli 1993, 106–11). Nonetheless, the editors chose to mark the developmental nature of this new set of textbooks by naming the entire series of textbooks *Revised Edition of the Provisional Textbooks for Colleges of Chinese Medicine*" (中医学院试用教材重订本). One of the most significant changes to the second edition of the national textbooks is that *bianzheng lunzhi* was officially incorporated into the textbooks as the organizing principle. Vice Minister of Health Guo Zihua, tasked with overseeing the national textbook editing process after the success of *Overview of Chinese Medicine*, has been credited with making the actual proposal to incorporate *bianzheng lunzhi* (at the time referred to by the synonymous term *bianzheng shizhi*) into the textbooks (See also Deng Zhongguang, Zheng Hong, and Chen Anlin 2004, 142).[14] I do not know what precisely inspired Guo Zihua's suggestion, but the term had been circulating since the mid 1950s. Moreover, it appeared in some of the experimental institutional textbooks of the late 1950s, where some editors described it as a "key characteristic" of Chinese medicine but did not discuss it in depth (Diagnosis Teaching and Research Group of the Jiangsu School of Chinese Medicine 1958, 6–7; Hu Guangci 1958, 1–4; Nanjing Zhongyi Xueyuan 1958, 152). The editors of the second edition of the national textbooks, however, decided to integrate *bianzheng lunzhi* into the content of the textbooks. This decision set the course for all subsequent editions of the texbooks. I believe the nature of these innovations, and perhaps the secret to the immense success of the concept, can be most fruitfully understood if we approach *bianzheng lunzhi* as a methodology that is described in the textbooks (and therefore clinically deployed) in two distinct modalities.

Dual Modalities of *Bianzheng Lunzhi*

It may seem surprising that the new concept *bianzheng lunzhi* was so readily accepted as a foundational concept upon which to organize the national textbooks. One important factor, in addition to the new social conditions of medical practice previously described, was that new term was not well defined initially. It was a flexible concept into which scholars could impute their preferred interpretations. The national textbooks only gradually refined the concept with each subsequent edition. The standardized interpretation of the concept would have been disseminated to students, but older doctors could claim to practice *bianzheng lunzhi* according to their own clinical proclivities. One example of an alternative interpretation of *bianzheng lunzhi* was promoted by the Republican-era innovator Ye Juquan, whom we encountered in Chapter 3. Ye published an article in the *Journal of Chinese Medicine* in 1958 entitled, "The Crux of *Bianzheng Lunzhi*—Presentation (*Zheng*) and Formula (*Fang*)." He argued that

> what is known as *bianzheng lunzhi* is not an amorphous concept. For definitive and widely applicable results, [one] must determine the main formula for treating the main cluster of symptoms *zhenghouqun* (症候群). . . . The classic formulas of Zhang Zhongjing most exemplify this approach (Ye Juquan 2014 [1958]).

In the remainder of this article, Ye Juquan gave numerous clinical examples of his approach to *bianzheng lunzhi* that were strikingly similar to the "formula presentation" methodology that was embraced by Cold Damage advocates in the Republican period and exemplified his clinical work at the Suzhou Hospital of National Medicine in 1939. In *Chinese Medicine in Contemporary China*, Volker Scheid has summarized attempts to systematize *bianzheng lunzhi* in other alternative ways, most notably by Qin Bowei in 1961 and Fang Yaozhong (方药中) in 1979 (Scheid 2002, 281–89). While I concur with Scheid's larger point that there are a diversity of clinical practices and methodologies that have been assembled under the unifying banner of *bianzheng lunzhi* (Scheid 2002, 263–73), I think it is essential to understand how *bianzheng lunzhi* was codified through the textbook editing process. As we will see, it not only provided organizational coherence to textbooks, it also established a framework for Chinese medicine hospital work and research agendas that needed to navigate between the worlds of Chinese medicine and Western medicine.

I believe that this remarkable achievement was possible because *bianzheng lunzhi* took on two forms, or two modalities. In other words, the national textbooks used the methodology of *bianzheng lunzhi* in two distinct and seemingly contradictory ways. These two modalities were never explicitly defined in the textbooks, but they first appeared in the second edition of the national textbooks. One modality is centered on the concept of *zheng* (证), in which *zheng* is transformed into a diagnostic category. Because the Republican-era connotation of "presentation" is no longer appropriate for this usage of *zheng*, I have adopted Ted Kaptchuk's gloss of "pattern" as the more appropriate translation for all writing on *bianzheng lunzhi* that follows the 1964 publication of the second-edition national textbooks (Kaptchuk 2000). The second modality is centered on the concept of *bing* (病). Within this modality, *bing* can easily slide between the Chinese medicine category and the biomedical concept of disease. It is my contention that these dual modalities of *bianzheng lunzhi* are the key to understanding the postcolonial character of contemporary Chinese medicine. On the one hand, the pattern-centered modality defines the uniqueness of Chinese medicine in opposition to the disease-based diagnostic practices of Western medicine. On the other hand, the *bing*/disease-centered modality offers a technology for blending the two medicines in clinical practice. As we will see in this chapter and in Chapter 5 on hospital practice, *bianzheng lunzhi* makes both purification and translation possible. Its emergence as a new concept, used in two forms, drives the emergence of our third dualism, transforming the *bing-zheng* dyad of the Republican period into the disease-pattern dualism of the Communist era.

As we explore the two modalities of *bianzheng lunzhi*, we will see that they are associated with two clusters of textbooks. The pattern-centered modality is laid out in four main textbooks, which students encounter in their first two years of coursework: *Basic Theory of Chinese Medicine*, *Chinese Medicine Diagnosis*, *Chinese Materia Medica*, and *Formulary*. These textbooks loosely correspond to some of the late imperial classics such as *Drug Property Verses*, *Formulas in Rhyme*, and *Binhu's Pulses*, which senior doctors such as Jiao Shude would have memorized in the Republican period.[15] The key innovation in the pattern-centered modality can be found in the second edition of *Chinese Medicine Diagnosis* (中医诊断学). The disease-centered modality of *bianzheng lunzhi* dominates in all the clinical textbooks, which students encounter primarily in their fourth year of medical school. They include *Chinese Internal Medicine*, *Chinese External Medicine*, *Chinese Gynecology*, *Chinese Pediatrics*, *Chinese Traumatology*, *Chinese Otorhinolaryngology*, and *Chinese Ophthalmology*. With regard to this modality, the key innovation occurred in the second edition of *Chinese Internal Medicine* (中医内科学). Beyond these two groups, there is another important cluster of textbooks introducing the medical canons. These textbooks consist of selections from the original texts, supplemented by classic commentaries and modern explanations on the selected passages. They include: *Lecture Materials on the Inner Canon*, *Lecture Materials on the Treatise on Cold Damage*, *Lecture Materials on the Essentials of the Golden Casket*, and *Warm Disorders*, which are all taught during the students' second and third years of medical school. The textbook versions of the classics tend to focus on key passages rather than the whole text. For this reason, they may be somewhat different than what a typical premodern apprentice would have encountered. But most significantly for the contemporary student, they do conspicuously address or incorporate the methodology of *bianheng lunzhi*.

First Modality: Pattern-Centered *Bianzheng Lunzhi*

If asked to describe *bianzheng lunzhi*, most doctors would probably describe something akin to what I call the pattern-centered modality. In *Knowing Practice*, her excellent ethnography of the clinical encounter in Chinese medicine, Judith Farquhar has described *zheng* as the "pivot," the crucial concept at the center of this methodology.[16] In fact, her ethnography can be considered a detailed exploration of what I call the pattern-centered modality of *bianzheng lunzhi*, as it was taught to her in the early 1980s at the Guangzhou College of Chinese Medicine. The distinguishing feature of this approach to *bianzheng lunzhi* is that one does not need to know (or is simply not influenced by) the diagnosis of the Chinese medicine *bing* or biomedical disease when determining a pattern and deciding upon a treatment. Farquhar's ethnography captures some of the essential features of this modality. The intellectual process takes doctors from concrete clinical presentations to an abstract statement of the pattern and back to concrete therapeutic interventions. The pithy summation of the pattern works as a pivot between the wordy statements of patient and the verbose (usually written) prescription of a therapy. Although her distinction among the three *zheng* (征, 症,证), which she glosses as "signs, symptoms, and syndrome," adds some unnecessary confusion to her analysis, her larger point about the intellectual trajectory of *bianzheng lunzhi* as a step-by-step methodology, moving from the concrete to the abstract and back again remains illuminating (Farquhar 1994).[17]

Farquhar's analysis is useful, in part, because the textbooks themselves are not explicit about the process. The best overview I have encountered in textbooks can be found in the sixth-edition version of the *Basic Theory of Chinese Medicine* textbook.

> *Bianzheng lunzhi* can be divided into two stages. In pattern discrimination, the information, symptoms, and signs collected through the Four Examinations (*sizhen*) (looking, listening/smelling, asking, and palpitation) are analyzed and synthesized to determine the cause, type, location, and relative strength of the pathogen and patient's own constitution (*xiezheng guanxi*). This culminates in the discrimination of a pattern. In treatment determination, a treatment principle is determined according to the results of pattern discrimination (Wu Dunxu, Liu Yanchi, and Li Dexin 1995, 7).

MEDICAL DISCOURSE   CLINICAL PRACTICE

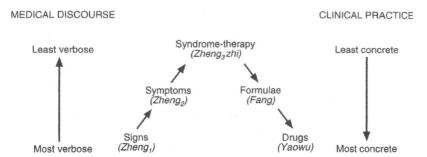

Figure 15. "Verbosity and Concreteness in the Clinical Encounter." Image from Judith Farquhar's *Knowing Practice* (Farquhar 1994, 205).

This statement gives some additional detail to the first stage of the process, but unfortunately, is quite vague about the treatment determination process.

Using Farquhar's diagram, however, we can flesh out this process and better understand the relationship to the textbooks to the methodology of *bianzheng lunzhi*. During "pattern discrimination," the first part of the process, the physician relies on material covered in the *Basic Theory of Chinese Medicine* and *Chinese Medicine Diagnosis* textbooks, such as viscera manifestation and the Four Examinations to guide the identification of a pattern. The pattern is expressed in very succinct, standardized phrases, usually four characters long, such as "phlegm and heat obstructing the Lungs" (*tanre yongfei*). In "treatment determination," the second part of the process, a treatment principle (*zhifa*) is established to counter the pathological propensities of the pattern— for example, clearing heat in the Lungs and transforming phlegm (*qingfei huatan*). In this stage the physician would then turn to material found in the *Formulary* and *Chinese Materia Medica* textbooks. He or she would select from among many hundreds of standard formulae to find one that best suits the treatment principle. (More experienced physicians may draw on several formulas or use formulas that they design themselves.) Then the doctor would modify this classic combination of herbs, adding or subtracting medicinals as needed, to craft a final prescription that best suits the individual needs of the patient. As Farquhar has noted, this description of *bianzheng lunzhi* is highly idealized, and clinicians often take "short cuts" or emphasize certain moments of the process over others (Farquhar 1994, 211–20).

As this summary suggests, the pattern-centered modality turns on having a recognized and standardized catalog of the most common patterns. This is precisely one of the new developments that appears with the second edition of the *Chinese Medicine Diagnosis* textbook. Chinese medicine diagnosis texts from the Republican period did not include such lists of patterns. In fact, Republican-era texts rarely addressed the goal of "diagnosis"—a *bing, zheng,* disease, of other nosological category—despite borrowing this biomedical term. Instead, these texts focused almost exclusively on the Four Examinations—looking (*wang*), listening/smelling (*wen*), asking (*wen*), and palpitation (*qie*). For example, Qin Bowei's *Principles of Diagnosis* in 1931 was devoted primarily to the pulse and tongue exam—specific techniques within the palpation and looking examinations—and gave only some limited attention to the asking and listening/smelling examinations (Qin Bowei 1955 [1931]). In 1933, Wu Keqian wrote a comprehensive text, *Practical Diagnosis for National Medicine,* which provided a detailed overview of the Four Examinations but also included some elements of the physical exam from biomedicine (Wu Keqian 1933). There was no defined list of the most commonly see patterns in either of these texts. Early textbooks from the Communist era were no different. A 1955 textbook, *Lecture Materials on Chinese Medicine Diagnosis,* produced for the Beijing Advanced Studies School of Chinese Medicine, did not go beyond the Four Examinations. Interestingly, it did briefly introduce the concept of holism and *bianzheng lunzhi,* stating that they represent the "basic spirit" (*jiben jingshen*) of Chinese medicine, without providing much explanation on practical implications of either concept (Diagnosis Teaching and Research Group of the Beijing Advanced Studies School of Chinese Medicine 1955).

A break with these conventions can be found in the first edition of *Chinese Medicine Diagnosis,* and it becomes more definitive in the second edition of the same textbook. There were two important additions to the first edition of *Chinese Medicine Diagnosis* that distinguish it from all prior Chinese medicine diagnosis texts. First, the editors included a chapter on the Eight Principles (*bagang*), which they called "one of the foundations of the *bianzheng shizhi*" (Guangdong College of Chinese Medicine 1960, 79). As Wang Yuchuan noted in his 1999 article, the term "Eight Principles" was coined by the famous Republican doctor Zhu Weiju, although the concept has roots that go back to the late imperial period. The Eight Principles summarize basic pathological processes in terms of four related dyads: Hot and Cold, Deficiency and Excess, Interior and Exterior, Yin and Yang. Second, the editors added another chapter called *Zhenghou Fenlei,* or "Classification of Presentations." Here the classification focused on the Six Jing of the *Treatise on Cold Damage,* the Four Sectors (*wei, qi, ying, xue*) of the Warm Disorders current, and the basic pathologies of the organs, channels, and external pathogens. Much of this material had previously appeared in the *Overview of Chinese Medicine,* published two years earlier. While the term *zheng* was used throughout

Table 1. First Modality of *Bianzheng Lunzhi* Emerges (author's emphasis)

Comparison of New Additions to *Chinese Medicine Diagnosis*	
First Edition	Second Edition
Chapter 2: Eight Principles	Chapter 3: Eight Principles
1. Yin and Yang	1. Yin and Yang
2. Exterior and Interior	2. Exterior and Interior
3. Cold and Hot	3. Cold and Hot
4. Deficiency and Excess	4. Deficiency and Excess
Chapter 3: Classification of Presentations (*zhenghou fenlei*)	Chapter 4: Classification of **Patterns** (*zhenghou fenlei*)
1. Six Jing	1. Patterns by Etiological Cause
2. Four Sectors and Three Burners	2. **Patterns by Organ and Channel**
3. Organs and Channels	3. Six Jing
	4. Four Sectors and Three Burners
	Chapter 5: Using Examination Methods
	1. **Summary of Pattern Discrimination**
	2. Writing Medical Records
Appendix 1: Patterns by Etiological Cause	Appendix 1: Selected Classical Texts
Appendix 2: Writing Medical Records	Appendix 2: Selected Verses

these two new chapters, I have continued to translate it as "presentation," since this material is not organized into the standardized patterns that subsequently become foundational to *bianzheng lunzhi* with the second edition of the *Chinese Medicine Diagnosis* textbook.

Important innovations are found in the second edition of *Chinese Medicine Diagnosis* that consolidate the shift in connotation of *zheng*, from presentation to pattern, from a description of clinical findings to an unmistakable diagnostic category. To mark this shift, I translate *zheng* as "pattern" in this and subsequent editions of the national textbooks. This shift is most apparent in two major changes. First, the editors significantly expanded the material on *Zhenghou Fenlei*, which is best translated as "Classification of Patterns." In particular, the editors focused on the pathologies of the organ systems, which had only received cursory attention in the first edition. Considerable space was given to naming the patterns associated with the organs. The editors identified roughly three to five main patterns for each organ; each pattern was defined by a standard constellation of symptoms, including a typical tongue and pulse presentation. In contrast to the first edition, the patterns associated with the Six Jing and the Four Sectors were clearly secondary to the organ-related patterns, a trend that has continued throughout the latter editions as well as in clinical practice.

Second, the editors made a concerted effort to explain the role of *zheng* in the diagnostic process and how it relates to the methodology of "pattern

discrimination and treatment determination." For example, at the beginning
of the "Classification of Patterns" chapter, they state:

> After completing the Four Examinations and determining the patterns
> (*bianzheng*) of Eight Principles, it is possible to make conclusions
> about exterior and interior, yin and yang, hot and cold, deficiency and
> excess, but this is still a preliminary notion, only indicating the general
> approach to treatment. No connection to the organs and channels,
> the cause and the pathomechanism of an illness has been established.
> The next step in pattern discrimination (*bianzheng*) is to rely on the
> "classification of patterns."
>
> The classification of patterns is not done by arbitrarily categorizing
> the symptoms of diseases. . . . The purpose of classifying patterns is . . .
> to develop a more concrete diagnosis (Guangzhou College of Chinese
> Medicine 1964, 117).

In this chapter, the editors then included a long list of etiological and pathological factors that enable one to go beyond a mere categorization of symptoms to an actual classification of patterns.

To further elaborate on the description, the editors also added a new chapter entitled, "Summary of Pattern Discrimination," which included a new
section, "The Essentials of Discriminating Patterns" (辨证要点). This section
contains one of the most detailed descriptions of how to carry out *bianzheng
lunzhi* that one can find in any edition of the textbooks. Students were instructed that good pattern discrimination required one to be "detailed and
accurate," "focused on the main presentation," and cognizant of the "course
of the illness," and were advised that "specific symptoms may be the key" to
one's pattern discrimination. The editors also tried to balance this new focus
on pattern with an exhortation to be aware of "the relationship between discriminating a *bing* and a pattern" (Guangzhou College of Chinese Medicine
1964, 144–49). In the following passage, the editors urged doctors to dialectically move between pattern discrimination and *bing* discrimination.

> [Because it is possible to have a sore throat due to many different
> *bing*,] one must both discriminate pattern and *bing*. Let's say that
> "discriminating a pattern" means: to use the results of the Four Exam-
> inations, together with internal and external causes and the location
> of the *bing*, to completely and concretely assess the unique qualities
> and contradictions of a given stage of disease. Then the difference
> with "discriminating a *bing*" is: to take the results of pattern discrimi-
> nation, compare it with multiple similar diseases, reflect on the special
> features of each related disease, and meticulously confirm the pattern

of the patient. In the process of advancing the pattern discrimination, one must consider the unique characteristics of this or that disease, eliminating them one by one until a final conclusion is reached. . . . And most importantly after determining the *bing*, the pattern discrimination can be more reliably integrated with the treatment principles, formulary, and herbs. This will elevate the clinical results and reduce one's missteps (Guangzhou College of Chinese Medicine 1964, 148).

Four decades later, Deng Tietao, one of the key figures in editing this textbook, would bemoan the fact that doctors had forgotten these lessons clearly laid out in the second edition of *Chinese Medicine Diagnosis* (Deng Zhongguang, Zheng Hong, and Chen Anlin 2004, 143). This entire section reappeared verbatim in the fifth edition of *Chinese Medicine Diagnosis*, for which Deng Tietao was the chief editor, but was removed from the sixth edition, for which Zhu Wenfeng was the chief editor (Deng Tietao and Guo Zhenqiu 1984, 142–45; Zhu Wenfeng 1995).

In this passage, we can clearly see that the relationship of *bing* and *zheng* has shifted profoundly since the Xie Guan definition of the Republican period. *Zheng* is no longer an external manifestation of an inner *bing* pathology. It has become a key diagnostic category in its own right. The editors of *Chinese Medicine Diagnosis* insisted that doctors must work dialectically between the two diagnostic categories of *bing* and *zheng* to avoid mistakes. When treating a patient who presents with a small amount of blood in the stools, treatment will be very different if one can confirm whether the *bing* is hemorrhoids or colon cancer. Likewise, when treating measles, it is easy to confuse the early presentation with other upper respiratory conditions. This mistake could cause complications in a measles treatment but would be easily avoided with a proper *bing* discrimination (Guangzhou College of Chinese Medicine 1964, 148–49).[18] Yet despite this insistence of moving between *bing* and pattern, negotiating between two levels of diagnosis, the overall result of the innovations in *Chinese Medicine Diagnosis* was to elevate *zheng* over *bing* in importance, making it the central diagnostic category of Chinese medicine. Perhaps one significant reason for this outcome was the emergence of a second modality of *bianzheng lunzhi*, which described the relation of *bing* to pattern quite differently.

Second Modality: Disease-Centered *Bianzheng Lunzhi*

What I call the second modality of *bianzheng lunzhi* would not necessarily be recognized as a distinct clinical methodology, yet it plays a crucial role in clinical practice. The second modality has become the primary means for negotiating the relationship between pattern and *bing* in hospital practice. Because of the linguist slippage between *bing* as a Chinese medicine concept and its use as "disease" in Western medicine, this modality has become, even more importantly, the primary means for negotiating the relationship between Chinese medicine and Western medicine in everyday clinical practice. The key elements of this modality were also firmly established through the writing of the first and second editions of *Chinese Internal Medicine*, but especially the latter. The key innovation in this textbook also involved the incorporation of *bianzheng lunzhi*. But unlike *Chinese Medicine Diagnosis*, which privileged the centrality of pattern to the diagnostic process and then suggested moving dialectically between pattern and *bing* discrimination to counter this new emphasis on pattern, this textbook formalized a different relationship between the two concepts, making pattern a subcategorization of *bing* and therefore ultimately of biomedical disease categories as well.

The innovations in *Chinese Internal Medicine* can be made clear by first comparing them briefly to classic internal medicine texts. By the late imperial period, internal medicine and other clinical texts, much like today's clinical textbooks, were organized around *bing* as a rubric. But in contrast to today's textbooks, there was no consistent organizational principle for the discussion of treatment. *Returning to Health from the Ten Thousand Illnesses* (萬病回春), the popular Ming dynasty internal medicine text by Gong Tingxian (龔廷賢) (1512–1619), provides a good example of the tendency. This text is organized around 195 *bing*. Each *bing* was divided into two parts. The first part, usually called "Pulses," provided a brief description of the overall clinical presentation, the underlying pathology, and related treatment principles. The second part consisted of a list of useful formulas and very brief descriptions of their therapeutic actions. In the case of "Sleeplessness" (不寐), one of his shorter *bing* entries, he recommended two formulas: "High Pillow and No Worries Powder" (*Gao Zhen Wu You San*) to treat "Heart and Gallbladder deficient timidity" and "Sour Jujube Seed Decoction" (*Suan Zao Ren Tang*), a classic formula from the *Essentials of the Golden Casket*, to "treat excessive sleep and inability to sleep" (Gong Tingxian 2007 [1588], 227). Even within these minimal treatment guidelines, Gong Tingxian's approach was inconsistent. The first formula was recommended for addressing a particular pathomechanism (similar to a "pattern" in today's textbook); the second formula was suggested for treating two seemingly contradictory symptoms. This same trend could also be observed in the work of Zhang Jingyue (1563–1640), one of the great medical scholars of the Ming. In *Complete Works of Jingyue* (景岳全書), he provided a more robust discussion on "Sleeplessness" than Gong Tingxian, but his treatment guidelines were nonetheless brief. At the end of the entry, he listed twenty-nine different formulas and six auxiliary formulas but provided no guidelines on using them to treat Sleeplessness (Li Zhiyong 1999, 1,103–4).

The first two editions of *Chinese Internal Medicine* formalized the presentation of *bing* entries and, most significantly, established a standard format for discussing treatment. The shift was most apparent in the second edition, in which *zheng* was used to clearly subdivide each *bing* into a small number of common patterns, each with a recommended formula for treatment. In Table 2, I have outlined the general structure of each *bing* entry in the first and second editions to help highlight this shift. The most striking difference between the two editions is the transformation of "Presentation Discrimination" (*bianzheng*) in the first edition to "Pattern Discrimination and Treatment Application" (*bianzheng shizhi*) in the second edition. In the first edition, "Presentation Discrimination" reviewed clinical presentations and underlying pathologies. Treatment strategies were placed in the following section. In the second edition, clinical presentations, underlying pathomechanisms, and recommended treatments were all integrated under "Pattern Discrimination and Treatment Application" (*bianzheng shizhi*). This change reflected Guo Zihua's call to incorporate *bianzheng lunzhi* (at the time called *bianzheng shizhi*) into the national textbooks.

While this development may strike some readers as too minor to mark what I have called a major transformation in the theory and practice of Chinese medicine, its effects became quite profound as this new standardization took hold and was implemented in clinical practice. Instead of lists of appropriate formulas, ranging from as few as two to more than twenty-nine, like our aforementioned Ming dynasty examples, this new approach to writing about internal medicine highlighted a small number of patterns and associated formulas. Moreover, each pattern was accompanied by a description of the "main presentation," "pattern analysis," "treatment principle," and "formula and herbs." This new way of discussing *bing* by breaking down each condition into its various patterns quickly became standard for all subsequent editions of the clinical textbooks, including the various subspecialties of gynecology, pediatrics, external medicine, and so on. One of the key effects of this approach was to suggest that each *bing* could be subdivided into so many subtypes or variants. Ultimately, it became quite common for doctors use this very language, often referring to the "pattern variants" of "pattern types" (证型) for a particular disease. This new relationship between *bing* and pattern is at the heart of what I call the second modality of *bianzheng lunzhi*. In contrast to the first modality of *bianzheng lunzhi*, which elevated a new connotation of *zheng* as the new diagnostic rubric of Chinese medicine, the second modality downgraded the

Table 2. Second Modality of *Bianzheng Lunzhi* Is Formulated (author's emphasis)

Comparison of *Bing* Entries in *Chinese Internal Medicine*

First Edition	Second Edition
Overview (*gaishuo*)	Overview (*gaishuo*)
Etiology (*bingyin*)	Etiology and Pathology (*bingyin bingli*)
Presentation discrimination (*bianzheng*)	**Pattern Discrimination Treatment Application** (***bianzheng shizhi***)
	• **Patterns**
	▪ **Main presentation**
	▪ **Pattern analysis**
	▪ **Treatment**
	▪ **Formula and herbs**
Treatment (*zhifa*)	Relevant formulas (*fufang*)
Conclusion (*jieyu*)	Archival Selections (*wenxian zhailu*)
Relevant formulas (*fufang*)	Sample Medical Cases (*yi'an xuan*)

concept of pattern somewhat. Pattern was reframed as a subtype of *bing*. In the first modality, the editors of *Chinese Medicine Diagnosis* urged their readers to refine their pattern discrimination by also determining a *bing*. In the second modality, the editors of *Chinese Internal Medicine* effectively asked their readers to refine their *bing* diagnosis with an additional pattern classification.

Integrated Medicine and the Second-Edition Textbooks

Mao Zedong's fascination with "integrated medicine," which had been proceeding along its own, somewhat separate, institutional track since the mid-1950s, had a surprising and important influence on the formalization of *bianzheng lunzhi* through the writing of the second edition of the textbooks. The faintest hint of this history can be found in a brief prefatory statement at the beginning of all the second-edition textbooks, titled "Publication Remarks for the Revised Edition of the Provisional Textbooks for Colleges of Chinese Medicine" (中医学院試用教材重訂本出版说明). In these remarks, the six participating colleges were acknowledged (Hubei College of Chinese Medicine had joined the Beijing, Shanghai, Guangzhou, Chengdu, and Nanjing colleges that produced the first edition), and several special participants were thanked. This latter group included four senior doctors, acting as advisors, and four recent graduates of "integrated medicine" programs, who were mentioned by name—Huang Xingyuan (黃星垣), Xu Zicheng (许自诚), Zhang Dazhao (张大钊), and Tan Jiaxing (谭家兴) (see, for example, Guangzhou College of Chinese Medicine 1964).[19] Given the strong emphasis on collectivism at this time, the acknowledgment of these individuals caught my attention. I had the good fortune to eventually meet and interview all four of these "integrated medicine" doctors. Through these encounters, I learned that they made important contributions not only to the second-edition textbooks, but also more broadly to the profession.

The crucial moment that catapulted these four doctors into prominence occurred in the summer of 1963 during the first of two textbook editing conventions. The *Chinese Internal Medicine* textbook, the only clinical textbook included in the first convention, was rejected by the academic review committee composed of the four senior doctors. The *Chinese Internal Medicine* textbook, which was originally written by professors from the Shanghai College of Chinese Medicine, was important because internal medicine was considered the most important of all the clinical specializations. It was expected to be the model for the other clinical textbooks, which were to be written at a second convention in the fall. According to my interviewees, none of the participating Chinese medicine doctors were willing to accept responsibility for revising this textbook, or perhaps they lacked ideas for how to improve it. Huang Xingyuan recalled, "No matter what they wrote, they always came back to *Overview of Chinese Medicine*. They couldn't get past it."[20] In other words, the Shanghai College representatives were unable to come up with a new format for the *bing* entries, which differed substantially from the *Overview* and therefore, by implication, the first edition of the national textbooks.

Guo Zihua, the vice minister of Health, who was running the convention, made the decision to give this task to the four young integrated medicine doctors, who had all recently completed three-year training programs in Chinese medicine. Each of these individuals had distinguished himself in some capacity during his respective training program. At the same time, the doctors were still inexperienced practitioners of Chinese medicine, and their inclusion in the textbook editing process surely reflected some political motivations, given Mao Zedong's enthusiasm for integrated medicine. Nonetheless, the four doctors were welcome participants in the conference and were generally regarded with some prestige, both because of their backgrounds in Western medicine and their strong interest in Chinese medicine. In addition, they were viewed as neutral participants, without any special allegiances to a master, lineage, or institution. It may have been for these reasons that Guo Zihua turned to them for help.

The first task was to establish a sample entry (*tili*) for the internal medicine textbook that was acceptable to the review board. Over an intense two-day period, the integrated medicine doctors worked together with a couple of Chinese medicine doctors handpicked by Guo Zihua to revise the *bing* entry for "Jaundice" (黃疸). When the revised Jaundice entry was ultimately found acceptable, this structure was extended to all the other *bing* entries. In short, these four integrated medicine doctors played a significant role in formulating what I have called the second modality of *bianzheng lunzhi*, establishing the standardized structure of the *bing* entries for the *Chinese Internal Medicine* textbook and all other clinical textbooks as depicted in Table 2.

The influence of these four doctors continued beyond the textbook editing conferences for the second edition of the national textbooks. Indeed, their other work may have been even more important. Huang Xingyuan became the most highly regarded of the four. He told me with pride that he was primarily responsible for writing the "General Overview" (总论) to the second edition of *Chinese Internal Medicine*. This discussion clearly and succinctly summarized the principles of *bianzheng lunzhi* that had been developed in both the diagnosis and internal medicine textbooks. Subsequently, he was invited to be one of seven editors of the highly influential reference text *Practical Chinese Internal Medicine* published in the mid 1980s (Fang Yaozhong et al. 1984). As I mentioned in Chapter 1, he devoted the latter part of his career to writing about and helping establish the new subdiscipline of Chinese emergency medicine. In the Epilogue, we will encounter one of his students, Fang Bangjiang (方邦江), who trained with Huang Xingyuan in the 1980s and has been vigorously trying to promote the use of Chinese medicine in emergency medicine care.

Zhang Dazhao and Xu Zicheng had both attended the integrated medicine program Hubei College of Chinese Medicine and collaborated on a famous article published in 1962, "Examining the Theoretical System of Our Motherland's Medicine from the Perspective of the Organ Systems Theory." This article was published in *Health News* and the *Guangming Daily*, two prominent newspapers, as well as in the 1962 sixth edition of *Journal of Chinese Medicine*. It stirred a flurry of debate about the centrality of the "organ systems," a more modern terminology for referring to what we have previously examined as "viscera manifestation," to the practice of Chinese medicine (China Association of Integrated Medicine 1998, 137–38). The prominence of organ-related patterns in second editions of both *Chinese Medicine Diagnosis* and *Chinese Internal Medicine*, which were not found in the first editions, may well have been a result of that influential article.

Tan Jiaxing may have quietly had the greatest influence of the four because he worked as an editor for both the third and fourth editions of internal medicine textbooks, published in 1974 and 1979, respectively. Both textbooks made a significant contribution to the development of the second modality of *bianzheng lunzhi*. Written during the Cultural Revolution and guided by

Mao Zedong's directive to "thoroughly reform education," the third edition introduced radical changes. First, the editors renamed it *Internal Medicine* (内科学), dropping the reference to Chinese medicine, and then split the textbook into two volumes, a Chinese medicine volume and a Western medicine volume. Tan noted that there were intense debates about these changes, as well as the requirement to include references to *Quotations from Mao Zedong* (known in the West as Mao Zedong's *Little Red Book*) (China Association of Integrated Medicine 1998, 140). I have never been able to locate a copy of this third-edition textbook in my archival searches, but Tan felt the radical leftism of the Cultural Revolution seriously tarnished the final product. He was, however, immensely proud of the accomplishments of the fourth edition.[21] This textbook built on the radical changes of the third edition, shed the extraneous references to Maoist thought, and greatly expanded the number of entries. Like the third edition, it was also called *Internal Medicine* and split into two volumes.[22] The first volume closely followed the model of the second edition, *Chinese Internal Medicine*. The second volume, however, was entirely organized around biomedical disease entries. Each entry included a biomedical description of the disease accompanied by the following sub-sections: overview, etiology and pathology, clinical presentation, diagnosis and differential diagnosis, and analysis of main symptoms. But unlike a biomedical textbook, the treatment section included both Chinese medicine and Western medicine therapies. The Chinese medicine therapies for each entry were organized under the rubric "*bianzheng shizhi*" and, just like the second-edition *Chinese Internal Medicine* textbook, described the most common patterns and their associated formulas (Shanghai College of Chinese Medicine 1979).

With the arrest of the Gang of Four in 1978 and the rise of Deng Xiaoping to CCP party secretary, the political winds shifted again, and the influence of integrated medicine waned. The fifth edition of *Chinese Internal Medicine* returned to the format of the second edition. Subsequent internal medicine textbooks — the sixth edition and more recent editions organized by publishing houses instead of the Ministry of Health — have carefully limited the inclusion of biomedical content. But the innovations of the third and fourth editions were far closer to the realities of clinical practice, where hybrid ways of blending Western medicine and Chinese medicine had already emerged by the 1970s and 1980s. The significance of these two textbooks is that they clearly extended the use of the second modality of *bianzheng lunzhi* to biomedical disease categories. Pattern could just as easily be a subcategorization of a Western medicine disease as a Chinese medicine *bing*. Indeed, I observed that most doctors of Chinese medicine are generally more interested in orienting their therapies to a biomedical disease than the Chinese medicine *bing*. In fact, *bing* generally plays only a very minor role in designing treatment plans in contemporary practice.[23]

With the third and fourth editions of the *Chinese Internal Medicine* textbook, the transformation of the Republican-era concepts of *bing* and *zheng* into the Communist-era dualism of disease and pattern was more or less complete. In this unpredictable epistemic journey, *bing* and *zheng* still existed in an intimate interior-exterior relationship in the 1920s. By the late 1920s and 1930s, that relationship had been to wobble as *bing* was weakened by the comparison to disease and *zheng* was elevated to new significance by the distinction with symptom. During the rapid transitions of the early Communist period, especially through the textbook editing process of the early 1960s, the purifying dynamics of this postcolonial moment helped to divorce *zheng* from *bing*, redefine it as pattern, and make it the key diagnostic category of Chinese medicine. Pattern, as found in the clinical methodology of *bianzheng lunzhi*, became the defining diagnostic category of Chinese medicine, just as disease defined the diagnostic procedures of Western medicine. At the same time, the hybridizing forces of this period simultaneously redefined pattern as a subclassification of disease, facilitating the clinical integration of the two medical practices. We will explore how these purifying and hybridizing dynamics shape contemporary clinical practice in Chapter 5.

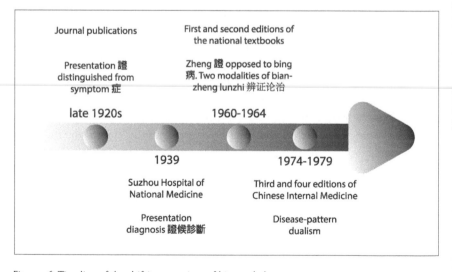

Figure 16. Timeline of the shifting meanings of *bing* and *zheng*.

Paradigm Shifts and Grease Spots

In this chapter's account, I have emphasized that *bianzheng lunzhi* is a recent, and indeed remarkable, invention of the Communist era. I consider it the ultimate postcolonial technology, enabling Chinese medicine to survive in a world dominated by Western medicine. Recalling the two histories of *bianzheng lunzhi* that I discussed at the beginning of the chapter, it should be clear that I am inclined toward the seventy-year-old model. But most doctors I have encountered, including many that participated in the editing of the first and second editions of the textbooks, would disagree with me, insisting that *bianzheng lunzhi* is two millennia old. I often wondered how to resolve this apparent paradox, until I eventually concluded that it is this paradox itself, the ability of *bianzheng lunzhi* to be both old and new, that has made it so successful.

The field of historical epistemology can help us appreciate the ability of *bianzheng lunzhi* to serve many purposes and exist within these multiple histories. At one extreme of this literature, Thomas Kuhn is the quintessential scholar of radical epistemic change. In *The Structure of Scientific Revolutions*, Kuhn argued that knowledge changes through "scientific revolutions" or "paradigm shifts." Although conventional historians present scientific change as part of a narrative of linear progress, Kuhn contends that these narratives are illusions, created by the work of what he calls "normal science" in the aftermath of a scientific revolution. The history of science proceeds in unexpected leaps and breaks with the past, he argues. Moments of radical change will produce a new "paradigm" and a shared vision of the world through which scientists operate over a sustained period of time (Kuhn 1970, 5). There is no directionality to a scientific revolution. A new paradigm cannot be predicted from a previous one. It is only the normalizing scientific work within a new paradigm that will obscure the epistemic break in the name of creating a linear history of progress.

Kuhn's vision of epistemic change is useful for understanding the significance of *bianzheng lunzhi* because it highlights two important characteristics of Chinese medicine in the Communist era. First, paradigms have totalizing effects. *Bianzheng lunzhi* has acquired precisely this characteristic. All previous medical theories, such as Cold Damage, Warm Disorders, and many others, can be knit together into a coherent whole that encompasses education, research, administration, and clinical practice. Second, Kuhn can help us understand the role of textbooks in creating *bianzheng lunzhi*. Kuhn has argued that textbooks are an "invariable concomitant of the emergence of a first paradigm in any field of science" (Kuhn 1970, 137). Textbooks codify a newly accepted body of theory, illustrate it with successful applications, and justify it by concealing its revolutionary nature.

> [Textbooks] have to be rewritten in the aftermath of each scientific revolution, and, once rewritten, they inevitably disguise not only the role but the very existence of the revolutions that produced them. . . . Textbooks thus begin by truncating the scientist's sense of his discipline's history and then proceed to supply a substitute for what they have eliminated. Characteristically, textbooks of science contain just a bit of history, either in an introductory chapter or, more often, in scattered references to the great heroes of an earlier age. From such references both students and professionals come to feel like participants in a long-standing historical tradition. . . . The scientists of earlier ages are implicitly represented as having worked on the same set of fixed problems and in accordance with the same set of fixed canons that the most recent revolution in scientific theory and method has made seem scientific.[24]

In contemporary Chinese medicine practice, the national textbooks have played a similar but more active role than the one Kuhn describes. They didn't just consolidate the scientific revolution; they actively pushed it forward. Isabelle Stenger's reflections on Kuhn helps to clarify this point. She notes that Kuhn's paradigm shift corresponded closely to the scientific activity carried on in the "context of modern universities, where research and the initiation of future researchers are systematically associated within an academic structure that took shape throughout the nineteenth century but that was previously nonexistent" (Stengers 1997). In similar fashion, it is difficult to imagine the emergence of *bianzheng lunzhi* outside of the state-run college system developed in the Communist era. Thus, it was textbooks produced in this context, as opposed to the ones written during the Republican era, that ultimately helped to create this new paradigm.

Yet none of the doctors I spoke with considered the textbooks to be revolutionary. All agreed that they were important achievements for the profession, but their value was in the fact that they "systematized" (*zhengli*) what came before.[25] Indeed, when comparing premodern texts with the textbooks, the changes can seem minor and would be easily missed by someone not intimately familiar with the contemporary education system for Chinese medicine. William James is the philosopher who can perhaps most readily help us counterbalance the radical leaps of Kuhnian paradigm shifts. He has argued that knowledge changes incrementally, imperceptibly, like the spreading of a grease spot.

> Our knowledge grows in *spots*. The spots may be large or small, but the knowledge never grows all over, some knowledge always remains what it was. . . .
> Our minds thus grow in spots; and like grease spots, the spots spread. But we let them spread as little as possible: we keep unaltered as much of our old knowledge, as many of our old prejudices and beliefs, as we can. We patch and tinker more than we renew. The novelty soaks in; it stains the ancient mass; but it is also tinged by what absorbs it. Our past apperceives and co-operates; and in the new equilibrium in which each step forward in the process of learning terminates, it happens relatively seldom that the new fact is added *raw*. More usually it is embedded cooked, as one might say, or stewed down in the sauce of the old (James 1995 [1907], 64).

If we borrow James's metaphor of the stew, we can perhaps better imagine how *bianzheng lunzhi* could represent both radical transformation and imperceptible change at the same time. The one new ingredient that confronted the editors of the early textbooks was the growing dominance of Western medicine. By stewing down this ingredient "in the sauce of the old," they produced a new form of clinical practice, centered on *bianzheng lunzhi*, that was imperceptibly different—at least to their minds—from the medical practice that they learned as teenagers and young adults. At the same time, this innovation made possible new understandings of the diagnostic process of Chinese medicine, allowing hybrid integrations with Western medicine and enabling doctors to work in the context of postcolonial power inequalities that had never existed before.

5

Chinese Medicine on the Margins

The fifth and final year of medical school consisted of a series of clinical clerkships at affiliated teaching hospitals. It was the first time we actively participated in patient care. In contrast to most of our clinical training in the third and fourth years, we were expected to use our knowledge of Western medicine in addition to our knowledge of Chinese medicine. This was the year when we realized just how important Western medicine was to hospital work. As Hu Yuning, a Dongzhimen Hospital attending physician that we encountered in Chapter 1, explained to me, "As soon as you start working at the hospital, you have to start cramming (*e'bu*) Western medicine."

I personally experienced this desperate desire to "cram" more biomedical knowledge during my own clerkship in the Dongzhimen Hospital Nephrology Department. I was assigned to train with a graduate student, Tao Yufang, who had already completed a year of residency prior to beginning his graduate training. Another graduate student, Huang Fan, who had no residency experience and was just beginning her first clinical rotation as a graduate student, was also temporarily assigned to work with Tao Yufang until she was ready to handle her own set of patients. Tao Yufang was put in charge of eight beds. My tasks as a medical student included conducting simple exams, writing medical notes, completing forms for medical orders, and fulfilling any other basic tasks Tao Yufang felt I could handle. Even though I was particularly focused on my primary goal of learning Chinese medicine, I always felt like my work as a fifth-year medical student, basic as it was, was impeded by my inadequate mastery of biomedicine.

For junior doctors, there is no easy way to balance the dual tasks of learning both Chinese medicine and Western medicine. This issue inadvertently became a topic of debate among Tao Yufang, Huang Fan, and me one after-noon during our nephrology rotation. About one week after the start of my clerkship, I was writing up the progress notes for one of our patients when I discovered that the previous entry by Tao Yufang described the patient's pulse as "deep and thin." I thought that I had felt a very different pulse during our rounds that morning, and I wanted to discuss this discrepancy with Tao Yufang before making an entry into the record. "Dr. Tao, yesterday you noted that this patient's pulse was deep and thin, but when I felt it today it seemed to be. . . ." He cut me off. "I didn't even take her pulse. I never do. The Chinese medicine pulse exam is quackery. I just make something up for the medical records. You can write whatever you think is appropriate." I was stunned by this incredibly frank and utterly heretical comment. The pulse exam is consid-ered an essential part of the Chinese medicine diagnostic process. I had never heard anyone seriously dismiss it like this. I made a lighthearted challenge. "Dr. Tao, the ancient doctors may have overly revered the pulse exam, but haven't you gone too far in the other direction?" Tao Yufang continued his diatribe. "The pulse exam should be eliminated. Not only that, but I think the *Inner Canon* and the *Treatise on Cold Damage* should be burned. What kind of science still relies on books 2,000 years old? This is one of the bad habits of Chinese people. These books need to be replaced." I thought I noticed a twinkle in his eye. Tao Yufang was enjoying his irreverence, but I could tell he was serious, too.

At this point, the debate had caught Huang Fan's attention. I countered, "If you 'burn' the *Inner Canon* and the *Treatise on Cold Damage*, where does your theory come from?" Huang Fan, pleased with an opportunity to rib Tao, chimed in, "That's right." Thinking I had another ally, I reached into my book bag and pulled out a small book on the pulse exam that I just happened to be reading at the time. Written by a contemporary clinician of some fame, it was my exciting new discovery from a recent bookstore venture. I thought it was an excellent guide to the subtleties of the pulse and enthusiastically showed it to Tao Yufang. He waved it away with his hand. "It's no use. The pulse exam is only good for deceiving people." I extended the book to Huang Fan, thinking she might be interested. She took it reluctantly, turned it over a couple times and then gave it back to me. Speaking with great earnestness, she said, "If you think this is a good book, you should read it." She paused. "Learning Western medicine is really our priority at this moment."

I already had great affection for Tao Yufang and Huang Fan at the time of this conversation, but I doubt that I was able to hide my dismay. This was cer-tainly not the first time I had heard these kinds of disparaging remarks about Chinese medicine. But I had never heard them made by doctors of Chinese medicine. My heart sank as I thought about the remainder of my rotation in the Nephrology Department. How much Chinese medicine could I expect to learn under this kind of tutelage?

As I tried to come to terms with my shock, my first thought, perhaps a defensive one, was to categorize these remarks as another example of the general postcolonial phenomenon of "worshipping the foreign" (*chongyang meiwai*). There have been many moments in China's tumultuous modern history in which the various nations of the West have been objects of scorn rather than reverence, but the power of the West has also had a tremendous allure in modern Chinese history. Were Tao Yufang and Huang Fan transferring their own geopolitical desires into the sphere of medicine? Was their preference for Western medicine analogous to the dreams of so many of my Chinese friends to study in the United States?

Over the ensuing weeks, I realized that the attitudes of Tao Yufang and Huang Fan toward Chinese medicine were not as simple as I imagined on that day. In some ways, their interest in Western medicine was no different than my own enthusiasm for Chinese medicine. Furthermore, they took their careers seriously and tried to teach me as much medicine—both Chinese and Western—as they could during my rotation. Huang Fan was a dedicated doctor; she meticulously attended to her patients and strove for excellence. Tao Yufang was keenly interested in herbal medicine, and, when not working at the hospital or doing his graduate school research, he was working on a contribution to a new publication on Chinese materia medica. But I was also aware that their skepticism toward Chinese medicine was a widespread phenomenon, especially among junior doctors. Wang Baokui, an accomplished Chinese medicine doctor at Beijing Hospital, recounted a similar event to me during an interview that took place not long after my exchange with Tao Yufang and Huang Fan.

I didn't have any influential teachers when I was doing my clinical training [in 1984–85]. Why? Upon reflection, I think it is because the supervising doctors that train students are usually residents. It is unusual to have an attending physician [as instructor]. . . . Chinese medicine theory [and]. . . its integration with clinical practice is loose. Western medicine theory and practice are integrated more tightly. Ultimately, theory cannot replace practice, and this is especially true for Chinese medicine. Therefore, if your teacher hasn't trained with a good teacher, then he probably won't be good at training you. I recommend that only doctors at the level of assistant professor train students. But this is very hard to achieve. At the time, I was trained by resident physicians. I thought they didn't know a thing, and looking back, I realize that they really didn't. But there is nothing you can do. This situation is caused by a lack of qualified teachers. . . . Among my teachers, there were two that actually asked me, "Does Chinese medicine work?" That is what they actually said to me as my teacher. But at the time, I liked traditional Chinese culture. I believed that Chinese medicine worked. But I believed blindly, religiously, and that allowed me to persevere. If I didn't have that blind faith, I would have slipped and probably have given up on Chinese medicine.[1]

Wang Baokui's account not only captures the skepticism of junior doctors who question the efficacy of Chinese medicine, but also offers insights into how these attitudes are reproduced through the institutional structures of Chinese medicine. He argues that the current system of hospital training fails to promote the effective transmission of Chinese medicine. Under the current system, where junior doctors train with other junior doctors who are marginally more experienced, only "blind faith" can keep one from turning away from Chinese medicine to Western medicine.

The skepticism among junior doctors is not only caused by a lack of qualified teachers; perhaps more importantly, it reflects the power asymmetries that operate within hospitals of Chinese medicine. Although Chinese medicine hospital policies are supposed to nurture and promote Chinese medicine, actual work requirements create a heavy reliance on Western medicine. When junior Chinese doctors like Tao Yufang and Huang Fan voice their skepticism toward Chinese medicine, they are also expressing their awareness of these power inequities. Their work demands skill in Western medicine but only adequacy in Chinese medicine. They actively use Western medicine in their everyday patient care and know that it works; they passively observe senior doctors using Chinese medicine and are less confident whether it can produce results. They need to acquire strong skills in Western medicine as quickly as possible, but they can often defer the mastery of Chinese medicine. Even as a fifth-year medical student, I was keenly aware of this pressure to improve my Western medicine skills so I could work more effectively in my limited role. Like Wang Baokui's teachers, my clinical teachers were junior doctors, with just one or two more years of experience than me. They were plagued by epistemological doubts. Huang Fan later confessed to me in an interview, "I don't trust Chinese medicine theory. I don't think you can use Chinese herbs effectively, if you don't know what is really going on in the body [according to Western medicine]."

In this chapter, I will explore how clinical work in a Chinese medicine hospital can often marginalize Chinese medicine, particularly for junior doctors who lack clinical experience. Deng Tietao has written that "one mistaken idea is that whatever problem Western medicine can resolve, Chinese medicine should stand to the side" (Zhu Liangchun 2005, 7). Examining a case study in detail, I will show how the disease-pattern dualism that emerged with the methodology of *bianzheng lunzhi* can result in precisely this phenomenon, inadvertently privileging Western medicine while diminishing the role of Chinese medicine. When the two medical systems are viewed as radically different and the epistemological authority of biomedicine is unquestioned, pattern discrimination becomes an impoverished version of disease diagnosis. Chinese medicine becomes useful only when one approaches the therapeutic limits of Western medicine. In the following case study, Tao Yufang, Huang Fan, and I all actively participated in caring for a patient whom I shall call Dong Chunhua. We will observe how *bianzheng lunzhi* was an essential tool for integrating her Chinese medicine and Western medicine treatments. But the power structures of the hospital were such that Chinese medicine treatments often had to "stand to the side."

The Chinese Medicine Case Record

On the morning of October 14, 1999, Dong Chunhua, a fifty-six-year-old woman, arrived at the Dongzhimen Hospital outpatient facility. She had been unable to eat solid food for the past month and was very fatigued. With the help of family members, she was able to register to see an internal medicine specialist, and they made their way through the large crowds to the second floor of the outpatient clinic. When her turn came, the consulting physician quickly realized that her condition might be serious and sent her to do some blood work. The results were problematic, and the doctor recommended that Dong Chunhua be admitted to the hospital for more comprehensive testing and treatment.

While Dong Chunhua was being seen in the outpatient clinic, I was doing rounds with Dr. Tao and Dr. Huang in the Nephrology ward. We had already finished rounds that morning and were writing up our medical orders when a nurse informed us that a new patient was being assigned to our section. The nurse handed the admissions slip for Dong Chunhua to Dr. Tao. It stated that the patient's chief complaint was "poor appetite and general fatigue for the past month," and her preliminary diagnosis was "idiopathic anemia and renal insufficiency." We glanced at the accompanying lab results, showing that Dong Chunhua had a very low hemoglobin count (75g/L), a slightly depressed white blood cell count (9.5 x 10^9/L), elevated neutrophil levels (82%), considerable electrolyte imbalances, elevated blood urea nitrogen (21.8 mmol/L), elevated serum bicarbonate (CO_2CP: 17.5 mmol/L), and some red blood cells in her urine (3–5/HP). Dr. Huang decided to handle this admission, and I joined her to help.

Dong Chunhua was lying on her bed when Dr. Huang and I entered her room. She told us that she had always been in good health, but about a month ago she started having sharp, burning pains in her side. A few days later, she developed blisters in this same area and started to ache all over, but most prominently in her legs. This was the beginning of all her other problems, she complained. Soon afterward she lost her appetite and became very fatigued. For the last month, she had only consumed a small amount of liquid each day.

Dr. Huang and I looked at each other, dubious that Dong Chunhua's initial problem, which sounded like a case of shingles, might have caused her later digestive problems and fatigue. We probed for more details, asking her about the medical attention she had gotten over the past month. She told us that she had first gone to a local health center. For ten days, she was given glucose injections, IV drips of cephradine (a first-generation cephalosporin), dexamethasone (a corticosteroid), vitamin B6, domperidone (to promote motility of the digestive tract), and Bufferin. She said these treatments helped the blisters but not her other symptoms. She subsequently went to the county hospital. The doctors took some X-rays and didn't find anything unusual. When she complained that it had been more than ten days since her last bowel movement, they gave her some laxatives. She was able to move her bowels once, but her overall condition did not improve.

So far Dong Chunhua's story did not sound like a classic case of renal insufficiency, usually marked by vomiting and reduced urination, as the preliminary diagnosis stated. When we asked her about these symptoms, Dong Chunhua told us that she had mostly just had a sense of abdominal fullness and no vomiting, except for one day recently when she vomited three times. She had not noticed anything unusual about her urine. When Dr. Huang pressed her, she said that she occasionally had some urgency and a slight burning sensation when urinating. If anything, the quantity had increased.

We were under some time constraints because new medical orders needed to be submitted to the nursing station by 11 A.M., so we pushed ahead, first checking the patient's tongue and pulse, iconic features of the Chinese medicine examination, then doing a full physical exam, an essential part of the biomedical assessment. Dong Chunhua's tongue appeared pale, suggesting a Spleen and Stomach deficiency, but had a thin, yellow coating, indicating that this deficiency was complicated by internal heat and possibly dampness. The pulse exam is one of the most difficult aspects of Chinese medicine, and

neither Dr. Huang nor I were confident of our skills. Nonetheless, we concurred that Dong Chunhua's pulse was wiry, thin, and rapid, the first quality
probably reflecting her continuing pain, the other characteristics indicating
deficiency and internal heat. Continuing with the physical exam, we found
that Dong Chunhua had a slightly elevated blood pressure of 145/70 mm Hg.
There were some superficial lesions on the left side and back at the level of
the fifth rib that had already healed over. We also discovered that she had a
third-degree thyroid goiter. Dong Chunhua told us that she had had this goiter
for more than twenty years and that it hadn't caused any problems in the past.

At the end of the consultation, Dr. Huang and I went back to the doctors'
office to write up our medical orders before the nurses left for lunch. Dr. Tao
came over to help, and together we issued fifteen "temporary medical orders"
that were to be carried out on that day only. Four of these were rush orders
for laboratory tests of the patient's blood, urine, serum electrolytes, and renal
function markers. The other tests included a stool analysis for occult blood,
erythrocyte sedimentation rate, hepatitis panel, full biochemical profile, thyroid screen, serum test for immunoglobulin G and complement C_3 and C_4
levels, electrocardiogram, full abdominal ultrasound, and posterior-anterior
and lateral chest X-rays. Lastly, Dr. Huang ordered a one-time IV drip with
10ml of 15% potassium chloride in 500ml of normal saline to address the patient's electrolyte imbalance.

We also issued ten "long-term medical orders" that were to be carried out
every day until the supervising physician put a stop on them. We ordered
Level One nursing care, a high-quality protein and high caloric diet, one
standard dose of Chinese herbal medicine per day (the actual prescription was
to be specified separately), and several Western medicine treatments to be administered every day. The Western medicine treatments follow. I've included
an explanation of the drug actions in paranthesis.

(1) 10 mg of benazapril, once daily (an ACE inhibitor for high blood
pressure)
(2) 500 ml of glucose 5% in water with 10 ml of 15% potassium chloride and 6 units of insulin, infused daily (to address the patient's
electrolyte imbalance)[2]
(3) 500 ml of Hartmann's solution with 0.1 g of Vitamin B_6, infused
daily (for nutritional purposes and electrolyte regulation)
(4) 1.5 g of cefuroxime, administered intravenously twice a day (a
second-generation cephalosporin)

Separately, on a standard herbal medicine prescription form, Dr. Huang
submitted a prescription for twelve herbs—a typical number—to be administered for one day.

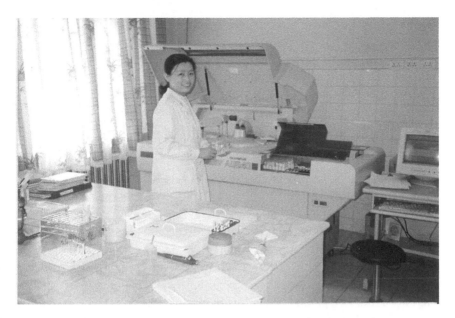

Figure 17. A lab technician operating a chemistry analyzer at Dongzhimen Hospital, 2002.

Chai Hu 10g	Huang Qin 10g	Bai Shao 10g	Bai Zhu 15g
Fu Ling 30g	Bai Mao Gen 10g	Lu Gen 10g	Ban Xia 10g
Chen Pi 10g	Sheng Gan Cao 6g	Zhi Shi 10g	Sha Ren 10g

As with most herbal prescriptions, these herbs were to be prepared by boiling them in water. The resulting decoction would be administered as half-doses in the morning and the evening. As Dr. Huang noted in the medical record, this combination of herbs was designed to clear heat, transform dampness, strengthen the Spleen, and regulate the Stomach. Because of the required preparation time, the Chinese medicine prescription would not be administered until the next day.

After lunch, Dr. Huang began writing up "the initial note" (or "initial progress note") (首次病程纪录), the first key text of the Chinese medicine case record. Later that afternoon, I wrote the more extensive "medical student admissions note" (住院病历), which serves as a training exercise for students and residents. The "initial note" has several basic components that must appear in the following order: basic patient information, history of present illness, past medical history, physical exam, laboratory and radiographic results (if available), Chinese medicine diagnosis, biomedical diagnosis, and a treatment plan that includes Chinese medicine and Western medicine therapies and the justifications for these treatments. Dr. Huang was to be totally responsible for the patient's treatment for the next twenty-four hours until a more senior physician would have the opportunity to see the patient. She worked hard all afternoon, preparing a draft of the initial note, writing an error-free final version in fountain pen as required by the Medical Services Department (医务处) and committing the text to memory. When admitting new patients to the Nephrology Department ward, doctors are expected to recite their initial note by heart at the 8 A.M. staff meeting for all the doctors and nurses. The next morning, Dr. Huang did her recitation flawlessly.

When a new patient is admitted to the ward and placed in a bed, the junior doctor responsible for that bed is immediately involved in a burst of activity, conducting an initial history and physical, issuing medical orders, commencing treatment. But by far the most time and energy are spent on writing up the medical record. Chinese medicine has a long history of case record scholarship, and by the sixteenth century it had become a vibrant medical genre (Cullen 2001). Classical case records contained a brief account of the patient's condition, perhaps just a line or two, as in Ye Tianshi's *Case Records as a Guide to Clinical Practice* (臨證指南醫案) and usually not more than a dozen lines, as in Xu Dachun's *Case Records of Swirling Creek* (洄溪醫案), followed by a treatment and almost inevitably a cure (Liu Gengsheng 1997). In the early twentieth century, doctors of Chinese medicine began to incorporate some of the organizational categories of the biomedical case record into their own record keeping (Andrews 2001). But with the development of Chinese medicine hospitals in the late 1950s, a new type of case record writing emerged, adapted to the institutional requirements of hospital care. Unlike the classic case records that showcased the skill of a master physician, these new hospital records were written collectively, usually by junior doctors, documenting chronologically and at great length the patient's changing condition and treatments.

When I was doing my medical training, active case records were kept in a metal clipboard with hinged cover and stored in a special filing cabinet at the nursing station. (Today hospitals have moved to fully digitized medical records.) As collectively produced documents, they were nodes that linked doctors, nurses, technicians, accountants, clerks, and so on, across the hospital and sometimes beyond its institutional borders. When the patient is actively being treated, the case record shuttles among the junior doctors, who record progress notes and paste lab results to it; the senior doctors, who reference it when making rounds; and the nurses, who update temperature charts and carry out medical orders. When the patient is discharged, hospital accountants produce a bill of services from it and store it in the case records room so it can be pulled if the patient returns to the hospital or if other doctors conducting research are interested in it. If there are also legal issues related to the patient's condition or treatment, the case record will be referenced in the court proceedings. Because of these multiple functions—medical, administrative, financial, and legal—doctors are required to follow very strict and detailed writing guidelines, including one of the most dreaded rules of the pre-digital age: all written entries were required to be made in fountain pen, completely free from errors and corrections. Occasionally, a doctor could get away with using a razor blade to scratch away a small mistake of the fountain pen. But if this trick failed, the doctor would have to copy the entire page (both sides). The Medical Services Division closely monitored the writing of medical records, sometimes fining departments for failing to adhere to their guidelines.

In many respects the contemporary Chinese medicine case record is very similar to its Western medicine counterpart. They both participate in the biopolitical operations of the nation state that manage bodies and populations. The Chinese medicine case record has adopted the categories and organizational format of its Western medicine counterpart: a cover sheet, medical orders, discharge summary, medical student admissions note, initial note, progress notes, lab reports, and so on. But the contemporary Chinese medicine case record must also mark its difference. This necessity is achieved through the addition of specific Chinese medicine content. Therefore, while the biomedical case record is written entirely in the idiom of Western medicine, the Chinese medicine case record is written in the language of *both* Western medicine and Chinese medicine. In other words, the Chinese medicine case record contains a linguistic doubling. This doubling is most striking in the medical student admissions note. For example, in the medical student admissions note for Dong Chunhua, I included two types of medical exams (the Chinese medicine Four Examinations and the Western medicine physical exam), two diagnoses (Chinese medicine and Western medicine), and two idiomatically appropriate justifications for these two diagnoses.[3]

At first glance, this doubling would seem to be a reasonable, albeit cumbersome, method for ensuring that both medical systems get equal representation in the Chinese medicine case record. But just as the medical student admissions note lacks any real clinical relevancy, this apparent evenhandedness proves illusory. The language of Western medicine dominates the remainder of the medical record. Western medicine documentation of the patient's condition and treatment operates as the baseline of information, to which Chinese medicine documentation is added as a supplement. When doctors emphasize the Chinese medicine therapy, Chinese medicine content increases. When doctors rely primarily on Western medicine therapy, the Chinese medicine content drops precipitously and may be eliminated altogether. During my clerkship in the Chinese External Medicine Department (*zhongyi waike*), I noticed that doctors often omitted, or perhaps just forgot, even the most distinctive markers of Chinese medicine, such as the tongue and pulse exams. These patients were usually slated for surgery, and a Chinese medicine assessment of the patient's condition was considered superfluous in these circumstances.

Double Diagnosis

The one area in which doubling always occurs is the diagnosis, and this is precisely where the key concepts of disease, *bing*, and pattern are deployed. According to hospital regulations, doctors must make a "double diagnosis" (*shuangchong zhenduan*; 双重诊断)—one in Chinese medicine and one in Western medicine—for each admitted patient. The "double diagnosis" can be found in multiple places in the medical records, such as the cover sheet (住院病案首业), the discharge summary (出院总结), the medical student admission note, the initial note, and some daily progress notes (病程记录). As Dong Chunhua's case demonstrates, the double diagnosis can often be a source of tension within the case record.

Before exploring the challenges of making a double diagnosis, it is important to remember that making a "single diagnosis"—in Chinese medicine or Western medicine—is always a tenuous endeavor. Doctors must balance the requirement to produce accurate, detailed, empirical observations of the patient's condition with the need to generate a particular "narrative" about the patient's illness—that is, a diagnosis that explains all the patient's signs and symptoms. As this excerpt from Dr. Huang's initial progress report shows, these two requirements do not necessarily align neatly.

> On September 12th, 1999, the patient experienced a sudden sharp pain in both flanks that had no apparent cause. It was followed by the appearance of blisters several days later, which subsequently burst and oozed a thin yellow liquid. Three days later, the same changes occurred on the left side of her back. These symptoms were accompanied by fever, and a generalized pain that was most noticeable at the skin lesions and in the legs. The patient also had some stomach discomfort, a loss of appetite, . . . and general fatigue. . . . [Following treatment at a local health station and then at the Luhe Hospital in Tong County], the patient's condition did not change. Her fatigue

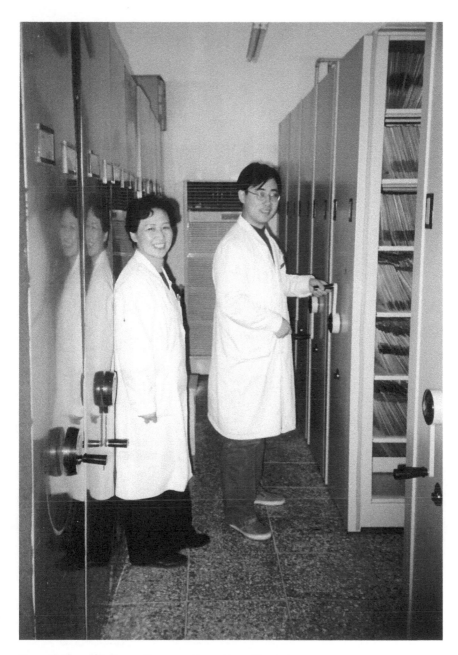

Figure 18. The medical records room at Dongzhimen Hospital, 2002.

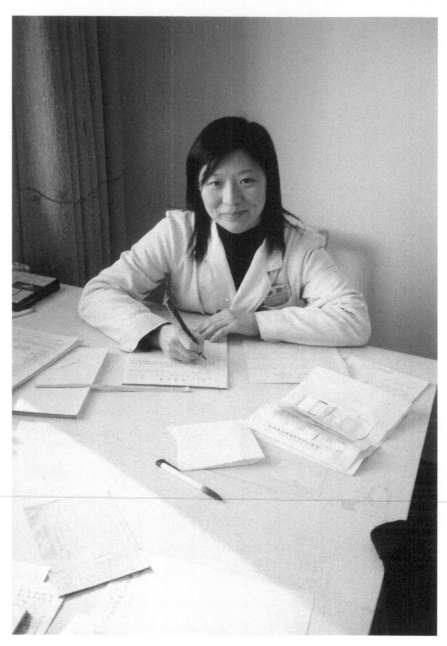

Figure 19. An attending physician making an entry into a medical record, Dongzhimen Hospital, 2002.

was severe. Several days ago, she vomited three times in one day. . . . The patient was admitted to our hospital on October 14th, 1999. Her current symptoms are: general fatigue, loss of weight, approximately ten kilos over the last month; sharp, burning pain in both flanks and the left side of the back that worsens at night; numbness, pain, and sense of coldness in the lower extremities, upper abdominal discomfort, loss of appetite, no vomiting. No bowel movements in the last ten days. Urination is frequent, occasionally urgent, painful, hot. Amount is copious. Sleep is restless.

This excerpt from the "history of present illness" section of the initial progress report illustrates some of the general intellectual challenges of making a diagnosis, regardless of the medical system. Does the sequence of events and symptoms point to one underlying problem, which manifests itself in multiple ways that change over time? Or does it reflect several underlying problems occurring in conjunction and in series, each one producing its own unique set of symptoms? For example, are the skin lesions and pain related to the patient's stomach discomfort, loss of appetite, and general fatigue? Furthermore, has the patient expressed herself in a manner that is consistent with or easily translated into the terminology of medicine? Dr. Huang's description of the patient's urination as occasionally urgent, painful, and hot was something that was later contested because it conflated ambiguous bodily sensations with precisely defined medical terms.

Like all doctors of Chinese medicine working in a hospital, Dr. Huang faced the additional challenge of making sense of this information in two ways—of producing a "double diagnosis." Both diagnoses would have to be not only faithful to the patient's presentation but also reasonably consistent with each other. Since it is this latter task that is unique to the Chinese medicine profession, we will examine it more closely by turning to Dr. Huang's diagnosis of Dong Chunhua. In her initial progress report, she proposed the following Chinese medicine and Western medicine diagnoses, presented in two successive lists.

Chinese medicine diagnosis:
1. Chronic Kidney Heat (慢肾热)
   Damp heat pouring down, qi and blood exhaustion (*shire xiazhu, qixue kuixu*)
2. Abdominal Fullness (痞满)
   Liver qi stagnation, Spleen and Stomach depletion (*ganyu qizhi, piwei xuruo*)

3. Fire Rash Encircling the Waist (缠腰火丹)
   Damp heat accumulating internally, qi and yin exhaustion (*shire neiyun, qiyun kuixu*)
4. Goiter (瘿瘤)
   Phlegm and blood stasis obstructing the collaterals (*tanre zuluo*)

Western medicine diagnosis:
1. Chronic renal insufficiency, non-compensatory stage
   Pyelonephritis?
   Acute glomerulonephritis?
2. Idiopathic anemia
   Malnourishment anemia?
   Renal anemia?
3. Shingles
4. Simple Goiter?

As we can see in Dr. Huang's initial diagnosis, the double diagnosis is further split into two levels. Within the Chinese medicine diagnosis, the first level is the Chinese medicine *bing*; the second level is the pattern (*zheng*). In Dong Chunhua's case, Dr. Huang diagnosed four different *bing*: Chronic Kidney Heat, Abdominal Fullness, Fire Rash Encircling the Waist, and Goiter. Each *bing* is followed by the pattern, a descriptive phrase four to eight characters long. For example, Dr. Huang determined that the relevant pattern for the Chronic Kidney Heat *bing* was "damp heat pouring down, qi and blood exhaustion."

In the Western medicine diagnosis, there are two levels as well—the "primary diagnosis" (*zhuyao zhenduan*) and "secondary diagnosis" (*congshu zhenduan*) (Wang Yongyan and Han Xiao 2000). Unlike the Chinese medicine diagnosis, these two levels are expressed in terms of a single concept: disease. Doctors distinguish between these two levels only if they want to indicate a relationship between two diseases. Therefore, the secondary diagnosis is usually a complication or variant of the primary diagnosis.[4] In Dr. Huang's primary diagnosis, she identified four diseases: chronic renal insufficiency, idiopathic anemia, shingles, and simple goiter. Only the first two diseases needed a secondary diagnosis, which she punctuated with question marks to indicate that the evidence was not yet conclusive.

In theory, the Chinese medicine diagnosis—the *bing* and *zheng*—and Western medicine diagnosis—the disease with its complications and variants—can vary independently of each other, since each has its own diagnostic criteria. But in clinical practice, doctors must nonetheless also try to make sense of these two diagnoses in terms of each other. Their mere juxtaposition seems to call for an attempt to reconcile them. However, there are considerable translational challenges to this task. The terms that most closely resemble each other, disease and *bing*, rarely correspond exactly. The relationship between pattern and disease is more indirect and complicated.

The urgency to seek convergence is so strong that doctors sometimes "bend the rules" to create equivalencies. One way, which is probably not too common, is to "fudge the data." I participated in one instance when I was writing the progress notes for a patient on the Acupuncture ward, a stroke victim with hypertension. This diagnosis was based on his blood pressure readings, but the patient's hypertension was asymptomatic, so there was no basis to suggest a corresponding Chinese medicine *bing* diagnosis. My supervising physician instructed me to write that the patient was suffering from the Chinese medicine bing of "Vertigo" (眩晕)—even though he did not have any dizziness, the necessary symptom for this diagnosis. In a similar fashion, some equivalencies have become so universally accepted that doctors seem to forgo, or perhaps just forget about, the justifications for a Chinese medicine *bing*. For example, I observed many doctors diagnose "Wasting Thirst" (消渴) as an equivalent for adult-onset type II diabetes, even though the presentation of this disease almost never corresponds to the definition of this *bing*—"increased thirst, increased eating, increased urination, and loss of weight." These symptoms do correspond well to juvenile-onset type I diabetes. Doctors have so universally accepted Wasting Thirst as the equivalent for type I diabetes that they readily extend the congruence to type II diabetes, even though its clinical presentation does not meet the definition of this *bing*.

First Disease

As these examples of "rule bending" show, the basic principle of finding a Chinese medicine *bing* that is a suitable equivalent for a biomedical disease is to privilege the latter. Dong Chunhua's case shows some of the typical ways in which Western medicine is given priority over Chinese medicine in everyday hospital work.

Hospital regulations state that all patients admitted to the in-patient wards must be seen by a senior physician within twenty-four hours. Since the senior physicians in the Nephrology Department were not scheduled to do rounds the day after Dong Chunhua was admitted, Dr. Huang and I tracked down Dr. He, assistant director of the Nephrology Department, and asked him to examine the new patient. The three of us found Dong Chunhua resting on her bed. Dr. Huang summarized her findings to Dr. He as he flipped through the metal clipboard holding Dong Chunhua's record, jumping back and forth between Dr. Huang's initial note and the lab results. He asked the patient a few questions, focusing on her urination. "How much burning and urgency do you have when you urinate?" "Just a little, maybe none at all," Dong Chunhua replied, "but I have to go often." Dr. He turned to Dr. Huang. "What's important here is that the patient can't hold her urine. This doesn't sound like a case of acute glomerulonephritis or pyelonephritis to me. Inability to retain urine is a sign of early-stage renal insufficiency. The renal insufficiency is also probably the source of her digestive troubles and anemia. So we will need to modify your diagnosis. . . ." He instructed her on which lab tests to do to confirm the biomedical diagnosis and modified the patient's biomedical therapies. Lastly, he looked at Dr. Huang's Chinese medicine prescription. "We can keep some of these herbs, but the Chinese medicine pattern should focus on turbid poison (*zhuodu*)," he said. Then he dictated a new prescription, trying to retain as many of Dr. Huang's original herbs as possible that were consistent with the new pattern he had diagnosed. He clapped the metal clipboard closed and handed it back to Dr. Huang with a gentle smile of encouragement.

That afternoon, Dr. Huang wrote the following progress notes: "The patient reports: general fatigue, abdominal fullness, stabbing pain in both flanks and the left side of the back, numbness, pain, and sensations of cold in both legs, no chills or fever, no nausea or vomiting, able to eat more today than yesterday but still less than normal, no bowel movements, urination frequent and copious, no pain or burning upon voiding, restless sleep. . . . Yesterday's rush lab tests indicate: routine blood examination: HGB [hemoglobin] 75 g/L, GRA [neutrophils] 82%, WBC [white blood cells] 9.5 x 10⁹/L; routine urine examination: PRO [protein]: 0.75 g/L, ERY [erythrocytes] 250 /uL, LEU [leukocytes] 25 /uL, red blood cells 3–5 [per high power field], white blood cells 0–1 [per high power field]; serum electrolytes: K⁺ 2.98 mmol/L, Na⁺ 130.8 mmol/L, Cl⁻ 97.5 mmol/L. GLU [Glucose] 7.3 mmol/L; [and renal function exam]: BUN [blood urea nitrogen] 21.8 mmol/L, CO_2CP [serum bicarbonate] 17.5 mmol/L. After finishing his consultation, Assistant Director He remarked that the patient is a middle-aged woman, previously in good health, but she now cannot retain her urine, which means that kidney function is already impaired. According to the patient's illness history, the cause of this damage is not clear; therefore, she is suffering from a glomerulopathy of unknown cause. Her Chinese medicine diagnosis is: 1. Chronic Obstruction and Retention (qi and blood deficiency, turbid poison accumulating internally); 2. Snaking Blisters (damp heat accumulating internally); 3. Goiter (phlegm and blood stasis obstructing the collaterals). The Western medicine diagnosis is: 1. chronic renal insufficiency non-compensatory stage, nephritis of unknown cause, anemia of renal origin, hypertension of renal origin; 2. shingles; 3. simple goiter? Complete all standard exams to confirm the diagnosis."

In this note, as with most Chinese medicine case records that I have seen, Dr. Huang followed the convention of presenting the Chinese medicine diagnosis first. But in this case, as with most cases, the Western medicine diagnosis comes first epistemologically. A close look at Dr. He's revisions of Dr. Huang's Chinese medicine diagnosis confirms this point.

Chinese medicine diagnosis:
  1. Chronic Obstruction and Retention (慢关格)
     Qi and blood deficiency, turbid poison accumulating (*qixue kuixu, zhuodu neiyun*)
  2. Snaking Blisters (蛇串疮)
     Damp heat accumulating internally (*shire neiyun*)
  3. Goiter (瘿瘤)
     Phlegm and blood stasis obstructing the collaterals (*tanre zuluo*)

Western medicine diagnosis:
  1. Chronic renal insufficiency, non-compensatory stage
     Nephritis of unknown cause
     Renal anemia
     Renal hypertension
  2. Shingles
  3. Simple goiter

Dr. He eliminated the first two *bing* in Dr. Huang's diagnosis, Chronic Kidney Heat and Abdominal Fullness, and replaced them with a single *bing*, "Obstruction and Retention (*guange*) (关格)." This major change to the Chinese medicine diagnosis was based on his new biomedical diagnosis of chronic renal insufficiency, for which he recommended *guange* as the corresponding Chinese medicine *bing*. *Guange* is generally defined as anuresis (no urination) and vomiting—literally obstruction above and retention below as the Chinese characters indicate.[5] As renal insufficiency progresses into renal failure, these two symptoms do indeed become the most prominent features of the patient's condition. But at the time of Dr. He's visit, the patient had only reported one episode of vomiting, and her urination was not diminished but rather increased. Therefore, *guange* would have been impossible to diagnose by Chinese medicine standards alone. The critical evidence for the Chinese medicine diagnosis came from the Western medicine lab chemistries, espe-cially the BUN and CO_2CP results, which suggested the biomedical diagnosis of renal insufficiency.[6] (This diagnosis was later confirmed when lab results showed that the patient had elevated serum creatinine [267 μmol/L] and uric acid levels [430 μmol/L].) Because renal insufficiency can often progress to renal failure, Dr. He used these biomedical test results as the basis for the new Chinese medicine diagnosis of Obstruction and Retention (*guange*).

The preeminence of the Western medicine diagnosis is further demon-strated by the word "chronic." Dr. He did not just diagnose the patient as having Obstruction and Retention but as having "Chronic Obstruction and Retention (*man guange*)." Biomedical diseases frequently distinguish between "acute" and "chronic" forms, but classically Chinese medicine *bing* did not. Indeed, most contemporary doctors of Chinese medicine have not adopted this hybrid convention. But the Nephrology Department frequently used these modifiers as one way to achieve a closer congruence between disease and *bing*. Dr. Huang, whose rotation in this department had only begun a few days earlier, had been trying to follow this departmental convention when she made her original diagnosis of "Chronic Kidney Heat" (Lu Renhe and Gao Jing).[7]

The very concept of Kidney Heat itself further highlights the hybrid predi-lections of the Nephrology Department. This term is not recognized in most contemporary Chinese medicine scholarship as a *bing* category. For example, the well-regarded *Concise Dictionary of Chinese Medicine* does not include a gloss on this term (Editorial Committee of the Comprehensive Dictionary of Chinese Medicine 1979). Although there are some references to Kidney Heat in classical scholarship, most ancient doctors were far more concerned with the effects of deficiency on the Kidneys. The lead doctors of the Nephrology Department had dusted off this forgotten relic and proudly revived this term as a highly useful clinical construct. But they had disposed of the classical understandings of Kidney Heat, which were fragmented and contradictory anyway, and made it a Chinese medicine equivalent for the biomedical dis-ease of glomerulonephritis. During his consultation, Dr. He pointed out that the patient's occasional discomfort during urination should not be miscon-strued as the painful burning of glomerulonephritis. Without any conclusive evidence to support this biomedical diagnosis, there was no basis to diagnosis the patient with Kidney Heat.

Dr. He also eliminated Dr. Huang's second Chinese medicine diagnosis of Abdominal Fullness. This diagnosis, he told Dr. Huang, properly refers to digestive tract disorders and should not be used as an equivalent for anemia, which is caused by a loss of blood or an inability to produce red blood cells.

Barring the discovery of some occult blood in the patient's stool, the most likely cause of the patient's anemia was her renal insufficiency. He pointed out that even though the patient's kidney damage had only come to light recently, the patient was probably suffering from an ongoing, gradual impairment that would have affected the kidneys' ability to produce erythropoietin, a hormone essential to the stimulation of red blood cell production. Therefore, he instructed Dr. Huang to modify the patient's diagnosis in the medical record to show her anemia as a complication of renal insufficiency and not an independent disease diagnosis. By eliminating anemia as a primary (biomedical) diagnosis, Dr. He had also eliminated the need to find a Chinese medicine equivalent.

The diagnostic privileging of disease over *bing* in this case is typical of Chinese medicine hospital care. Like Dr. Huang and Dr. He, all hospital physicians of Chinese medicine that I observed put a great deal of emphasis on achieving consistency in their Chinese medicine and Western medicine diagnoses. In some instances, this process requires some intellectual fudging, as the previous example demonstrates. But at other times, achieving equivalency is relatively straightforward. The patient's last two diagnoses are an example where the disease and *bing* definitions are so close that there was little debate over congruence. Although Dr. He revised Dr. Huang's terminology in the third diagnosis, changing Fire Rash Encircling the Waist to the more standard term Snaking Blisters, they both agreed, as most doctors of Chinese medicine would, that this *bing* is a good equivalent for shingles. Likewise, Goiter overlaps with simple goiter, and this diagnosis was also unproblematic.

These examples prompt the question of what is gained and lost through these conventions of equivalency. On the one hand, doctors produce a document that is logically consistent, an important goal in medical recordkeeping in general. Dr. Huang's original assessment, despite her best efforts, had suggested conflicting interpretations of the patient's condition. Dr. He was able to impose intellectual rigor on this case by bringing the disease and *bing* in line and showing how the patient's major ailments could all be explained by renal insufficiency. On the other hand, doctors may have to sacrifice certain principles of the Chinese medicine diagnosis to achieve congruence. This gentle bending of the rules is an everyday necessity for doctors in Chinese medicine hospitals. As one might expect, this practice undermines the analytical strength of the concept of *bing* by making it derivative of disease.

At first glance, one might think that the weakening of a diagnostic category like *bing* would have disastrous consequences for the practice of Chinese medicine. When the Institute of National Medicine issued a proposal for the "unification of disease names" in 1933, many leading doctors of Chinese medicine were up in arms about the damage it would cause to the theoretical foundations of the medical system (see Chapter 3). But contemporary doctors perform a version of this unification with every patient. Moreover, they have a popular maxim for dealing with a situation that once seemed to portend terrifying epistemological ramifications: "First diagnose a disease, then determine a pattern" (*xian bianbing, zai bianzheng*).[8] As this aphorism suggests, biomedicine predominates in the first stage of the diagnosis. But once this stage has been completed, doctors make a methodological shift from disease/*bing* diagnosis to *bianzheng lunzhi*. This shift creates a space in which doctors can practice Chinese medicine with greater freedom from the influence of Western medicine. The degree of freedom, however, depends to a large extent on the clinical skills of each individual physician.

Coming Last

Dr. He continued Dr. Huang's Western medicine regimen, with a small modification to the potassium chloride IV infusion, and added three new treatments. He prescribed: (1) 500ml of glucose 10% in water with 10 ml of 15% potassium chloride, infused daily (to address the patient's electrolyte imbalance); (2) 500ml of glucose 10% in water with 100ml of 50% glucose solution, and 8 units of insulin, infused daily (to increase caloric intake); (3) 0.5 µg of alfacalcidol daily (a form of Vitamin D used to compensate for the calcium metabolism abnormalities associated with renal failure); (4) 10 mg of cisapride, three times per day (to increase gastrointestinal motility). Dr. Huang noted all these changes in the progress notes. In the last sentence of this page-long note, she made an idiomatic switch to the language of Chinese medicine. "Based on the tongue and pulse, [the patient] clearly has damp heat in the Middle Burner, impeding the transportation and transformation of the Spleen and Stomach and causing Stomach Qi not to descend. Treat by dredging the Liver, clearing heat, transforming dampness, strengthening the Spleen, and harmonizing the Stomach." The note concludes with Dr. He's new prescription of sixteen herbs—a modification of Dr. Huang's prescription with three of the original herbs removed and seven new ones added—to be taken for the next four days.

Chai Hu 10g	Huang Qin 10g	Huang Lian 10g	Bai Shao 10g
Bai Zhu 15g	Fu Ling 30g	Zhi Shi 10g	Pei Lan 15g
Gua Lou 30g	Sha Ren 6g	Chen Pi 10g	Ban Xia 10g
Shou Jun 10g	Jiao Shan Zha 10g	Jiao Lai Fu Zi 10g	Jiao Mai Ya 10g

The linguistic shift that takes place at the end of this progress note is typical of most progress notes. In general, doctors begin their notes in the language of Western medicine, reporting changes in the patient's presentation and re- cording new lab results, and end them in a brief idiomatic flourish of Chinese medicine. If the patient is due for a new Chinese medicine prescription, gen- erally once every three or four days when senior doctors make rounds, then junior doctors will note the pathomechanism of the illness, the treatment principle, and the new prescription in the case record, such as in the previous example. On other days, doctors will abbreviate or even omit this aspect of the progress note. I stress this linguistic shift in the progress note because I find it emblematic of the epistemological challenges that doctors face in trying to deploy two medical systems simultaneously. Chinese medicine comes last because it is figuratively and literally practiced on the margins of an epistemo- logical space determined by biomedicine.

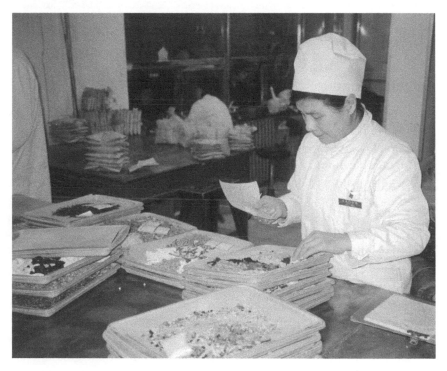

Figure 20. A senior pharmacist at Dongzhimen Hospital checking an herbal prescription to make sure it has been prepared correctly, 2002.

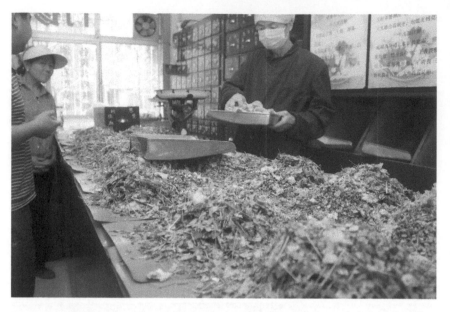

Figure 21. The pharmacist at Zhou Xinyou's private clinic (see Chapter 1) preparing a prescription. Lanzhou, Gansu Province, 2011.

Double Therapies

This marginalization has important consequences for therapy. As Dr. Huang's and Dr. He's treatments show, almost all patients in the wards received a combination of Chinese medicine and Western medicine therapies. In contrast to the "double diagnosis," hospital policy does not require the use of double therapies; rather, administrators exhort doctors to use Chinese medicine therapies whenever possible and resort to Western medicine only when needed (*neng zhong bu xi*). In practice, the reverse is more often the case. Chinese medicine is the therapy of last resort when there are no good options with Western medicine. This therapeutic imbalance is the result of the diagnostic imbalance. Since the Western medicine diagnosis comes first epistemologically, Western medicine therapies also come first. When a diagnosis indicates a biomedical treatment with well-known efficacy, it is easy for doctors to forgo an earnest attempt to treat this ailment with Chinese medicine.

Dr. Huang's use of cefuroxime exemplifies this problem. Dong Chunhua was admitted to the hospital with elevated neutrophil levels, suggesting a possible bacterial infection. The evidence for infection was not strong because her white blood cell count was in the normal range. Nonetheless, concerned that Dong Chunhua's renal insufficiency might be caused by glomerulonephritis, Dr. Huang decided, in consultation with Dr. Tao, to play it safe and prescribed a broad-spectrum antibiotic. Eight days later, Dr. Jin, one of the senior physicians in the department, became suspicious that Dong Chunhua was unnecessarily taking antibiotics and ordered new bloodwork. When the results showed no change in Dong Chunhua's white blood cell count and neutrophil levels that had dropped to normal levels at 68%, he stopped the order.

The privileging of the Western medicine diagnosis makes it not only hard, but even legally risky, to ignore the indicated Western medicine therapies. I asked many of my clinical teachers working in the inpatient wards what would happen if they decided to rely on Chinese medicine alone and a patient's condition subsequently deteriorated seriously. One of my teachers in the Gerontology Department put it most succinctly: "Oh, it would definitely be bad." Of course, nobody knew for sure because they had never seen it happen. But they all agreed that if a patient receiving standard biomedical care deteriorated seriously or even died, the doctor would be entirely blameless. The situation would be deemed beyond the reach of modern medicine. In this case, Dr. Huang unnecessarily hedged her bets. But had there been a true glomerulonephritis, perhaps only a few highly skilled clinicians would have dared to rely exclusively on Chinese medicine therapies.

This privileging of the biomedicine diagnosis does not mean Chinese medicine therapies are always marginalized. But it circumscribes their relevance to situations where there is no Western medicine therapy with recognized clinical efficacy. In fact, Dong Chunhua's main illness, renal insufficiency, is a good example of just such an illness. Her various biomedical treatments were mostly supportive in nature.[9] As Dr. He and many other doctors in the Nephrology Department told me, Chinese medicine frequently offers the best possibility for halting or even reversing the progress of renal insufficiency. But even when doctors perceive Chinese medicine to have advantages over Western medicine, they must still carefully negotiate the relationship between the two medical systems.

Because of the predominance of biomedicine in contemporary Chinese medicine practice, therapies have increasingly been limited to the areas where Western medicine is perceived to be weak—the chronic, the functional, and the hard to treat. But even this space is perceived to be under threat. Many junior doctors believe that "range of therapy" (zhiliao fanwei) is shrinking with every advance of Western medicine. At the same time, it is arguably shrinking if the clinical skills of the younger generations of Chinese medicine doctors are diminishing.

Although the practice of double therapies can undermine the status of

Chinese medicine, it is important to point out that most doctors consider it a great asset. Not only does it give a doctor more tools to work with, but it also invites doctors to coordinate both types of therapies in strategic ways. At the same time, combined therapies make it difficult to evaluate the efficacy of their Chinese medicine prescriptions. Doctors feel reasonably confident that they know what to expect from biomedical treatments, which are well studied and standardized. But young doctors who lack clinical experience struggle to assess Chinese herbal therapies, which are tailored to a patient's unique presentation. If a patient starts to feel better, it is often assumed that it is because of the biomedical treatment.

To counter the ambiguity inherent in double therapies, Chinese medicine clinics and hospitals will try to promote the "special characteristics of Chinese medicine" (*zhongyi tedian*) — that is, the areas in which they believe they have a therapeutic advantage over Western medicine. One way in which the Nephrology Department at Dongzhimen Hospital was starting to do this during my clinical clerkship was through the work of one of its attending physicians, Yu Xiuchen. She had developed a reputation for effectively using herbal treatments to treat gangrene caused by diabetes or peripheral vascular disease. As a result, she was being allotted an increasingly share of the departmental beds for this work. Most of her patients had been slated for amputation surgery at other hospitals. After several weeks or months of treatment, many of her patients had indeed been spared the most radical surgeries, perhaps losing two toes instead of half a foot, or half a foot instead of the whole foot, and so on. During our fourth year of medical school, Xuanwu Chinese Medicine Hospital, in southwest Beijing, became the site of our clinical and classroom training for a semester. This hospital also had an excellent reputation for its expertise in gangrene therapies. This "special characteristic" has become an essential way for this small, local hospital to compete with larger Chinese medicine and Western medicine hospitals in Beijing. They have established a Vascular Disease Department (脉管炎科) and credit their late departmental chief, Shi Jinghua (石晶华), for developing their unique therapeutic approach to this disease.[10] These treatments were so important to the livelihood of the hospital that our teachers would not divulge the entire contents of the various formulas they used.

Deferring Chinese Medicine

The potential for marginalizing Chinese medicine inherent in the practice of double therapies is further exacerbated by hospital training regimens and career trajectories of junior doctors. Double therapies are practiced throughout the hospital, but the relative emphasis on Chinese medicine and Western medicine depends very much on one's location within the hospital. Some departments rely primarily on Western medicine; such is obviously the case with the Dongzhimen Surgery Department, which was designed to provide a Western medicine service and has a considerable number of doctors on its staff who have never studied Chinese medicine. Other departments that are ostensibly Chinese medicine in orientation may also rely heavily on Western medicine. On the first day of my rotation in the outpatient clinic for the Cardiovascular Department, one of the doctors counseled me. "You are a foreign student, so I assume your goal is to really learn Chinese medicine. I recommend that you transfer to the outpatient clinic of a different department where you can really observe some of the special characteristics of Chinese medicine, such as the Gastroenterology or Gynecology departments. We use a lot of Western medicine pharmaceuticals and Chinese patent medicines (*zhongchengyao*) [premade herbal pills] in this clinic." Although the Cardiovascular Department is a bit anomalous, the great dividing line in hospital care is between the inpatient wards and the outpatient clinic. In the former, the emphasis is on Western medicine treatments; in the latter, it is Chinese medicine treatments. As many Chinese medicine doctors intone, "The inpatient wards are the realm of Western medicine; the outpatient clinics are the realm of Chinese medicine."

The training of junior doctors, however, does not generally take place in the outpatient clinics, where Chinese medicine is most emphasized. Like hospitals of Western medicine, new doctors enter the hospital as "resident physicians" (*zhuyuan yishi*) and work primarily in the inpatient wards. After five years of work as a resident, doctors are evaluated and must advance to the rank of "attending physician" (*zhuzhi yishi*) to continue working as a doctor. Upon attaining this rank, doctors continue to work in the inpatient wards but will be assigned consultation hours in the outpatient clinic of their respective department. As doctors gain in experience and rank, the number of outpatient hours will increase, and so will the doctor's consultation fees. After five years as an attending physician, doctors are eligible for promotion to "assistant chief physicians" (*fuzhuren yishi*); in another five years, they can be considered for the highest rank of "chief physician" (*zhuren yishi*). Only doctors that meet a specific set of criteria, which includes research and publications requirements, can be promoted above the rank of attending physician.

As doctors progress in rank and experience, they spend less time in the inpatient wards and more time in the outpatient clinics. Like a hospital of Western medicine, junior doctors   the residents and attending physicians — shoulder most of the labor-intensive burden of inpatient care. Senior doctors — the assistant chief and chief physicians—conduct rounds twice a week. They supervise junior doctors, especially with regard to serious and difficult patients. As their workload diminishes in the inpatient wards, it increases in the outpatient clinics, where the doctor's greatest asset, his or her clinical experience, is put to its greatest use. The doctor, the patient, and the hospital all profit from this arrangement. Because "registration fees" increase with rank and reputation and doctors receive a portion of these fees, the most famous doctors of Chinese medicine will continue seeing patients in the outpatient clinic for many years after they have retired, sometimes well into their eighties and even nineties.[11]

This sort of career trajectory of slowly progressing from inpatient to outpatient care, from predominantly Western medicine care to predominantly Chinese medicine care, is certainly one very reasonable way of structuring the division of labor in the Chinese medicine hospital. It offers a pragmatic solution to the multiple demands that confront the hospital. First, it provides competent training for its junior doctors and efficiently distributes the burdens of institutional medical care. Junior doctors learn both Western medicine and Chinese medicine under the tutelage of senior physicians. They master Western medicine first, making them far less likely to "misdiagnose" a patient, one of the greatest fears of a young Chinese medicine practitioner. As attending physicians, junior doctors begin to develop more competency in Chinese medicine. They are given more responsibility for the Chinese medicine prescriptions in the inpatient wards and are scheduled to work in outpatient clinics. At the same time, senior doctors are relieved of the more intensive daily labor of caring for patients in the wards. They supervise the junior doctors and focus on the critically ill and hard-to-treat patients. They devote more time to research and the more lucrative work of the outpatient clinic.

Second, the standard career trajectory also satisfies the demands of the patients and the needs of the healthcare system in general. Not every patient comes to a Chinese medicine hospital seeking Chinese medicine care. Some have simply come to the nearest hospital covered by their insurance plans. Even those that come for Chinese medicine care still want a Western medicine diagnosis. As one teacher told me, a biomedical diagnosis was still necessary in the outpatient clinic, even if not strictly required by the hospital. "You must give patients an explanation [of what is going on clinically]" (*yao gei yige jiaodai*). Only a biomedical diagnosis was considered sufficient to this task.

Although there is much pragmatism embodied in the current institutional structures of Chinese medicine hospitals, the power structures of these institutions are such that they defer rather than promote Chinese medicine. To paraphrase my teacher Dr. Sun Pei, Chinese medicine hospitals produce good doctors, but not necessarily good doctors of Chinese medicine.

Accelerating Careers

The patterns of deferral that are built into the typical career trajectory of a hospital doctor are being exacerbated by the growing opportunity and perceived need to pursue an advanced graduate degree in Chinese medicine. Young doctors like Tao Yufang and Huang Fan who have tested into graduate programs can accelerate their rise through the ranks of physicians. Chinese medicine graduate school degrees are part of a growing emphasis on professionalism in the field of Chinese medicine. Before the end of the Cultural Revolution, there were no graduate degrees offered to Chinese medicine doctors. Furthermore, during the Cultural Revolution, the undergraduate system of medical education that was established in the 1950s and 1960s was dramatically reoriented toward the more pragmatic needs of workers and peasants. In the countryside, barefoot doctors were trained in short three- to six-month courses. In the cities, medical college curriculums were reduced to three years, with a strong emphasis on learning through practice. In 1978, Deng Xiaoping's reform of the education system restored competitive undergraduate programs and introduced graduate programs into Chinese medicine education.

The emphasis on professionalism over egalitarianism in the post-Mao era has led to a growing emphasis on educational degrees as a way to achieve higher professional rank but has not necessarily elevated the clinical skills of young doctors. During one of our first clinical observation assignments during our third year of classes, I witnessed an example of this contradiction at Gulou Chinese Medicine Hospital, a small district hospital in one of the old parts of Beijing. As students in the outpatient clinic of the Acupuncture Department, it was easy to see that Dr. Ge was the most popular doctor in the clinic. From the moment he walked into the clinic at 8 A.M. until his lunch break, he treated a continuous stream of devoted patients, sometimes more than thirty individuals in a morning. While Dr. Ge was quickly moving from one patient to the next, his colleagues stood idly by. Dr. Zhang, the next-most-popular doctor, would see a handful of patients in a morning, and the other young doctors typically didn't have any at all. In his early fifties, Dr. Ge was not only the best and most experienced acupuncturist, but also the most senior member of the department. Yet despite all these attributes, he had not been selected as the chief of the department. Dr. Zhang, who was just thirty-nine years old at the time, held that title. Dr. Zhang openly recognized Dr. Ge as the superior clinician and the rightful chief. But because he lacked a formal medical degree, new hospital rules prevented him from attaining this position. Like many youths during the Cultural Revolution, Dr. Ge had only finished middle school and had later learned medicine as a barefoot doctor, gradually acquiring his skills through practice in accordance with the prevailing educational doctrines of the time. In contrast, Dr. Zhang came of age after the Cultural Revolution, when higher educational degrees had been restored. She had a bachelor's degree in Chinese medicine from the Beijing University of Chinese Medicine, which ultimately helped her secure her professional rank.

Although Dr. Ge's case is tied to the unique events of the Cultural Revolution, it is instructive for the challenges of professionalization that I witnessed during my training. One of the main enticements of a graduate school degree, especially a Ph.D., was that it allowed students to join hospital staff at the level of attending physician. Thus, with six years of graduate studies, a doctor could attain the same rank as his or her counterparts who have worked their way up the hospital career ladder. In addition, Ph.D. holders are also well positioned for rapid promotions because of their new research and publication skills. At Dongzhimen Hospital, I heard a good deal of resentment about attending physicians who had attained their rank though this kind of "shortcut," the most common retort being that these doctors have little or no clinical experience. On a return visit to the Gerontology Department at Dongzhimen Hospital in 2002, I discovered that established attending physicians were responding to this trend by enrolling as "part-time graduate students," completing Ph.D. degrees while they continued working their day jobs. In the two years since I had trained in the department, three of the attending physicans in the department had become advisees to the department chair, Tian Jinzhou.

One of the important and potentially positive consequences of this emphasis on postgraduate degrees is that it is producing new networks of doctors and students. The impact on students can vary widely depending on their advisor. Because of the growing emphasis on professionalism, advisors will recruit graduate students into their research programs. The students rarely pursue their own research topics but rather are enlisted in the collective research enterprises of their advisors. These research projects tend to be dominated by the methodologies of Western science and medicine, focusing on clinical trials or laboratory research. If, however, the student's advisor is a clinician, the student will also have an invaluable opportunity to learn some of the advisor's clinical expertise by assisting in the clinic. Reputable and energetic doctors may train large networks of students, constituting something akin to the premodern lineages of masters and disciplines. As they rise to ever higher and more prestigious positions, they inevitably bring their new lineages of advisees and graduate students with them. The late Dong Jianhua (董建华), one of the leading physicians who helped to establish Dongzhimen Hospital, successfully trained a large number of graduate students in this way. Many of them had become the leading doctors and administrators at the hospital when I was doing my training there. I frequently heard these doctors speak in glowing terms about their former advisor.

Although a large and growing number of elite physicians at Chinese medicine institutions are actively involved in medical research, there are a considerable number of doctors who question the merits of current research protocols for Chinese medicine. Indeed, they suggest that current graduate school training often takes young doctors away from the more important task of developing solid clinical skills. While I was doing my clerkship in the Emergency Medicine Department at Dongzhimen Hospital, I once heard Dr. Liu Qingquan, head of the department, scold a group of the young graduate students about the merits of their research with the following sarcastic harangue.

> Transmitting [experience] is extremely important to Chinese medicine. The older generation of doctors [the first generation of academytrained physicians], like Tian Delu [a student of Dong Jianhua] and Lu Renhe, really have a good foundation in Chinese medicine. They pass a portion of their knowledge on to their graduate students. Because their graduate students lack that same solid foundation in the theory of Chinese medicine, they can only pass on a portion of their knowledge to the next generation. The result is: the first generation passes on two formulae to the second generation; the second generation passes on one formula to the third; and the third generation just passes on one herb! How many graduate students incorporate the *Inner Canon* or *Essential Prescriptions Worth a Thousand Gold* (千金要方) into their research?

At the moment, I was standing next to a Ph.D. student, who was studying with Tian Jinzhou, who in turned had trained with Dong Jianhua. She listened nervously to this gloomy assessment and seemed to be calculating what percentage of Dong Jianhua's famous clinical skills might be passed on to her. "Dr. Liu, when you put it that way, you make me tremble with anxiety."

Healthy Skepticism

This chapter began with a vignette about two young Chinese medicine doctors and their skepticism toward Chinese medicine. They questioned some of its most cherished practices (pulse taking), its most revered texts (*Inner Canon* and *Treatise on Cold Damage*), and openly expressed their preference for Western medicine. These attitudes are to a great extent the result of the unique postcolonial context of contemporary Chinese medicine practice, in which elite institutions of Chinese medicine, despite their best intentions, marginalize and defer the practice of Chinese medicine. Given the current conditions under which doctors learn and practice Chinese medicine, it is hard to imagine how young doctors could not be infected with a certain amount of skepticism about their own profession.

Not long after finishing my rotation in the Nephrology Department, I had the honor of interviewing the renowned senior physician Yin Huihe (印会河). He surprised me with his critical reflections on the nature of Chinese medicine, but his sharp remarks made me rethink my encounter with Dr. Tao and Dr. Huang. Could their doubts about their own profession be productive, perhaps even important to the future of Chinese medicine? Yin Huihe was the son of a well-known doctor in Jingjiang, Jiangsu Province. He started practicing medicine at age seventeen in 1940. In the mid-1950s, he tested into the Jiangsu School for Advanced Studies in Chinese Medicine, where he became involved with editing *Overview of Chinese Medicine*. Later he became the chief editor of *Basic Theory of Chinese Medicine* for the third (the first time this textbook was published), fourth, and fifth editions of this national textbook. During his career, he taught at the Beijing College of Chinese Medicine and worked at the affiliated teaching hospital, Dongzhimen Hospital. In the early 1980s, he was transferred to the Sino-Japanese Hospital, a new hospital that was supposed to have both cutting-edge Chinese medicine and Western medicine services. This hospital was originally designed to be a second affiliated hospital to the Beijing College of Chinese Medicine, but not long after completion it was "taken over" administratively by the Ministry of Health, and its orientation gradually shifted toward Western medicine.

In the 1990s, Yin Huihe and Jiao Shude were the two most prominent doctors of Chinese medicine at the Sino-Japanese Hospital. Both had national reputations as physicians and had made significant contributions to their shared profession. At the same time, they were clearly competitors. Jiao Shude presented himself as a traditionalist, the ultimate champion of a pure Chinese medicine theory and practice, as we saw in Chapter 2. "Nothing is above *bianzheng lunzhi*," he told me. Yet he had also trained as a Western medicine doctor and graduated in 1958 from the prestigious first "integrated medicine" class at the China Academy of Chinese Medicine. Yin Huihe was from a well-known family of Chinese medicine doctors. Despite his very traditional training, he caused considerable controversy when he later declared that integrated medicine was the only way forward for Chinese medicine. I conclude this chapter with excerpts from my interview with Yin Huihe because of the striking similarity of his views to those of Tao Yufang and Huang Fan. Like Tao and Huang, Yin Huihe was extremely skeptical of many of the traditions within Chinese medicine. But unlike Tao and Huang, he had a lifetime of clinical experience behind him. Despite publicly proclaiming his allegiance to integrated medicine, he privately told me that he had never prescribed a single Western medicine drug in his life. Of all the many doctors I had the honor of interviewing, there was probably no one with a more remarkable pedigree in Chinese medicine who expressed such contrarian opinions about his own profession. His words remind us of the complicated ways in which doctors must negotiate the relationship between Chinese and Western medicine in contemporary China.

> YHH: Actually, I began by studying the *Inner Canon*. But now I don't consider the *Inner Canon* to be a Chinese medicine book. It's an encyclopedia. It contains a lot of things, including Chinese medicine . . . which later generations advanced. The *Inner Canon* that you see [in textbooks] is basically selections, an excerpt from here, an excerpt from there. . . . Nobody teaches the entire *Inner Canon*. This shows that my opinion is not necessarily wrong.

A quick smile broke through his scowl.

I had not been prepared to hear these kinds of heretical claims from a renowned doctor. I wondered how he could have been the chief editor of *Basic Theory of Chinese Medicine*, the essential first textbook for every student of Chinese medicine, while also having such a critical attitude toward the *Inner Canon*. That textbook was to a large extent a distillation of concepts and principles found in the *Inner Canon*. I asked him to explain the apparent contradiction, and he shrugged his shoulders. "[That work was just] editing a textbook." I pressed further.

> EIK: When you were editing *Overview of Chinese Medicine* and *Basic Theory of Chinese Medicine*, you were not relying entirely on the *Inner Canon*, were you?
> YHH: Of course, not. You can't depend entirely on the *Inner Canon*.
> EIK: If you can't rely on the *Inner Canon*, what texts can you rely on?
> YHH: The supplementary scholarship of the later generations. . . .
> The *Inner Canon* was the earliest. But without the developments of the later generations, it is not worth a cent. How could there not be developments? Science moves forward. Some people think the four canons are the highest. That's nonsense. . . . *Essentials of the Golden Casket* is one of the four canons. . . . You have read three volumes. There are another three volumes that you haven't read. I have read them. They are even more atrocious [than the other

canons]. For example, "crown of heavenly efficacy" (天靈蓋), the skull of a corpse, is considered a medicine. . . . The rope used to hang a man is considered a medicine. That's ridiculous, not even worth discussing.

Yin Huihe also placed a great value on the role of Western medicine in clinical work.

> YHH: The reason I took the path of integrating Chinese and Western medicine is that I was forced to take it. I was the first director of the Internal Medicine Department and Medical Affairs Division at the Beijing College of Chinese Medicine. When patients are admitted [to the hospital], it is not like the outpatient clinic. In the outpatient clinic, they can walk away. In the wards, they come looking for you, if you don't help them. Every day, they come looking for you. What can you do? If you depend entirely on what the ancestors have left us, it is not enough. Besides, there are many illnesses that don't even have symptoms, and they are serious illnesses. . . . The only thing you can do is take the path of Western medicine. So, I studied some. Not enough to be a Western medicine doctor. But it is much better if you know some. At least, you know which illnesses are serious and can stay out of trouble.

On October 30, a little more than two weeks after she was admitted to this hospital, Dong Chunhua had an unexpected episode of heart palpitations. Her heart rate raced to 190 beats per minute, and her blood pressure fell to 90/60 mm Hg. Because Dr. Huang had been assigned to a new section of beds, Dr. Tao was the responsible physician when this event took place. Scrambling to bring the situation under control, he called an attending physician for help, who in turn administered a 40ml IV infusion of glucose 25% in water with 5ml of verapamil hydrochloride (a calcium channel blocker) and gave Dong Chunhua an oxygen mask. Although Dong Chunhua's vital signs soon returned to normal, her confidence had been broken. At the urging of her family but against the recommendations of her doctors, she requested to be discharged from the hospital that day. During her short stay in the hospital, there had been some slight improvements in her condition. But these changes were too preliminary to know whether she might have benefited from a longer stay. Ironically, it is quite possible that the heart palpitations that cut short her hospital stay may have been caused by one of her Western medicine therapies. In July 2000, just a few months before Dong Chuanhua was admitted to the hospital, Janssen Pharmaceutica, the makers of cisapride, voluntarily removed this drug from the U.S. pharmaceutical market because the FDA had issued a warning letter that this drug could cause cardiac arrhythmias in some patients. Cisapride is still used in many countries for promoting digestion, but doctors in China now use it much more conservatively.

Dong Chunhua's case is a typical example of medical care in a Chinese medicine hospital. Like many stays in hospitals around the world, it came to an ambiguous conclusion. The medical attention she received was good but could have been better, especially since her doctors never fully accounted for her sudden weight loss (10 kilograms in a month). It is possible that a more systematic approach to this problem may have led to treatments, perhaps Chinese medicine treatments, which did not include the use of cisapride and might have avoided the unfortunate incident of cardiac arrhythmias.

This case illustrates how contemporary doctors of Chinese medicine have adopted their craft to the power asymmetries of the Chinese medicine hospital. Today Chinese medicine physicians must learn two types of medicine; Western medicine physicians are required to master only one. Since the 1950s, there has been a steady trend for Chinese medicine doctors to achieve ever-greater competency in Western medicine, even at the cost of sacrificing skills in Chinese medicine. *Bianzheng lunzhi* is the methodology that emerged together with the disease-pattern dualism in the Communist era. Doctors use *bianzheng lunzhi* not only for prescribing Chinese medicine therapies (what I have called the pattern-centered modality), but also as a technology for negotiating the relationship with Western medicine therapies (the disease-centered modality). In the case of Dong Chunhua, we can see how *bianzheng lunzhi* serves to integrate Chinese medicine into the conventions of inpatient care in a Chinese medicine hospital. This integration is achieved, perhaps ironically, by privileging Western medicine and marginalizing Chinese medicine.

When considered from the perspective of the disease-pattern dualism, we can see how *bianzheng lunzhi* is an invaluable tool for organizing patient care and translating between the worlds of Western medicine and Chinese medicine. At the same time, the practice of double diagnosis and double therapies has pushed the "therapeutic range" of Chinese medicine to the margins—to the chronic, the functional, and the hard to treat. Wherever effective biomedical therapies exist, Chinese medicine must seemingly "stand to the side." That does not mean that Chinese medicine is a mere bystander, however. In fact, it is quite possible that Dong Chunhua could have benefitted considerably from Chinese medicine therapies. But the marginalization and deferral of Chinese medicine in the inpatient wards meant that she never got to experience these potential benefits before her stay was cut short. Nonetheless, one might reasonably ask whether *bianzheng lunzhi*, the methodology that all doctors of Chinese medicine celebrate as the quintessence of their practice, leads to an impoverished form of clinical medicine. In Chapter 6, we will turn to the role of clinical virtuosity, showing how *bianzheng lunzhi* can also form the basis for innovative, dynamic forms of clinical practice.

6

Prescriptions for Virtuosity

Bianzheng lunzhi is one of the key innovations in contemporary Chinese medicine practice. That Chinese medicine exists as a major healthcare institution in mainland China and as alternative means of health care in numerous countries around the globe is in no small part because of the development of *bianzheng lunzhi* as the central clinical methodology of Chinese medicine. The claim that *bianzheng lunzhi* is the "essence" of Chinese medicine is perhaps not historically accurate, but it does indeed capture its paramount significance to contemporary practice. But at the same time, *bianzheng lunzhi* is also a problematic clinical methodology. In the inpatient wards of Chinese medicine hospitals, *bianzheng lunzhi* defers the use of Chinese medicine until a Western medicine diagnosis and therapy have been carried out first. The therapeutic range of Chinese medicine seems to be increasingly limited to the marginal areas of medical care not yet dominated by Western medicine. As a result, junior doctors feel that it is more important to learn Western medicine than it is to master the diagnostic and therapeutic subtleties of Chinese medicine. How can we reconcile these two contradictory assessments of *bianzheng lunzhi*? What does this postcolonial predicament mean for the future of Chinese medicine? In this chapter, I will explore these questions through a case study that was recounted to me by Dr. Sun Pei, the same teacher that we encountered in the Introduction.

This case study is a story of two doctors, the first a respected senior physician, the second a young, inexperienced doctor, who both struggle over the correct way to treat a patient. Although there are many possible ways to analyze this story, I have chosen to emphasize two themes of particular relevance to this narrative. First, this is a story of the transformation of contemporary

Chinese medicine practice. The unique clinical dynamics of this case pit two doctors of different generations with different clinical methodologies against each other. At the risk of being too simplistic, I have characterized the older doctor as representing a "canonical approach," a style of medical practice still prevalent in the Republican era. In contrast, I depict the younger doctor as representing a "textbook approach," using the Communist-era methodology of *bianzheng lunzhi*. Neither of these characterizations is entirely accurate, but they do capture an important difference between the two doctors. My purpose is to further highlight the uniqueness of *bianzheng lunzhi*. But unlike the discussion of Chapter 5, in which *bianzheng lunzhi* seems to participate in the marginalization of Chinese medicine, this case study illuminates some of the innovative potentials of this methodology.

Second, this is a story of clinical virtuosity, of how practice always surpasses the practitioner, of how certain small actions can have surprising, even exhilarating effects. While virtuosity is valued in any medical practice, it is particularly cherished in Chinese medicine (Farquhar 1994). Yet for most practitioners, virtuosity is elusive, hard to obtain, and beyond understanding. It is thought to be ineffable, and its results are imagined to be magical. But if we think of virtuosity as simply a special form of "action," it becomes less mysterious, although no less wondrous. As Bruno Latour has argued, there is always "a slight surprise to action."

> Whenever we make something, *we* are not in command, we are slightly *overtaken* by the action: every builder knows that. . . . That which overtakes us is *also*, because of our agency, because of the *clinamen* of our action, slightly overtaken, modified. . . . I never *act*; I am always slightly surprised by what I do. That which acts through me is also surprised by what I do, by the chance to mutate, to change, and to bifurcate. . . . We are surprised by what we make even when we have, even when we believe we have, complete mastery [original emphasis] (Latour 1999, 281{nd}83).

In the following case, we are confronted with the inherent limitations of any clinical methodology. The direct application of medical theory to individual patients may work on occasion, but it is rarely sufficient in complex cases. No matter how extensive one's knowledge of medicine may be, the successful treatment of a patient is never guaranteed and is always unexpected to some degree. As the two main characters of our story remind us, clinical efficacy is never merely a matter of correct theory. It is always the result of surprising action, and sometimes of virtuoso practice.

Dr. Sun, the young, inexperienced doctor that represents the "textbook approach" in this particular case, was one of my professors at the Beijing University of Chinese Medicine. At the time this story took place, however, he had not yet received his formal training in a college of Chinese medicine. This fact would seem to make him a poor example of textbook Chinese medicine, but as we will see, the conditions of his early medical education were such that he could not have reasonably known any alternative form of Chinese medicine practice. Dr. Sun began practicing medicine during the Cultural Revolution when higher education institutes were either closed or only open to a select number of students with the proper class background. He happened upon another avenue of development during this tumultuous time, becoming a "barefoot doctor."

> I really began to practice medicine after I joined a brigade. I happened to finish middle school after the Cultural Revolution had already begun, and I was sent to the countryside to join a brigade. My Chinese medicine practice really began in the countryside, where I was a barefoot doctor. I was part of the brigade for seven, nearly eight years. The entire time I treated the local folks, practicing and studying medicine at the same time.[1]

Although the Communist state had been quite successful in making basic public health services available to a wider populace in the early years of the People's Republic, the preponderance of healthcare resources—schools, hospitals, research institutes—remained concentrated in urban centers. The barefoot doctor program was an attempt to ameliorate this imbalance by rapidly training a new corps of healthcare workers to provide the rudiments of basic medicine to the rural population. The basic administration and socioeconomic unit of the Chinese countryside during this period was the commune, the rough equivalent of several villages today. Each commune selected a small number of individuals to receive the standard three to six months of medical training for the barefoot doctor program. Affluent communes might be able to afford more, but the poorest failed to provide even the minimum. In keeping with the prevailing Maoist ideology of the era, training emphasized practice over expertise.

Dr. Sun was a more well-rounded and capable physician than the average barefoot doctor. In his work, he was aided by the fact that both his father and grandfather were Chinese medicine practitioners. His father, in particular, was an important influence, providing guidance during this period, usually by correspondence. Standard training for barefoot doctors emphasized the importance of "integrated medicine" and was taught through special hybrid manuals that blended the basics of both Western medicine and Chinese medicine. But Dr. Sun's father instructed him to rely on Chinese medicine texts such as the *Overview of Chinese Medicine*. During our interview, Dr. Sun repeatedly claimed his clinical style was learned (*zuchuan*) from his father. But during this early stage in his career, when he was separated from his father, the *Overview* was a much more important influence for his everyday clinical work. For this reason, I have designated Dr. Sun's approach in the case below as a standard "textbook approach."

> At the time the book that was most influential for me was *Overview of Chinese Medicine*. It was a general summary of many aspects [of Chinese medicine]. But it was an introductory book (*qimengshu*). My father told me to study this book in order to get a general understanding of Chinese medicine. I also read many other books. But I always felt like I was missing the point. The more books I studied, the less I knew how to treat my patients. This was the situation in my early years of study. As a result, whenever I was unsure how to treat a patient, I would write a letter to my father for advice. My father would tell me the [treatment] method and where to find a discussion of this method. It was very strange. The book would be lying right in front me, but for some reason I hadn't realized that the theoretical or therapeutic references that it contained were just the ones I had been looking for.[2]

Written in 1958, the *Overview of Chinese Medicine* was the first textbook of Chinese medicine designed for use in nationwide medical curriculums. Designed for "courses of Chinese medicine in colleges of Western medicine, for review by less advanced doctors of Chinese medicine, or to show young enthusiasts for Chinese medicine the correct path forward" (Nanjing Zhongyi Xueyuan 1958, 1), Sun Pei very much fit its intended audience. Although simpler than the national textbooks, the *Overview* was certainly more sophisticated than barefoot doctor manuals of that era. It is also likely that Sun Pei may have actually been reading the *Revised Overview of Chinese Medicine* (新编中医学概论), which was published during the Cultural Revolution in 1972. If so, this version would have even more an exemplar of the emergent paradigm of *bianzheng lunzhi*.

In spite of the attempts to make this textbook accessible to the nonspecialist, the young Dr. Sun still encountered many frustrations. His confusions were probably similar to those of my classmates, who often felt the world of Chinese medicine foreign and the presentations of the textbooks formulaic. But Dr. Sun's father encouraged his son to continue working with this textbook. He explained that confusion was normal, perhaps even intrinsic to the study of Chinese medicine. In order to overcome one's confusion one had to learn how to achieve virtuosity.

When I finished my stint with the brigade and returned to Beijing, I asked my father [about my problems with the *Overview*]. My father said, "This [book] is just to build a foundation. A real Chinese medicine doctor can't be made with this book. You have read much, but clinically don't know how to use it. That's normal. Only with practice, can you make it your own (*bian wei ziji de*; 变为自己的). Because you haven't made it your own, you don't know how to find the appropriate information [in this book]. But reading is essential. You can't make something your own, if you don't know of it or have never heard of it."[3]

To become a virtuoso Chinese medicine doctor is to learn how to "make a text your own." The problem is not in the text itself, but in how one reads it. For Dr. Sun's father, the *Overview*, as well as any other important Chinese medicine text, cannot be read as a transparent medium of knowledge, as a vehicle of medical information that can be applied directly to each individual clinical situation. The act of reading cannot be divorced from practice. To grasp an important text is to "make it one's own," to embody it through practice, to allow it to act through you. But it is not until Dr. Sun encounters the other main character in this story, Dr. Song, that he fully comprehends this lesson.

Dr. Song worked in the Chinese medicine department of a small street-level Western medicine hospital, Guangnei Hospital (广内医院), in the Xuanwu District in the southeast of Beijing. He was well known in this district as a specialist in the "Cold Damage School" and would often lecture locally on the *Treatise on Cold Damage*. After returning to Beijing at the end of the Cultural Revolution, Dr. Sun was assigned to the Chinese medicine department of Guangnei Hospital, where he worked for the next two years under the supervision of Dr. Song. The two doctors would sit across from each other at a large consultation table, permitting both doctors to see patients individually, while also allowing Dr. Song to offer guidance to Dr. Sun when needed. This close spatial proximity, which I also observed in the outpatient clinics of Dongzhimen Hospital, was one of the essential ingredients in this case. It allowed both doctors to see the same patient, take turns treating her, and observe each other's treatments.

Dr. Sun remembers his two years of working with Dr. Song as one of the most fruitful learning experiences of his life. But it was also one of the most challenging because of Dr. Song's different clinical style. As a specialist in the *Treatise on Cold Damage*, Dr. Song relied primarily on the "canonical formulas" that are found in this text and Zhang Zhongjing's other treatise, *Essentials from the Golden Casket*. Dr. Sun himself had not even read the canons at this time and was unsure of how to use "canonical formulas." In his eight years of work as a barefoot doctor, Dr. Sun had learned to practice Chinese medicine through the guidance of his father and standardized textbooks, such as the *Overview*. Moreover, his father was partial to "contemporary formulas" (时方), popular formulas from the Tang dynasty and later that do not derive from Zhang Zhongjing. While textbooks do use some of the canonical formulas alongside the most popular of the "contemporary formulas" from the late imperial period, they do so within the framework of *bianzheng lunzhi*. The formulas are divorced from their presentations in the canons themselves.

Dr. Sun's father was clearly aware of these differences in clinical approach. Although he had previously not allowed his son to read the canons, he now encouraged it. Dr. Sun recalled his struggles with these difficult texts.

> The old doctor . . . often mentioned the *Treatise on Cold Damage* and the *Inner Canon*. But I had never really read these two books before. So at this time my father said to me, "You can now read these two books. But don't ask questions. First read them through and try to understand them yourself. When you really can't understand, then you can ask Dr. Song or come back to ask me. That's how you should study." I did what he said, . . . but to be honest the more I read, the harder it got. . . . Why? Because the language is abstruse and because they didn't seem to correspond to [the reality of] clinical practice. In particular, I couldn't find any actual medical cases . . . that seemed to match the descriptions in *Treatise on Cold Damage*. I had spent all this time reading it, but I couldn't find any appropriate patients, so I couldn't use it.

Like many contemporary students of Chinese medicine, Dr. Sun found reading the canons a difficult, even unrewarding, task. Whereas he had once struggled with the clinical relevance of the *Overview*, he now faced a challenge of even greater magnitude with the canons. Although Chinese medicine textbooks appear foreign to the novice, they are nonetheless well-organized, systemic presentations in modern vernacular Chinese. The canons, as we will see, have a looser framework and a far more difficult writing style. They are open to and have been subject to wide-ranging interpretations by generations of scholars.

> The strange thing was that Dr. Song used the prescriptions from the *Treatise on Cold Damage*, but not according to the diseases described in the *Treatise*. He used the *Treatise* to treat all kinds of internal diseases, to treat anything, including some contagious diseases. To me, this was very peculiar. According to my understanding at the time, the

Treatise was a book about the treatment of contagious, febrile disease.
I thought this is what it claimed to be. There were parts that addressed
internal disease, but they were secondary. Yet the old doctor used it to
treat all kinds of internal diseases. He treated everything with the *Treatise* formulas. It seemed what the book said and what he did were not
the same. . . . I couldn't understand what the old doctor was doing, so I
went to ask my father. My father said, "Chinese medicine is profound.
Any single book summarizes the experiences of a doctor's entire life.
Don't limit yourself to thinking that it is specific to the treatment of a
certain disease. In one book, a doctor must touch upon all his practical
experience. As long as you embody (*tihui*; 体会) it properly, a single
book can make you into a doctor." At the time, I didn't really understand what he was saying.

Dr. Sun made these observations about his own training, the clinical practice of Dr. Song, and his father's advice, independently of the clinical case
we are about to explore. I have recounted his reflections at length because
they illuminate the challenge of learning Chinese medicine in contemporary
China and remind us of the hard work required to "make a text one's own,"
to achieve understanding through embodiment. The following case is unique
not because it describes a pioneering treatment for a rare and hard-to-treat
disease but because it involves two doctors using two completely disparate
treatments for a rather mundane medical problem. Confronted with the same
patient, Dr. Sun adopted a "textbook approach," and Dr. Song adhered to his
"canonical approach."[4] The unfortunate patient, who was buffeted back and
forth, had no choice in the matter. Cultural Revolution regulations intended
to suppress "individualism" prevented her from choosing one doctor over another. Strict limitations on the amount of medicine that could be prescribed
at any one time (a maximum of three days' worth) meant that the luck of the
draw sent her alternately back and forth between the two doctors. Dr. Sun saw
the patient first.

One of the cases [that influenced me most strongly] occurred when
I was working with Dr. Song. . . . This patient was a woman, twenty-
three years old. Her illness was what in Western medicine is called
an acute suppurative tonsillitis. In Chinese medicine, it is called
"Milk Moths" (乳蛾), because the purulent tonsils look like white
moths[5]. . . . I was sitting opposite the old doctor. We were both calling
numbers and seeing patients. On the first occasion, this patient ended
up on my side [of the consultation desk] Because of my family background, I had some experience with this disease. I knew how to treat

it. I wrote her a prescription based on [the formula] Lonicera and Forsythia Powder (*Yin Qiao San*), adding a few more herbs to clear and
relieve the throat. . . . Much in the same way that we use Lonicera and
Forsythia Powder to treat Gan Mao (感冒) [the Chinese medicine *bing*
roughly equivalent to the common cold] . . . with a wind heat pattern
and a sore throat. In fact, this kind of Gan Mao is just an early stage [of
acute suppurative tonsillitis] that hasn't become purulent yet.[6]

Although Dr. Sun credits his father as the inspiration for his choice of formula, Lonicera and Forsythia Powder is a standard textbook recommendation
for the treatment of acute suppurative tonsillitis and a famous Warm Disorders
formula created by Wu Jutong, one of the founding figures of the current
(Scheid et al. 2009 [1990], 36–38). In the *Revised Overview of Chinese Medicine*, Lonicera and Forsythia Powder was the indicated formula for both the
wind heat pattern of Gan Mao and the wind heat pattern of acute tonsillitis
(Guangzhou Army Rear-Service Unit Health Department 1973, 402, 679).
Compared to the original *Overview*, the *Revised Overview* is a more explicitly
"integrated medicine" text, combining Western medicine disease categories,
such as acute tonsillitis, and Chinese medicine patterns and formulas in its
therapy section. Although Dr. Sun's choice of formula may indeed reflect
family traditions, it was also completely consistent with the standards of institutionalized Chinese medicine at the time.

On the patient's second consultation, she happened to draw Dr. Song's
number. His approach to her illness could not have diverged more drastically
from the standard textbook approach of Dr. Sun. If the patient had responded
poorly to Dr. Sun's initial treatment, it would have been considered appropriate for any doctor to attempt a new approach. But on her second consultation
three days later, the patient appeared to be responding well to Dr. Sun's therapy. Nonetheless, Dr. Song chose to diverge from Dr. Sun's treatment and
follow his usual approach.

> Three days later, blood work showed that the patient's white blood
> cell count had dropped from over 12,000 to 11,000 plus.[7] Her primary
> complaint of throat pain had clearly diminished. There was also less
> pus. Originally, the patient had come early [in the disease process]
> and there had not been lot of pus, only spots not entire patches. After
> having taken three days of my Lonicera and Forsythia Powder prescrip-
> tion, the pus had been clearly reduced but the tonsils were still red.
> But on this second visit, it just so happened that when her number
> was called it was the old doctor's turn. At that time, patients were not
> allowed to select physicians. Not like today when you can take any-

one's number you want. At that time, the nurses assigned the numbers. Whoever got your number that was who treated you. Promotion of the individual was not permitted, so randomness was emphasized. Even though she was assigned to the old doctor, I was of course still very interested. The changes I just mentioned were the ones that I saw when the old doctor did his exam. He intentionally let me see them because he was also my teacher.

Now, can you guess what the old doctor prescribed? Ephedra, Aconite, Asarum Decoction (*Ma Huang Fu Zi Xi Xin Tang*)! Except he replaced Ephedra (*Ma Huang*) with Pinellia (*Ban Xia*), making it Pinellia, Aconite, Asarum Decoction (*Ban Xia Fu Zi Xi Xin Tang*)! And remember Pinellia and Aconite are "opposed herbs (反药)" . . . so the old doctor had to put a special signature on the prescription because of it! This was the first time I had seen the old doctor use "opposed herbs." My father had made me memorize the "eighteen oppositions" (十八反) and "nineteen antagonisms" (十九畏) [He told me that] it doesn't matter whether my treatments are good or bad, don't risk causing problems by using opposed herbs together.[8]

We can't know why Dr. Song chose to abandon the treatment plan initiated by Dr. Sun. Perhaps, he was simply more confident using "canonical formulas"; maybe he intended his change of course as a lesson for his young student. Regardless of the reasons, Dr. Song's prescription was shocking to Dr. Sun for several reasons that need to be explained in some detail.

First, Dr. Song had indeed chosen to treat the patient with a canonical formula, but it was a surprising if not perplexing choice. In the *Treatise on Cold Damage Disorder*, the one passage that discusses the use of Ephedra, Aconite, Asarum Decoction, gives no indication that it would be suitable for the Western medicine disease of acute tonsillitis. Line 301 reads:

Minor yin condition, just contracted, unexpectedly feverish, sinking pulse. Manage it with Ephedra, Asarum, Aconite Decoction.[9]

We do not have to delve into the great intricacies of *Treatise* scholarship to quickly grasp that the illness described in this passage is quite remote from the conditions of the twenty-three-year-old patient. She was feverish as most acute tonsillitis patients are, but not "unexpectedly" so. She had recently contracted her illness, but she had not "just contracted" it, a state that the *Treatise* distinguishes from a patient's condition after treatment. Her pulse, not mentioned by Dr. Sun, was most likely fast because of the acute, febrile nature of her illness and probably not "sinking," which would suggest the illness had moved to the interior. Lastly, "minor yin condition" is associated with profound constitutional weakness and serious deficiencies. But the patient's constitution seemed robust. Her main symptoms—sore throat and swollen, red, purulent tonsils—together with her response to the two different treatments reflect the response of a healthy individual, not the weakened state one of someone with "minor yin condition." Not a single one of the four main symptoms for Ephedra, Aconite, Asarum Decoction seemed to correspond to the patient's condition. No wonder Dr. Sun found Dr. Song's use of *Treatise* formulas bewildering!

Second, Dr. Song had modified this prescription in an apparently dangerous way. By replacing Ephedra with Pinellia, he was using a formula that had two "opposed herbs"—Pinellia and Aconite. The concept of "opposed herbs" refers to specific pairs of herbs—known as the "eighteen oppositions" (and to a lesser degree the "nineteen antagonisms")—that when used in combination are thought to seriously endanger the health of a patient. As Dr. Sun also noted in the interview, not all doctors agree on the actual dangers of these prohibitions, but most would only defy them in special situations, if at all.[10]

Lastly and perhaps most importantly, Dr. Song's choice of formula and herb modifications seemed to contradict the conventional Chinese medicine diagnosis of this illness. Dr. Sun had identified the patient as having a pattern of wind and heat, which would normally be treated with "pungent," "cold" herbs, such as Lonicera and Forsythia Powder. The positive results from the first three days of treatment suggest that Dr. Sun's diagnosis had been correct. Therefore, anything more than a slight modification of the prescription at this point would have been superfluous and potentially counterproductive. Dr. Song's Pinellia, Aconite, Asarum Decoction contained "pungent" and "hot" herbs. It had completely altered one of the key properties of Dr. Sun's Lonicera and Forsythia Powder. Dr. Song was apparently using heat to treat heat, defying one of the core principles of the *Inner Canon* that heat should be treated with cold (热者寒之). One could only expect that Dr. Song's formula would exacerbate the patient's primary symptoms of heat—fever, sore throat, and swollen tonsils.

On the third visit, the patient was once again assigned to Dr. Song. Her condition had indeed worsened. Dr. Sun felt his original diagnosis and treatment had been proven correct.

> Three days later, the patient returned for her third consultation. At that time, we were only allowed to write prescriptions for 3 days, not like today where you can write them for 7 days should the patient's condition call for it. . . . The patient ended up with the old doctor

again. Her white blood cell count was 15,000; the tonsils were fully purulent. Previously, there had only been spots of pus, but now they were
covered in pus. During the last 3 days, the patient had had moments
of intense pain, although it had not been too bad the last two days. But
the fever was higher. On the first visit, her fever had just been a little
over 37°C, 38°C at the highest. It hadn't reached 38°C after taking
my prescription. Now the basic temperature was 38°C, occasionally
spiking to 39°C. Naturally, I assumed the old doctor had made a mistake, right? The illness was getting worse! I thought the old doctor had
made a mistake. But in front of the patient, and considering that he
was my teacher, I couldn't say anything. So, I just watched, as the old
doctor said to the patient: "This is the inevitable course of the illness.
Don't worry. I will write a prescription for another 3 days. The fever
will go down and you will feel better." Saying this, the old doctor wrote
out the exact same prescription and the patient left.[11]

With this third consultation, Dr. Sun's assessment seemed to be confirmed.
By all objective measures, his treatment had been correct, and the patient had
improved. Dr. Song's treatment had been wrong, and the patient had gotten
worse. Yet Dr. Song confidently forged ahead with the very treatment that had
caused the patient's condition to worsen, oblivious to the patient's apparent
risk of developing an abscess or other more serious complication.

On the patient's fourth visit, she was randomly assigned to Dr. Sun. But
on this occasion, the patient's condition had not worsened but rather showed
signs of improvement, just as Dr. Song had predicted. All of Dr. Sun's assumptions about this case began to crumble.

On the next visit, the patient was assigned to me. . . . I took a look
to see how she was doing. The white blood cell count was down to
13,000, slightly lower than the last time, but still not as low as it had
been after my first consultation. Her temperature was down, below
38°C. She opened her mouth, and I saw that the large area of pus had
been reduced in half. This improvement had to be due to the last 3
days of herbs. Now, what was I supposed to do? The old doctor was
watching me, but he couldn't say anything, because the rules required
that the patient be seen by whomever she was assigned to see. Furthermore, it was customary among Chinese medicine doctors to never
discuss a treatment in front of a patient in order to avoid animosity or
suspicion among doctors. If you don't understand, you can discuss it
afterwards, but not in front of the patient. What was I supposed to do?
"Opposed herbs," I had never used them before. Did I dare to use the

old doctor's formula? Even if I had known it was all right to use, I still wouldn't have dared to sign for it. I couldn't write the prescription and then ask him to sign it for me. That would be outrageous. Besides I was confused. At first, I thought he had made a mistake, and she should have been getting worse and worse. But the reality was different. She worsened for a bit, but then improved. At last, with no other options, I prescribed Lonicera and Forsythia Powder again. That was all I knew how to do. I wasn't good enough to do anything else, and besides Lonicera and Forsythia Powder was safe. . . . When I finished writing this prescription, I looked up and saw the old doctor just shaking his head.[12]

Torn between two radically different ways of treating the patient, both of which seem to produce positive clinical results, Dr. Sun was confronted with a crisis of scientific authority. In the patient's previous visits, he had applied his textbook approach to this case. His diagnosis of "Milk Moths" (or acute suppurative tonsillitis) caused by wind and heat and his treatment with the cold, pungent Lonicera and Forsythia Powder had been totally consistent with national standards. The patient's response—positive to his treatment and initially negative to Dr. Song's opposing treatment—had demonstrated that his approach was correct. On the other hand, Dr. Song had adopted a canonical approach, although it had been anything but conservative. In fact, everything about it seemed to flout the most basic principles of clinical care. He had used a canonical formula but not according to the indications of the canons. He had then modified this formula in such a way to make it potentially toxic. And lastly, he had ignored a fundamental treatment principle by treating heat with heat. But the patient's response—initially negative but subsequently positive—seemed to also corroborate Dr. Song's approach. At this moment, there was no empirical standard by which to assess these two approaches. In fact, both treatments seem to be correct. Too young and inexperienced to take the risks of his teacher (or perhaps secretly clinging to the hope that his approach was still right), Dr. Sun stuck with his previous course of action. But when the patient returned for the fifth treatment, this crisis of authority had reached an impasse.

Three days later, the patient returned. How was she doing? After taking my Lonicera and Forsythia Powder for 3 days, her white blood cell count was unchanged at 13,000. The pus on her tonsils was improved, but the redness and swelling were much worse. Originally, the redness and swelling had improved together with the pus. But after my last treatment, the white blood cell count was unchanged, the pus was reduced slightly, and the swelling was severe. The patient said that the pain in her throat was excruciating. Her temperature wasn't high, still in the 37–38 degrees Celsius range. Now, it seemed to me that my 3 days of medicine had not had any appreciable effect. This made me even more confused. When I had first treated her with Lonicera and Forsythia Powder, the results were obvious. Somehow it had lost its efficacy after the old doctor's treatment. Could it be that the patient was not a Lonicera and Forsythia Powder pattern? Was it possible that the symptoms of throat pain and swelling were not caused by wind and heat? Why wouldn't it work? Furthermore, I had increased the dosage of Lonicera and Forsythia Powderthis time. In particular, I had used 30 grams of Lonicera, compared to the first time when I had just used the standard amount of 10 grams or so.[13]

At this point, the clash between Dr. Sun's textbook approach and Dr. Song's canonical approach had become so convoluted that it seemed unresolvable. What was originally a simple problem now appeared infinitely complex. The cooling properties of Dr. Sun's Lonicera and Forsythia Powder apparently had been rendered ineffective, if not counterproductive by the warming effects of Dr. Song's Pinellia, Aconite, Asarum Decoction. Likewise, Dr. Song's unconventional "warming" formula now seemed like an even more dangerous choice after Dr. Sun's latest treatment had made the patient's swollen tonsils and throat pain even more intense. With the previous visit, we had arrived at a curious moment in the patient's treatment where the two opposing approaches and formulas seemed equally appropriate. With this visit, we found ourselves in a distressing dilemma where both formulas seemed potentially dangerous. Dr. Sun's intellectual resources had already been exhausted by this point. Fortunately, Dr. Song was given the opportunity to resolve the impasse on this visit.

This time, it just so happened that the patient did not end up with me but with the old doctor. . . . The old doctor looked at me and laughed. Then he closed he eyes and thought and thought. Can guess what prescription he finally wrote? Was it Pinellia, Aconite, Asarum Decoction or Lonicera and Forsythia Powder? One hot, one cold, two diametrically opposed formulas. . . . That's right, he wrote the exact same prescription as me, without changing a single herb or even a single dosage. He sent her away with one day's worth of medicine. On the next visit the pulse was calm, the body cool, the fever down, the white blood count had dropped to 11,000. She was basically better This time, she was assigned to me, and I knew how to wrap things up.

My father had told me that when treating contagious, febrile diseases to finish up with Modified Fragrant Solomonseal Decoction (*Jia Jian Wei Rui Tang*).[14]

At this critical juncture, when the patient's treatment had reached an impasse and the efficacy of both the canonical approach and the textbook approach seemed in doubt, the only solution was not to change a thing. With this intervention, Dr. Song gave the "slight surprise of action" its greatest possible amplitude. He transformed the case from therapeutic impasse to clinical success with the smallest of acts—the same prescription, one more day.

When Dr. Sun finally had a chance to ask his teacher what really was the best approach to treating this case, Dr. Song replied, "Your method could have worked, and my method could have worked." The problem had not been which treatment was right and which was wrong; they were both right, and it was the oscillation back and forth between two completely different treatments that had been nearly disastrous. For Dr. Sun, this case expressed a central truth of Chinese medicine: there is never just one way to treat an illness. There will always be "different paths, different points of attacks, different methods, including diametrically opposed methods for curing an illness." The key is to "seize hold of a single thread, to stick to one theory" and see it through.

But we also need to recall his father's advice about virtuosity. Not only is it essential to realize there exists a multiplicity of approaches to any one illness, but that each approach itself is also a multiplicity. There can be no simple application of a clinical text, whether textbook or canon, because the outcome is always unexpected. The text, the treatment, the formula, the herbs are always transformed in the process. When the practitioner has the ability to "make it one's own," then the slight surprise of action becomes the exhilarating magic of virtuosity. In the same way that Dr. Song reinvented the Ephedra, Aconite, Asarum Decoction from the *Treatise on Cold Damage* to make it into a formula suitable for acute tonsillitis, he also the transformed the Lonicera and Forsythia Powder from the *Revised Overview of Chinese Medicine* into a solution for a condition much more complicated than a simple case of acute tonsillitis.

Perhaps the same can be said for *bianzheng lunzhi* and the future of Chinese medicine as a whole. Throughout this text, I have traced the postcolonial dualisms that have redefined contemporary Chinese medicine, along the axes of therapeutic action, bodily knowledge, and diagnostic strategies. In the latter half of the twentieth century, doctors of Chinese medicine have struggled against various purifications, which suggest that this practice is only suitable for chronic, functional, and hard-to-treat disorders. Against great odds, doctors have built the institutions of Chinese medicine—the schools, the textbooks, the hospitals, research centers—and the intellectual apparatus—*bianzheng lunzhi*—for responding to these challenges. These are impressive achievements, a courageous response to the postcolonial predicament of Chinese medicine. But these hybrid innovations may be analogous to Dr. Sun's Lonicera and Forsythia Powder, adequate to the straightforward, "textbook" problem of perpetuating Chinese medicine, but not necessarily to keeping Chinese medicine vibrant in China's complex world of medical practice today. No amount of standardization, scientization, or modernization—choose your favorite term—can enable *bianzheng lunzhi* to resolve the crisis of authority that confronts contemporary Chinese medicine today. Rather, it is only through the arduous task of "making it one's own," of sticking with *bianzheng lunzhi* to the end, perhaps until it has been transformed into something completely different, that this impasse will be overcome.

Epilogue

In late March 2020, less than two weeks after the World Health Organization declared COVID-19 a global pandemic, the Chinese government held several news conferences that seemed significant at the time but have been largely forgotten since. The outbreak had already been brought under control in China, just as many nations around the world were beginning to implement versions of the stay-at-home orders and quarantine measures that had been put in place roughly two months earlier in China. The reason for these news conferences was that the Chinese government wanted to bring attention to what it referred to as a "bright spot" and "important weapon" in the management of the epidemic—the positive role played by Chinese medicine professionals in treating and managing cases of COVID-19. In an attempt at some soft power influence, the State Council Information Office Press Conference reported that "Chinese Medicine is a Bright Spot of the Epidemic Prevention Efforts. China Is Willing to Share Its Experience with the World." These and other press releases included vague but impressive claims that over 90 percent of COVID-19 patients in China had received some form of Chinese medicine therapy. More notably, two specific clinical trials were discussed that included 564 and 1,265 patients, respectively, in which no patients receiving traditional therapies died or even became critically ill. A few Western media outlets reported on these new conferences, but there was little international interest in the apparent promise of Chinese medicine. As the pandemic quickly spun out of control in the rest of the world, relations between China and many other nations soured, and the Chinese government did not publicly repeat these tentative diplomatic overtures to share Chinese medicine with the world

These media events, together with other intriguing reports that were trickling out of China through Chinese medicine networks, became a catalyst for me and three Chinese colleagues to begin a collaborative investigation into the role of Chinese medicine during the COVID-19 outbreak in China. We sought to understand the actual clinical dimensions of Chinese medicine treatments for COVID-19 and the popular response to the new visibility of the Chinese medicine profession in an epidemic outbreak. Because of travel restrictions and funding limitations, we conducted most of our research virtually. Through the late spring and summer, we surveyed over 800 laypersons and interviewed roughly thirty respondents through internet calling technologies such as WeChat. Two of my colleagues, Lai Lili and Yang Huiyu, were also able to travel to Shanghai to interview six doctors of Chinese medicine who had volunteered to work on the clinical front lines during the height of the outbreak. They subsequently interviewed two biomedical doctors who were also on the clinical frontlines in Wuhan. Among our layperson interviews, we found a wide range of views on whether Chinese medicine contributed to the treatment and prevention of COVID-19. Most participants found the government press conferences unreliable and based their responses on their own personal encounters with Chinese medicine. A majority were unsure whether Chinese medicine doctors had been effective in treating COVID-19. A minority were deeply skeptical that Chinese medicine had any health benefits at all. A third group, also a minority, were enthusiastic users of Chinese medicine. They believed that Chinese medicine might be effective for treating COVID-19 but awaited more reliable reporting on this issue. Almost of all our respondents were generally ignorant of the basic principles of Chinese medicine, particularly as it related to treating COVID-19. For example, both enthusiasts and skeptics debated whether Chinese herbal remedies, such as Forsythia Epidemic Clearing Capsules (*Lian Hua Qing Wen Jiao Nang*), the patent medicine in most demand during the pandemic, had antiviral properties. They seemed unaware that Chinese medicine does not have a theory of microbes and treats infections through the alternative logic of pattern discrimination.

Among doctors of Chinese medicine, however, we encountered a much less ambiguous story. There was a palpable energy about the clinical contributions of Chinese medicine to controlling the pandemic. That excitement began with the fact that government included Chinese medicine professionals in its COVID-19 response, in contrast to the 2003 government response to SARS. The central government and multiple provincial governments issued—and then updated several times—"Diagnostic and Treatment Protocols" (诊疗方案) that gave significant space to suggested Chinese medicine treatments. On the national stage, some leading doctors of Chinese medicine, such as Zhang Boli (张伯礼), became recognizable figures on TV newscasts around the country. Most importantly, Chinese medicine professionals joined other volunteer biomedical healthcare workers to "assist Hubei" on the clinical front lines during the height of the crisis. While their numbers were only a fraction of their biomedical counterparts, roughly 4,000 compared to 42,000, their clinical results were notable. In Wuhan, the Jiangxia field hospital, one of sixteen field hospitals established across the city to handle patients with mild to moderate symptoms, was managed solely by Chinese medicine professionals. It successfully treated 564 patients—one of the figures featured in later press releases—with no reported deaths (Ochs and Garran 2020). Through our interviews, we learned that Chinese medicine doctors were also given a prominent role at Leishen Shan Hospital (雷神山医院), one of two facilities built rapidly in early February to handle severe and critical cases of COVID-19. Our interviewees explained that Chinese medicine doctors managed four wards at Leishen Shan Hospital out of thirty-two wards in total, with each ward containing forty-eight beds. Our interviewees worked in two of the Chinese medicine wards for a ten-day period beginning on February 19, 2020, the first day the hospital opened. We learned that they relied primarily on Chinese medicine therapies and confidently took most of their patients off antiviral medications, since they believed that Chinese medicine therapies would be more effective without the risk of side effects. They also found innovative ways to support patients on ventilators, administering Chinese medicine herbal therapies through nasalgastric tubes and intravenous infusions, while also providing acupuncture and other external treatments. Doctors from the Western medicine wards invited them to consult for their intubated patients as well. They collectively treated about 200 patients over a ten-day period and did not have a single death under their watch.

By the fall, diplomatic tensions were rising as the pandemic deepened in most parts of the globe and political pressures were intensifying within China. It became impossible to conduct any additional interviews about what transpired on the clinical front lines. Nonetheless, we were left with a surprisingly robust image of the role of Chinese medicine in this public health emergency. Our interviews with biomedical doctors confirmed that there was indeed widespread use of the patent medicine Forsythia Epidemic Clearing Capsules (*Lian Hua Qing Wen Jiao Nang*) by biomedical doctors. Although our interviewees were hesitant to comment on its therapeutic benefits, they were willing to use it because they believed it had minimal side effects and provided significant psychological benefits for patients desperate for any kind of remedy. They noted that it was used more widely than any single biomedical drug. The general willingness of biomedical doctors to prescribe a Chinese medicine therapy, even if there was no consensus on whether it had any therapeutic benefits, suggested a softening of long-standing prejudices toward the Chinese medicine profession.

We were also struck by the innovative approaches of our Chinese medicine interviewees. One physician, Fang Bangjiang, who had trained with the famous integrated medicine doctor Huang Xingyuan (see Chapters 1 and 4), has been part of the small revival of Chinese Emergency Medicine at Longhua Hospital, a leading hospital of Chinese medicine in Shanghai. He emphasized that COVID-19 should be considered an "acute deficiency pattern" (急性虚证) and needed to be managed by using treatment principles such as "double release of the exterior and interior" (表里双解), "interrupt and reverse" (截断扭转), "supplementation throughout" (全程补虚), "draining throughout" (全程泻下), and "treatment through the intestines" (从肠论治). These principles were quite distinct from the ones suggested in the various editions of Diagnostic and Treatment Protocols or the most popular Chinese medicine therapies, know as the "three formulas and three drugs" (三方三药) (Ochs and Garran 2020). Instead, they reflected the hard-earned experience of Fang Bangjiang and other colleagues in the Chinese Emergency Medicine Department at Longhua Hospital. In recent years, they have been using Chinese medicine therapies to help manage patients with sepsis, the life-threatening inflammatory response that can lead to shock and death if not controlled quickly. Fang Bangjiang believed that the therapeutic principles he had developed for treating sepsis could be readily adapted to the hyperinflammatory immune responses of severe and critical COVID-19 patients.[1]

Even if the public remained unclear about the efficacy of Chinese medicine for treating COVID-19, our research showed that Chinese medicine doctors were feeling empowered by their clinical contributions and the recognition of government officials. If the SARS epidemic was a small turning point for the Chinese medicine profession, then it seems like the COVID-19 pandemic could become a more significant inflection point. Is it possible that the public health crises of 2003 and 2020, both caused by related forms of the coronavirus, might lead to a renaissance for Chinese medicine? It is still too early to predict the effects of these two events, but the key themes of this book point to a nuanced path forward. On the one hand, we should not expect a moment of "liberation." Contemporary Chinese medicine is a postcolonial form of medical practice that was produced through decades of power inequalities vis-à-vis the global dominance of biomedicine and its central place in the biopolitical operations of the modern Chinese state. The hegemonic status of biomedicine and its place in the modern political order are unlikely to change soon. On the other hand, there is a growing embrace of Chinese medicine, as well as other ethnic healing systems, by political elites in China (Farquhar and Lai 2021). This more welcoming political climate will create new opportunities for doctors of Chinese medicine, such as we saw with the COVID-19 crisis, to continue to develop their craft and expand their range of practice.

The central goal of this book has been to describe the postcolonial transformation of contemporary Chinese medicine. I have shown that Chinese medicine no longer exists in its premodern forms. A diversity of healing practices has been replaced by an institutionalized form of medicine that is profoundly conditioned by its relationship to biomedicine. Contrary to many historical accounts, I have argued that Chinese medicine was perceived to be a clinically superior form of medicine in the Republican period. Skilled doctors of Chinese medicine of this era treated acute infectious diseases, borrowed liberally from European anatomy, debated how to reform their practice, and did not feel constrained by the encounter with biomedicine. It was only during the Communist era, when the profession was confronted by a highly centralized state supporting the rapid expansion of the Western medicine, that Chinese medicine began to change dramatically.

Drawing on Bruno Latour's analysis of the Modern Constitution, I have argued that the postcolonial transformation of Chinese medicine can be best understood through the dual dynamics of purification and hybridization. During the Communist era, Chinese medicine has come to be defined in opposition to Western medicine along the axes of the acute-chronic, structure-function, and disease-pattern dualisms. These purifying postcolonial dynamics have often limited Chinese medicine, defining it as inadequate for treating acute diseases, inappropriate for treating lesions of the anatomical body, and superfluous for any disease with an established Western medicine treatment protocol. At the same, doctors of Chinese medicine have also become remarkably adept at negotiating these postcolonial power inequalities, working across these same dualisms to produce hybrid innovations. In doing so, they have enabled the profession to survive against improbable odds. Indeed, compared with the fate of traditional healing systems and other non-Western forms of knowledge around the globe, the accomplishments of the Chinese medicine profession in the twentieth and twenty-first centuries have been remarkable.

I have also argued that "pattern discrimination and treatment determination" (*bianzheng lunzhi*) is the ultimate postcolonial technology. This clinical methodology emerged with and through the disease-pattern dualism. It has become a powerful tool with which to navigate the power inequalities that confront doctors of Chinese medicine in every clinical encounter. Doctors loudly proclaim *bianzheng lunzhi* as the quintessential feature of their practice, while they tacitly use it to integrate Chinese medicine with Western medicine. I have argued that *bianzheng lunzhi* should be celebrated for providing the organizing principle for contemporary textbooks, hospital record keeping, and research protocol design. It has been essential to the creation of an institutionalized form of Chinese medicine. But on its own, *bianzheng lunzhi* is not a solution to the postcolonial predicament. In hospital practice it can easily be marginalized by the need to privilege Western medicine. Yet throughout this book, we have seen that the best doctors, the ones who made *bianzheng lunzhi* "their own," have been able to transcend the limitations of the postcolonial moment. It is their virtuosity that offers hope for a renewal of this healing tradition.

At the beginning of this book, I discussed my interest in writing for multiple audiences. I hope that, for fellow practitioners of this healing tradition, my efforts to describe the social, political, and historical dimensions of the postcolonial transformation of Chinese medicine will bring a new appreciation of the work already done to preserve and invigorate this practice. For other readers, I hope that this book has introduced you to the richness of a medical system that continues to flourish despite numerous obstacles. Most importantly, I hope that all readers can draw lessons from the endeavors of Chinese medicine doctors. Perhaps their hybrid innovations and quest for virtuosity can provide guidance for other peoples caught in their own postcolonial power struggles.

Acknowledgments

For more than twenty-five years, I have had the privilege and great joy to be traveling through the world of Chinese medicine in China. Along the way, I studied with many wonderful teachers, met extraordinary doctors and scholars, and learned to practice this unique healing system. This brief acknowledgment cannot begin to express my gratitude to all the acquaintances that made this journey, and ultimately this book, possible.

Looking back at how *Prescriptions for Virtuosity* came together, I am increasingly aware of how improbable a project it was. This book pulls together multiple research stints in China that begin in the mid-1990s and stretch into the 2020s. It combines both ethnography and historical research and has been enriched by my own practice as a doctor of Chinese medicine. The core fieldwork experience that is described in this book was based on the five years from 1995 to 2000 that I spent studying at the Beijing University of Chinese Medicine and its affiliated hospitals. My experience as a full-time student in a standard university-degree program provided invaluable insights into China's medical institutions. I want to thank the officials and staff at both the university and its affiliated hospitals that supported me during this period. I am deeply grateful to Chen Hao and Wu Gang at the State Administration for Traditional Chinese Medicine and Zhang Ming at the Beijing Municipal Government. Without their support, I would not have been able to complete my clinical training and finish my education. Most importantly, to the dozens of professors and doctors who taught me, whether in the classroom or the clinic, there is no way to express my gratitude for all that you shared with me.

During my stay at the Beijing University of Chinese Medicine, many individuals helped me to learn about Chinese medicine outside of my training program. Hu Weiguo graciously shared his passion for this medical system, introducing me to many of his colleagues at the China Academy of Chinese Medical Sciences, including Wang Xiufu and Xue Ligong, who both became wonderful clinical mentors for me. I am grateful to Professor Yan Jianhua at the Beijing University of Chinese Medicine, whose curiosity about anthropology flowered into a collaborative research project, where I worked closely with his graduate student, Guo Hua, and my research assistant, Lai Lili. In retrospect, the interviews that we conducted together marked a key turning point in my research. When I originally met Lai Lili, she was hoping to switch careers, from Chinese medicine to anthropology. While I tried to help her with this transition, she ultimately did far more for me, guiding me through all kinds of research challenges. I was thrilled to see her later join the Ph.D. program for Anthropology at the University of North Carolina, eventually returning to China to become a professor at the Peking University School of Health Humanities.

My years at the Beijing University of Chinese Medicine were mostly self-funded, and I was often unsure if I would be able to complete the five-year program. Fortunately, Beijing was still a relatively inexpensive city in the late 1990s, and many generous and resourceful people kept me moving forward. I could not have asked for a better start to my time in Beijing than living with Lin Siao Fou-Menuhin, who put me up for many months and got me on my feet. Work at the Australian Trade Commission financed my medical school training in the initial years. The Chinese Ministry of Education generously deferred a year of tuition through the Chinese Cultural Studies Award. Occasional freelance writing gigs for the Economist Intelligence Unit done through Nick Driver and his consulting company, Clear Thinking, helped to cover my daily expenses. During my final two years, I relied on a small inheritance from my beloved grandfather, Louis A. Fine, to complete my studies and research. Wu Gang and Liang Juanjuan were incredible neighbors and landlords; Ji Yonghong brought a ray of sunshine to our shared courtyard compound. David Spindler taught me how to navigate Beijing's library system. Micah Truman and Wang Fang gave me a home away from home. Alex Graf connected me to a remarkable network of people through his sharp wit. After his tragic passing in 2003, his friends from the film industry would play an instrumental role in my later research. Many aspects of my research were also inspired by fellow anthropologist Jay Dautcher, who was doing his own fieldwork in Xinjiang in the late 1990s. His keen attention to language, music, and the craft of ethnography guided my own methodologies, and I deeply regret that he passed away before the publication of this book.

After I graduated from the Beijing University of Chinese Medicine in

2000, I returned to the U.S. to open my own Chinese medicine clinical practice and focus on my anthropological writing. Over the next few years, I made occasional short trips back to Beijing for additional clinical training at Dongzhimen Hospital and Guang'anmen Hospital. I want to thank all the doctors who welcomed me into their outpatient practices during this period, especially Sun Pei and Han Fei, whose clinical work inspired sections of this manuscript. The next stage of my research was unexpectedly sparked by one of these trips, when I had the good fortune to interview the famous doctor and scholar Deng Tietao in 2005. This conversation led to a successful grant application (American Research in the Humanities in China) with the American Council of Learned Societies (ACLS), which brought me back to China in 2008 for a year-long stay. Luo Hongguang, at the China Academy of Social Sciences, generously arranged for me to be affiliated with his institute. During this incredible year of research, I had the honor to interview over forty senior doctors of Chinese medicine about the early years of their clinical training and practice before or around the time of the Communist Revolution in 1949. These interviews are discussed in Chapter 1, but their influence was far greater, helping me frame the entire argument of the book. I am deeply indebted to all these doctors for welcoming me into their homes and clinics. My dear friends Li Qiao and Huang Fan took time off from their work in the film industry to arrange these visits. Without their persistence and charm, most of the interviews would have never happened.

Because these interviews had such a major influence on the book manuscript, it is important to clarify here how I have dealt with personal names in the text. I have used the real names of all doctors who were formally interviewed in the course of researching this book. That includes doctors interviewed as part of the ACLS grant, but also doctors interviewed at other stages of research. I have changed the names of other individuals— doctors, patients, classmates, and friends— who were involved in events described in the text but from whom it was not possible to obtain consent.

After the completion of the ACLS grant, I was fortunate to continue my research and writing through several other opportunities. In 2009, I made important progress on this manuscript through the support of a Wenner-Gren Foundation writing fellowship. Subsequently, I continued my research through a Wellcome Trust History of Medicine Project Grant for collaborative research on the history of East Asian medicine with Volker Scheid (principal investigator), Soyoung Suh, and Keiko Daidoji. Our project began in 2010 and officially ended in 2012, but the rich dialogue with these three colleagues continued for many years and helped to round out the historical writings in this book. I am especially indebted to Keiko Daidoji, with whom I collaborated most directly. Her excellent research and insights on Kampo medicine contributed directly to parts of this manuscript. During this period, I also had the good fortune to work briefly with Wang Xiaobin, an excellent videographer, who contributed some of the photos in the book. Since the outbreak of COVID-19, I have been collaborating with Lai Lili, Yang Huiyu, and Zhao Xiaopeng on research that contributed to the material in the Epilogue. I want to especially thank Yang Huiyu, who was instrumental in helping me acquire the premodern acupuncture images featured in Chapter 2. Lastly, the final revisions for this book were completed while I was conducting new research as a Fulbright Scholar at China Medical University in Taichung, Taiwan. I want to thank the Fulbright program and my gracious Taiwanese hosts, especially Yen Hung-Rong and Wang Lu-Hai, for their wonderful support during this time.

The central argument of this book about the postcolonial struggles of Chinese medicine were shaped by many wonderful scholars. Peter Redfield helped me to relate my observations about medical practice in China to larger debates within anthropology. Jim Hevia's innovative research on colonialism in China was an essential reference for my understanding on how this phenomenon affected Chinese medicine. Barry Saunders's work as an emergency medicine doctor and religious studies scholar helped me to understand the work of ritual in clinical medicine. Margaret Weiner was a meticulous reader of the manuscript and lifted me with her enthusiasm for the postcolonial framework of the project. Drafts of this manuscript were circulated amongst many amazing colleagues over the years, including Alison Greene, Jennie Burnett, Michelle Cohen, and Maya Parsons. I am particularly indebted to the invaluable help of Hilary Smith and Jia-Chen Wendy Fu during my final stages of writing. Undoubtedly, my greatest influence was Judith Farquhar, who first kindled my passion for Chinese medicine with a long letter written from Guangzhou in 1991 before I had even begun my research. I cannot thank her enough for all the years of mentorship and inspiration. It is not an exaggeration to state that her scholarship, critical insights, and intellectual passion have been with me, in some fashion, on every step of my journey.

I first met my spouse, Dana Powell, in 2003, when I was frustrated with the progress of my research and was wondering whether I could ever complete this book. She somehow forgave my moodiness, and we eventually had three beautiful boys together. I could not have completed the last and most difficult stage of the book manuscript without her help. Many significant parts of this manuscript were written after my family moved to Boone, North Carolina, in 2011. Dana started teaching in the Anthropology Department at Appalachian State University that fall, and I subsequently joined the department in

2013. Our second son was born in January 2012 with a life-threatening congenital heart defect that required immediate surgery. Following a successful surgery, he subsequently developed a rare form of epilepsy that we battled for six long years before finally bringing it under control. Although we relished the sweetness of our kids' early years, the physical exhaustion of navigating two academic careers, raising three children, and managing the health and special needs of our second son was often overwhelming. We are grateful for the kind support of Diane Mines, the chair of the Anthropology Department at Appalachian State University, who helped us navigate our early years in the department. Our dear friend Wang Junxia provided love and care for our young children for many years. My wife and I could not have both kept our jobs at Appalachian State without her help. My mother-in-law, Ellen Powell; my parents, Barbara and A. W. Karchmer; and many other family members pitched in to give us crucial support during these challenging years.

Lastly, I want to thank Tom Lay, Eric Newman, Aldene Fredenburg, and their colleagues at Fordham University Press for their embrace of this manuscript and hard work to make its publication possible. I hope the events, stories, and analysis found in this book will help others on their own journeys through the worlds of Chinese medicine, traditional healing, postcolonial knowledges, and medical anthropology.

Unless otherwise indicated, all photos were taken by the author.

Notes

Introduction

1. Elisabeth Hsu has explored this issue more systematically in her research at the Yunnan College of Chinese Medicine, conducted in the late 1980s. She also documented "widespread disillusionment" among the undergraduate students. Many students admitted that they wished they could have pursued another career, but they chose Chinese medicine because they felt that their exam scores were too low to test into these more desirable fields (Hsu 1999, 150–53).

2. Chapter 9 of *Essentials of the Golden Casket* is called "The Disorders, Pulses, Presentations, and Treatments of Chest Blockage, Heart Pain, and Shortness of Breath" (胸痺心痛短氣病脈證治第九).

3. Stacey Langwick's ethnography on traditional medicine in Tanzania, *Bodies, Politics, and African Healing: The Matter of Maladies in Tanzania,* is an excellent example of scholarship that explores the postcolonial impacts of biomedicine in Tanzania (Langwick 2011).

4. High school students in China are divided into a math-and-science track and a humanities track. Applicants to universities of Chinese medicine in the 1990s were selected only from the math and science track.

5. Lai Lili later became an invaluable assistant in some of my research activities. She eventually went to study for a Ph.D. in Anthropology in the U.S. and has written quite sensitively about Chinese medicine and other ethnic medicines in China.

6. I thank Shelley Ochs for sharing with me some of the popular articles that circulate among Chinese social media users related to this topic.

7. This claim would seem to omit the diverse medical traditions practiced among China's ethnic minorities. But Judith Farquhar and Lai Lili's new work on minority medicine in China shows that these practices get administered through the government agencies responsible for Chinese medicine, and their development is

strongly shaped by the social and political history of Chinese medicine in the China (Farquhar and Lai 2021).

8. Judith Farquhar has shown that the divide between the two professions is not absolute. Market reforms have allowed a modest return of diversity since the beginning of the reform era. These noninstitutional healing practices are always in danger of official sanction, however, if they are seen as embracing "superstition" (Farquhar 1996).

9. A similar argument could be extended to other aspects of contemporary social life in China. See Stacy Leigh Pigg's work for an example of a Latourian analysis of shamanism in Nepalese society (Pigg 1996).

10. One dualism not addressed in this work is the dichotomy between root and branch, usually heard in the expression "Western medicine treats the branch; Chinese medicine treats the root" (*xiyi zhi biao; zhongyi zhi ben*). This comparison also operates according to the twin processes of purification and hybridization. It would seem to represent a more favorable claim about the benefits of Chinese medicine than the other three dualisms, but that is not entirely true in the case of acute conditions. I choose not to feature it in my analysis because I found questions of root and branch to be more important *within* Chinese medicine, as a means for devising treatment strategies, than as a way of relating Chinese medicine to Western medicine.

11. In 2008–9, I was able to return to Beijing with the support of the American Council of Learned Societies to collect oral histories with senior doctors of Chinese medicine. From 2011 to 2012, I was fortunate to have the financial support of the Wellcome Trust for a collaborative project with Volker Scheid, Soyoung Suh, and Keiko Daidoji, exploring the history of East Asian medicine. This grant allowed me to conduct an additional year of archival research in Beijing.

12. In the early twentieth century, anthropology had been a burgeoning, vibrant field in China. Most ethnographers worked in the Chinese countryside, where they hoped to find inspiration for the renewal of Chinese society (Litzinger 2000). After the Communist revolution, the field was reorganized around the Stalinist model of ethnology (*minzu yanjiu*) in the 1950s, emphasizing the classification of ethnic groups to serve the political needs of the state. It was later repressed as bourgeois discipline in the 1960s and 1970s. In the 1980s, anthropology programs reemerged but remain tucked away in much larger departments of sociology (Wang 2005).

1. Efficacies of the State

1. Huang Xingyuan originally trained as a doctor of Western medicine and later enrolled in the experimental "doctors of Western medicine study Chinese medicine" program. He was well respected among his Chinese medicine colleagues, and his dual training made him an ideal figure to advance Chinese emergency medicine.

2. During the 2000s and especially the 2010s, granulated herbal formulas and single herbs have become a well-established aspect of Chinese medicine clinical

practice in mainland China. These products can be quickly dissolved in water and have the potential to speed up the delivery of herbal medicine to patients considerably.

3. Personal interview with Wang Juyi, Beijing, October 2008.

4. Personal interview with Zhou Zhongying, Nanjing, January 16, 2009.

5. Personal interview with Zhu Liangchun, Nantong, December 22, 2008.

6. Personal interview with Shen Fengge, Nanjing, March 15, 2009.

7. Because only a small number of doctors from this era were still alive at the time, I traveled to many of the major geographic regions of China, including northern China, the northeast provinces, the lower Yangtze delta, central China, Sichuan, and Guangdong to conduct these interviews. Some doctors grew up in large cities, but many began their careers in the countryside.

8. Personal interview with He Ren, Hangzhou, April 2, 2009.

9. Personal interview with Deng Tietao, Guangzhou, March 19, 2009.

10. Personal interview with Zhang Jin, Harbin, March 25, 2009.

11. Personal interview with Jin Shiyuan, Beijing, April 3, 2009.

12. Personal interview with Lou Duofeng, Zhengzhou, March 31, 2009.

13. Personal interview with Li Jinyong, Wuhan, April 1, 2009.

14. This 2:1 ratio should not be seen as a reflection of the population of doctors as a whole but of the success of these private schools. School-trained doctors were a far smaller percentage of the total, but the success of these graduates allowed me to track them down decades later.

15. Personal interview with Yan Runming, Beijing, December 16, 2008.

16. Personal interview with Deng Tietao, Guangzhou, March 19, 2009.

17. The precise role of the union clinics in the transmission of Chinese knowledge remains unclear. Xiaoping Fang also reports that potential disciples in Jiang Village in suburban Hangzhou had less patience or interest to withstand the hardships of this kind of training (Fang 2012, 44, 49). Anecdotally, my interviewees also corroborate this finding. For example, Li Jinyong reported that many of this father's disciples in rural Hubei also quit before finishing their apprenticeships (personal interview with Li Jinyong, Wuhan, April 1, 2009).

18. Personal interview with Deng Tietao, Guangzhou, March 19, 2009.

19. Personal interview with Li Jinyong, Wuhan, April 1, 2009.

20. This talk eventually became the basis for a paper of the same name (Karchmer 2015b).

21. Personal interview with Li Jinyong, Wuhan, April 1, 2009.

22. Personal interview with Deng Tietao, Guangzhou, March 19, 2009.

23. Personal interview with Deng Tietao, Guangzhou, March 19, 2009.

2. Geographies of the Body

1. Ironically, it was the lesser therapeutic techniques that Turner described that resonate the most with Chinese medicine. For example, Turner dismissed the herbs

used in the Ihamba performance, saying, "It is doubtful that the [herbal] medicines have any pharmaceutical value at all" (Turner 1967, 370). Likewise, he viewed cupping and bloodletting as a mere "sleight of hand" (Turner 1967, 366). While Chinese medicine has little to say about healing the "social body," all doctors would agree that herbal medicine, cupping, and bloodletting are clinically effective and essential aspects of Chinese medicine therapies.

2. I have translated the term *jiangyi* in the title of this textbook somewhat literally as "lecture notes" to emphasize the less formal nature of this textbook, especially when we compare it to the Communist-era textbooks. These latter textbooks only occasionally use the term *jiangyi* and more commonly use the more formal designation of *xue* (学), in the sense of "studies" or "-ology."

3. "National medicine" was a popular name for Chinese medicine in the Republican era (see Introduction). For a detailed analysis of the significance of this term, please see Sean Hsiang-lin Lei's *Neither Donkey nor Horse* (Lei 2014).

4. The conventional reference to the organs in Chinese medicine is "five viscera and six bowels" (*wuzang liufu*; 五臟六腑), "viscera" referring to "solid organs" and "bowels" indicating "hollow organs." Bao Tianbai dropped the pericardium in this passage, reducing the number of "bowels" (*fu*) to five.

5. The consensus that acupuncture channels lack an anatomical substrate may contribute to the popularity of this sort of hybrid image. In other aspects of Chinese medicine, perhaps where it is harder to disentangle the structural and functional, it is rare to find images at all. For example, in the *Basic Theory of Chinese Medicine* textbook, there are no images of the human body other than the drawings of the meridian channels, all produced in the same style as the 1959 image (Wu Dunxu, Liu Yanchi, and Li Dexin 1995).

6. Following Anne Marie Mol in *The Body Multiple*, we could argue that multiple bodies—for both medical systems—were really at stake in this dilemma (Mol 2002). But in adjudicating the claims of modern anatomy, Chinese doctors have tended to reduce the possibilities to one or two bodies.

7. Camillo Golgi and Santiago Ramón y Cajal shared the Nobel prize in 1906 for their research, which showed the nervous system to be a network of innumerable independent neurons.

8. By the 1970s, the structure-function dualism was already making its way into the English-language scholarly literature on Chinese medicine. In his summary of the relative strengths and weaknesses of two medical systems, Manfred Porkert relies entirely on the concepts of structure and function to make his assessment. "What is true of Chinese thought in general holds equally true for its practical applications in Chinese medicine: It is primarily interested in function as opposed to substratum." This claim is intimately connected to his work to define the unique characteristics of the body of Chinese medicine, as seen at the beginning of the chapter (Porkert 1976).

3. Frail Bodies and the Problem of Diagnosis

1. The section of the chapter draws from a research project done in collaboration with my colleague Keiko Daidoji. We have published a much lengthier exploration of the origins and significance of the Suzhou Hospital of National Medicine (Daidoji and Karchmer 2017).

2. While Yumoto was very careful in his use of the two orthographic variants for shō/zheng, the Chinese translator Zhou Zixu (周子敘) was not. Zhou used the same character, 證, for both expressions, suggesting that a semantic distinction between these two characters had not been well established in Chinese medicine discourse at this point in time (Yumoto Kyūshin 2007 [1930], 22).

3. Chinese readers will notice that I have translated *zheng* (症) as "presentation" in this passage. The context clearly indicates that Ye Juquan intended this connotation. In general, the editors of the journal were not as meticulous as Yumoto Kyūshin and Ōtsuka Keisetsu about policing the use of the different orthographic variants of *shō/zheng*. As I have argued elsewhere (Daidoji and Karchmer 2017), this slippage between the characters suggests that the distinction between "presentation" and "symptom" was still emerging for Chinese doctors in the Republican period. A contemporary doctor would never use the two characters (证 and 症) interchangeably, in part because their meanings are so different now.

4. New Textbooks, New Medicine

1. In the late 1990s, a textbook usually cost about 15 RMB, or roughly US $2 to $3 dollars, depending on the exchange rate.

2. Personal interview, Xiao Chengzong, Beijing, Winter 1999.

3. Zhu Weiju indeed coined the term "Eight Principles" but did not associate it with "pattern discrimination." He was famous for his clinical methodology called "Five Stages and Eight Principles" (*wuduan bagang*) (see Zhu Weiju 2005).

4. Personal interview, Zhang Jingren, Shanghai, 2000.

5. Personal interview with He Ren, Hangzhou, April 2, 2009.

6. Personal interview with Wang Juyi, Beijing, October 2008.

7. Personal interview, Zhu Liangchun, Nantong, December 22, 2008.

8. Personal interview, Jiao Shude, Beijing, Spring 1999.

9. Personal interview, Meng Jingchun, Nanjing, March 16, 2009.

10. Based on current library catalogs, at least 172 different textbooks were produced during the Republican period (Deng Tietao and Cheng Zhifan 2000, 215–19; Library of the China Academy of Chinese Medicine and Xue Qinglu 1991). These textbooks were highly individualistic and varied greatly according to the viewpoints of the author.

11. Decades later, senior doctors of Chinese medicine still decry the destructive influence of "Wang Bin thought," which they believe continues to pollute

the thoughts of everyday citizens and even doctors of Chinese medicine (Zhu Liangchun 2005, 27). When I visited with Li Jinyong to interview him, I found that he was so adamant about the continuing dangers of Wang Bin thought that he took the time to locate some of the original newspaper publications that he had personally clipped and saved in order to photocopy them for me.

12. In the early years of the new colleges, professors generally relied on their own lecture materials. Wang Juyi recalled that many of his professors at the Beijing College of Chinese Medicine would mimeograph their lecture notes and distribute them to the students in those early years (personal interview with Wang Juyi, October 2008). Some institutions, however, were further along in developing their lecture materials and published their own textbooks in the late 1950s, either under an individual author's name or the work unit's name.

13. Kim Taylor reports that Yin Huihe claimed to be the chief editor of this textbook in an interview that she conducted with him in 1997. This report may be incorrect. He was indeed the chief editor of a different textbook, *Basic Theory of Chinese Medicine*, published in 1984. But he was probably only one of many contributors to the *Overview*. In the prologue to the "revised edition" of the *Overview*, published in 1994, he was listed as one of the many contributors to the original publication (Meng Jingchun and Zhou Zhongying 1994, 1).

14. Deng Tietao further emphasized this point to me in person (personal interview with Deng Tietao, 2005).

15. *Basic Theory of Chinese Medicine* only first appeared (originally titled *Fundamentals of Chinese Medicine*) with the third edition of the national textbooks. The content for this textbook would have been mostly found in *Lecture Notes on the Inner Canon* in the first two editions of the textbooks.

16. Farquhar often translates *zheng* as "syndrome." I prefer not to use this gloss to avoid confusion with the biomedical use of that term.

17. I concur with Farquhar's general point about the first two *zheng*. Doctors are already processing and manipulating a patient's "raw" clinical presentation ($zheng_1$), as they choose what to record and how to record it ($zheng_2$). But her use of "signs" and "symptoms," respectively, for these two terms can be misleading because the terms derive from Western medicine, where they have different connotations. Her third term ($zheng_3$) refers to "pattern" (or syndrome, as she often calls it) and is the one Chinese medicine concept of the three terms. Keiko Daidoji and I have presented a history of how the three *zheng* of Farquhar's argument emerged in the medical discourse of the Republican era (Daidoji and Karchmer 2017a).

18. As this statement and the previous passage indicate, the editors used the term *bing* loosely, referencing both medical systems.

19. The only other individuals mentioned by name are four senior doctors who advised the process—Lu Zhenqiao (陆真翘), Wu Zhaoxian (吴棹仙), Qin Bowei (秦伯未), and Wu Kaopan (吴考槃).

20. Personal interview, Huang Xingyuan, Chongqing, 1999.

21. Personal interview, Tan Jiaxing, Changchun, 1999.

22. I was unable to locate a copy of the third edition despite many visits to various archives.

23. An example of the continuing influence of the third and fourth editions of the Chinese internal medicine textbook was the mammoth 2,500-page, two-volume set *Clinical Chinese Internal Medicine*, published in 1994. When I was a student, this text was considered the most authoritative Chinese internal medicine reference book available. Part One, nearly three-fifths of the text, was structured around Chinese medicine *bing*; Part Two, approximately one-third of the text, covered Western medicine diseases; Part Three summarized the latest research findings regarding Chinese medicine (Wang Yongyan, Li Mingfu, and Dai Ximeng 1997).

24. Kuhn 1970, 137–38.

25. Personal interview, Deng Tietao, Guangzhou, March 19, 2009.

5. Chinese Medicine on the Margins

1. Wang Baokui, personal interview, Beijing, Spring 2000.

2. When administering glucose drips for elderly patients, doctors in China will often include small amounts of insulin to aid with glucose metabolism.

3. Our case records were written according to guidelines outlined in a little blue book that could usually be found in the doctors' office on most wards. Some of the redundancy in the medical student admissions note was eliminated in the medical record reforms of 2000. (See State Administration of Traditional Chinese Medicine 2000.)

4. It is possible that this emphasis on the primary and secondary diagnosis reflects doctors' desire for parallelism in the double diagnosis. Biomedical doctors in the U.S. have told me that they usually do not distinguish between these two levels of diagnosis.

5. In some classical accounts, constipation was also considered another feature of *guange*. The Chinese Internal Medicine textbook has eliminated this symptom, most likely in an attempt to bring the definition of this *bing* in closer alignment with the biomedical disease of renal failure. The Nephrology Department also did not include constipation in its own definition of *guange*.

6. Urea is one of the metabolic end products of protein metabolism. Because the kidneys regularly expel it, blood urea nitrogen concentration is measured at an indicator of filtration rate. The kidneys are one of the main regulators of the pH level in the body. They excrete H^+ and recycle bicarbonate HCO_3^-, which acts as a buffer for H^+ in the bloodstream. Lowered CO_2 levels suggest that H^+ excretion and bicarbonate recycling is impaired, also an indication of potential kidney damage. The patient's electrolyte concentrations of potassium, as well as sodium and chlorine, were all low, further suggesting kidney dysfunction.

7. Lu Renhe and Gao Jing, leading physicians in the Neprhrology Department, wrote a textbook that is used for their graduate students. It includes many Chinese medicine *bing* categories not found in other clinical texts. Like Kidney Heat, many

of these diseases are neologisms that relate classical references to a Western medicine pathology.

8. Because of the linguistic overlap between disease and *bing*, some doctors interpret this maxim to be a statement about Chinese medicine alone: first diagnose a Chinese medicine *bing*, then determine a pattern. But in my experience, the vast majority of doctors invoke this aphorism as a statement about the relationship between Western medicine and Chinese medicine.

9. The one exception was the ACE inhibitor benazapril, which has known benefits for renal insufficiency caused by hypertension. In this case, however, it was used as a prophylactic. Dong Chunhua's hypertension was only slightly above normal and did not seem to be the cause of her condition.

10. See the hospital website, http://www.xwzy.com.cn/, where they promote the treatment of vascular disease as the hospital's number-one "specialty therapy."

11. In 2002, outpatient fees at Dongzhimen Hospital were: attending physicians, 5 RMB; assistant chief physicians, 7 RMB; chief physicians, 9 RMB or 14 RMB. In the "special outpatient clinic" (*teshu menzhen*), where only the most famous physicians in the hospital are invited to have consultation hours, the fees jump to 100 RMB. Since that time, all these fees have increased. The "special outpatient clinic" fees have jumped to several hundred RMB for the most famous doctors.

6. Prescriptions for Virtuosity

1. Personal interview, Sun Pei, Beijing, 2000

2. Personal interview, Sun Pei, Beijing, 2000.

3. Personal interview, Sun Pei, Beijing, 2000.

4. Unbeknownst to Sun Pei (and to me when I conducted this interview), the two doctors are also re-enacting the struggles between the Cold Damage and Warm Disorders schools that was so vehement in the Republican period (see Chapter 3).

5. Gan Zuwang has argued that a more historically accurate understanding of this disease name would translate as "Silkworm Chrysalis" (Gan Zuwang 1996, 198).

6. Personal interview, Sun Pei, Beijing, 2000.

7. Normal range is 4,000–10,000 white blood cells/μL.

8. Personal interview, Sun Pei, Beijing, 2000.

9. I have used the word "condition" as a translation for *bing* (病) in this passage. The connotations of *bing* in the *Treatise* are more expansive than its use as a nosological category in late imperial and modern Chinese medicine writings. The original line from the *Treatise* in Chinese is: 少陰病，始得之，反發熱，脈沉者，麻黃細辛附子湯主之。

10. Dr. Sun also pointed out that, strictly speaking, Pinellia is opposed to Aconite Root (*Wu Tou*) and not Prepared Aconite, the herb that Dr. Song actually used. But since the two herbs come from the same plant, the former being the untreated main root and the latter the treated branch root, Prepared Aconite is generally considered to be opposed to Pinellia as well.

11. Personal interview, Sun Pei, Beijing, 2000.
12. Personal interview, Sun Pei, Beijing, 2000.
13. Personal interview, Sun Pei, Beijing, 2000.
14. Personal interview, Sun Pei, Beijing, 2000.

Epilogue

1. This brief summary reflects some of the preliminary efforts of our small research collective. My collaborators are Lai Lili, associate professor at Peking University School of Health Humanities; Yang Huiyu, associate professor at the School of Law and Public affairs in the Nanjing University of Information, Science, and Technology; and Zhao Xiaopeng, a Ph.D. student at the Beijing University of Chinese Medicine. For more details on this topic, please see our coauthored, forthcoming essay, "Bricolage for a Troubled World: Chinese Medicine and the Response to COVID-19."

References

Acupuncture and Moxibustion Teaching and Research Group of the Nanjing College of Chinese Medicine (南京中医学院针灸学科教研组). 1959. *Concise Acupuncture and Moxibustion Studies* (简明针灸学). Nanjing: Jiangsu People's Publishing House.

Anderson, Warwick. 2014. "Making Global Health History: The Postcolonial Worldliness of Biomedicine." *Social History of Medicine* 27 (2): 372–84.

Andrews, Bridie J. 2001. "From Case Records to Case Histories: The Modernisation of a Chinese Medical Genre, 1912–1949." In *Innovation in Chinese Medicine*, edited by Elizabeth Hsu, 324–41. Cambridge: Cambridge University Press.

———. 2014. *The Making of Modern Chinese Medicine, 1850–1960.* Vancouver: University of British Columbia Press.

Bao Tianbai (包天白). 1937. *Lecture Notes on Anatomy* (解剖學講義). Edited by Wu Keqian (吳克潛). *Fourteen Lecture Notes from China Institute of Medicine* (中國醫學院講義十四種). Shanghai: China Institute of Medicine.

Barlow, Tani E. 1997. "Colonialism's Career in Postwar China Studies." In *Formations of Colonial Modernity in East Asia.* Durham, N.C.: Duke University Press.

Beijing College of Chinese Medicine Inner Canon Department (Beijing Zhongyi Xueyuan Jiaoyanzu), ed. 1960. *Lecture Notes on the Inner Canon.* Beijing: People's Medical Publishing House.

Bhabha, Homi K. 1994. *The Location of Culture.* London and New York: Routledge.

Bol, Peter. 2008. *Neo-Confucianism in History.* Cambridge, Mass.: Harvard University Asia Center.

Cai Jingfeng (蔡景峰), Li Qinghua (李庆华), and Zhang Binghuan (张冰浣), eds. 2000. *Comprehensive History of Medicine in China* (中国医学通史). Vol. 3, *Modern Volume.* Beijing: People's Medical Publishing House.

Cao Dongyi (曹东义), ed. 2008. *Getting to Know the Great Chinese Medicine Master Zhu Liangchun* (走近中医大家朱良春). Beijing: Chinese Medicine Press of China.

Cao Lijuan (曹丽娟), and Wang Ti (王体). 2014. "Tenth Anniversary of the Defense against SARS at the China Academy of Chinese Medical Science" (中国中医科学院放空SARS十周年纪念). *Asia-Pacific Traditional Medicine* (亚太传统医药) 10 (1): 1–3.

Cao Yingfu (曹颖甫). 2004 (1936). *Records of Experiments with Canonical Formulas*. Edited by Wang Zhipu (王致谱). Fuzhou: Fujian Science and Technology Press.

Chakrabarty, Dipesh. 2000. *Provincializing Europe: Postcolonial Thought and Historical Difference*. Princeton, N.J.: Princeton University Press.

Chen Houcheng (陈厚诚). 1996. "The Dissemination of Postcolonial Theory in China" (后殖民主义理论在中国的传播). *Social Science Research* (社会科学研究) 6: 125–31.

China Academy of Chinese Medicine (中国中医研究院). 2003. *Research on The Prevention and Treatment of SARS with Chinese Medicine. Vol. 2*. (中医药防治非典型肺炎(SARS)研究) (二). Beijing: Ancient Literature of Chinese Medicine Press.

China Association of Integrated Medicine (中国中西医结合学会), ed. 1998. *My Career in Integrated Medicine* (我与中西医结合事业). Beijing: Beijing University of Medicine and Peking Union Medical University United Press.

Cohen, Paul. 1984. *Discovering History in China: American Historical Writings on the Recent Chinese Past*. New York: Columbia University Press.

Croizier, Ralph C. 1968. *Traditional Medicine in Modern China: Science, Nationalism, and the Tensions of Cultural Change. Harvard East Asian Series 34*. Cambridge, Mass.: Harvard University Press.

Cui Yueli (崔月犁), ed. 1993. *Founder of the Chinese Medicine Profession in New China: The Collected Writings of Lu Bingkui's Sixty Years in Medicine* (新中国中医事业奠基人: 吕炳奎从医六十年文集). Beijing: Huaxia.

Cullen, Christopher. 2001. "*Yi'an* (醫案) (Case Statements): The Origins of a Genre of Chinese Medical Literature." In *Innovation in Chinese Medicine*, edited by Elizabeth Hsu, 297–323. Cambridge: Cambridge University Press.

Daidoji, Keiko, and Eric I. Karchmer. 2017. "The Case of the Suzhou Hospital of National Medicine (1939–1941): War, Medicine, and Eastern Civilization." *East Asian Science, Technology, and Society: An International Journal* 11 (2): 161–83.

Davidson, Arnold. 2001. *The Emergence of Sexuality: Historical Epistemology and the Formation of Concepts*. Cambridge, Mass., and London: Harvard University Press.

Deng Tietao (邓铁涛). 1995. *Collection of Deng Tietao's Medical Writings* (邓铁涛医集). Sanhe: People's Health.

———, ed. 1999. *The Early Modern History of Chinese Medicine* (中医近代史). Guangzhou: Guangdong Higher Education.

Deng Tietao (邓铁涛), and Cheng Zhifan (程之范), eds. 2000. *Comprehensive History of Medicine in China* (中国医学通史). Vol. 2, *Early Modern Volume* (近代卷). Beijing: People's Medical Publishing House.

Deng Tietao (邓铁涛), and Guo Zhenqiu (郭振球), eds. 1984. *Chinese Medicine Diagnosis* (中医诊断学). *Textbooks for Higher Education Medical Institutions* (高等医药院校教材). Shanghai: Shanghai Science and Technology Publishing House.

Deng Zhongguang (邓中光), Zheng Hong (郑洪), and Chen Anlin (陈安琳), eds. 2004. *Deng Tietao's Words to the Youth of Chinese Medicine* (邓铁涛寄语青年中医). Beijing: People's Medical Publishing House.

Diagnosis Teaching and Research Group of the Beijing Advanced Studies School of Chinese Medicine (北京市中醫進修學校診斷學教研組). 1955. *Lecture Notes for Chinese Medicine Diagnosis* (中醫診斷學講義). Beijing: Beijing Association of Chinese Medicine.

Diagnosis Teaching and Research Group of the Jiangsu School of Chinese Medicine (江苏省中医学校诊断教研组), ed. 1958. *Chinese Medicine Diagnosis* (中医诊断学). Shanghai: Shanghai Health Press.

Dongzhimen Hospital Gazette Office (东直门医院办公室). 1997. *Beijing College of Chinese Medicine Dongzhimen Hospital Gazette (1958–1992)* (北京中医学院东直门医院志).

Duara, Prasenjit. 1995. *Rescuing History from the Nation: Questioning Narratives of Modern China.* Chicago: University of Chicago Press.

Dumit, Joseph. 2012. *Drugs for Life: How Pharmaceutical Companies Define Our Health.* Durham, N.C.: Duke University Press.

Editorial Committee of the China Medical Yearbook (中国卫生年鉴编辑委员会). 2001. *The China Medical Yearbook 2001* (中国卫生年鉴 2001). Beijing: People's Medical Press.

Editorial Committee of the Comprehensive Dictionary of Chinese Medicine (中医大词典编辑委员会). 1979. *The Concise Dictionary of Chinese Medicine* (简明中医词典). Beijing: People's Medical Publishing House.

Editorial Department for the Compilation of Chinese Medicine Work Documents (中医工作文件汇编编辑部). 1985. *Compilation of Chinese Medicine Work Documents 1949–1983* (中医工作文件汇编 1949–83 年). Beijing: People's Republic of China Ministry of Health Chinese Medicine Division.

Elman, Benjamin A. 1984. *From Philosophy to Philology: Intellectual and Social Aspects of Change in Late Imperial China.* Cambridge, Mass.: Council on East Asian Studies, Harvard University.

Escobar, Arturo. 1995. *Encountering Development: The Making and Unmaking of the Third World.* Princeton, N.J.: Princeton University.

Fang, Xiaoping. 2012. *Barefoot Doctors and Western Medicine in China.* Rochester, N.Y.: University of Rochester Press.

Fang Yaozhong (方藥中), Deng Tietao (邓铁涛), Li Keguang (李克光), Chen Keji (陈可冀), Jin Shoushan (金寿山), Huang Xingyuan (黄星垣), and Dong

Hanliang (董汉良), eds. 1984. *Practical Chinese Internal Medicine* (实用中医内科学). Shanghai: Shanghai Science and Technology Press.

Fang Zhouzi (方舟子). 2007. *Criticizing Chinese Medicine (批评中医): The Great Debate on Chinese Medicine in the New Century* (中医新世纪大论战). Beijing: Peking Union Medical College Publishing House.

Fanon, Frantz. 1963. The Wretched of the Earth. New York: Grove Press.

———. 2008 (1952). Black Skin, White Masks. New York: Grove Press.

Farquhar, Judith. 1994. *Knowing Practice: The Clinical Encounter of Chinese Medicine*. Boulder, Colo.: Westview.

———. 1996. "Market Magic: Getting Rich and Getting Personal in Medicine after Mao." *American Ethnololgist* 23 (2): 239–57.

———. 1998. "Chinese Medicine and the Life of the Mind: Are Brains Necessary?" *North Carolina Medical Journal* 59 (3).

———. 2014. "Reading Hands: Pulse Qualities and the Specificity of the Clinical." *East Asian Science, Technology, and Society: An International Journal* 8 (1): 9–24.

Farquhar, Judith, and Lili Lai. 2021. *Gathering Medicine: Nation and Knowledge in China's Mountain South*. Chicago: University of Chicago Press.

Finkler, Kaja. 1985. *Spiritualist Healers in Mexico*. Salem, Wisc.: Sheffield.

Foucault, Michel. 1971. *The Order of Things: An Archaeology of the Human Sciences*. (1st American ed.) New York: Pantheon.

Gan Zuwang (干祖望). 1996. *Medical Discourses of Gan Zuwang* (干祖望医话). Beijing: People's Medical Publishing House.

Gong Tingxian (龚廷贤). 2007 (1588). *Returning to Health for Ten Thousand Illnesses* (万病回春). Beijing: People's Health Publishing House.

Gordon, Deborah R. 1988. "Tenacious Assumptions in Western Medicine." In *Biomedicine Examined*, edited by Margaret M. Lock and Deborah R. Gordon, 19–42. Boston: Kluwer Academic.

Grosz, Elizabeth. 1994. *Volatile Bodies: Towards a Corporeal Feminism*. Bloomington and Indianapolis: Indiana University Press.

Guangdong College of Chinese Medicine (广东中医学院), ed. 1960. *Lecture Materials for Chinese Medicine Diagnosis* (中医诊断学讲义). Beijing: People's Medical Press.

Guangzhou Army Rear-Service Unit Health Department (广州部队后勤部卫生部组织), ed. 1973. *Revised Overview of Chinese Medicine* (新编中医学概论). Beijing: People's Medical Publishing House.

Guangzhou College of Chinese Medicine (广州中医学院), ed. 1964. *Chinese Medicine Diagnosis (中医诊断学讲义)*. Revised Edition of the Provisional Textbooks for Colleges of Chinese Medicine (中医学院试用重订本). Shanghai: Shanghai Science and Technology Press.

Gupta, Akhil. 1998. *Postcolonial Developments: Agriculture in the Making of Modern India*. Durham, N.C.: Duke University Press.

Hanson, Marta (E). 1998. "Robust Northerners and Delicate Southerners: The Nineteent-Century Invention of a Southern Medical Tradition." *Positions* 6 (3): 515–50.

———. 2010. "Conceptual Blind Spots, Media Blindfolds: The Case of SARS and Traditional Chinese Medicine." In *Health and Hygiene in Chinese East Asia: Publics and Policies in the Long Twentieth Century*, edited by Angela Ki-Che Leung and Charlotte Furth. Durham, N.C.: Duke University Press.

———. 2011. *Speaking of Epidemics in Chinese Medicine: Disease and the Geographic Imagination in Late Imperial China*. London and New York: Routledge.

Hao Guangming (郝光明). 2001. "The Lonely Century of Chinese Medicine" (孤独的百年中医). *Medical World*: 22–30.

Haraway, Donna. 1988. "Situated Knowledges: The Science Question in Feminism and the Privilege of Partial Perspective." *Feminist Studies* 14 (3): 575–99.

He Lianchen (何廉臣). 2003 (1927). *Classified Cases of Efficacious Treatments by Famous Doctors of the Nation* (全国名医验案类编). Edited by Wang Zhipu (王致谱). Fuzhou: Fujian Science and Technology Press.

Hebei Province Association of Public Health Work (河北省卫生工作者协会). 1956. *Chinese Medicine Treatment Methods for Japanese B Encephalitis* (流行性乙型脑炎). Baoding: Hebei People's Medical Press.

Hevia, James L. 2003. *English Lessons: The Pedagogy of Imperialism in Nineteenth-Century China*. Durham, N.C.: Duke University Press.

Hsu, Elizabeth. 1999. *The Transmission of Chinese Medicine*. Cambridge Studies in Medical Anthropology. Cambridge: Cambridge University Press.

Hu Guangci (胡光慈), ed. 1958. *Chinese Internal Medicine: New Interpretations of Treatments for Miscellaneous Disorders* (中医內科雜病証治新义). Chongqing: Sichuan People's Press.

Hu Xianglong (胡翔龙), and Cheng Shennong (程莘农). 1997. *Soul of the Golden Needle: Meridian Research* (金针之魂: 经络研究). Changsha: Hunan Science and Technology Publishing House.

Huang Xingyuan (黄星垣), ed. 1985. *Emergency Care in Chinese Internal Medicine* (中医内科急症证治). Beijing: People's Medical Publishing House.

James, Willliam. 1995 (1907). *Pragmatism*. New York: Dover.

Janzen, John H. 1978. *The Quest for Therapy: Medical Pluralism in Lower Zaire*. Berkeley: University of California Press.

Kaptchuk, Ted J. 2000. *The Web That Has No Weaver: Understanding Chinese Medicine*. Chicago: Contemporary Books.

Karchmer, Eric I. 2010. "Chinese Medicine in Action: On the Postcoloniality of Medicine in China." *Medical Anthropology* 29 (3): 1–27.

———. 2013. "The Excitations and Suppressions of the Times: Locating the Emotions in the Liver in Modern Chinese Medicine." *Culture, Medicine, and Psychiatry* 37 (1): 8–29.

———. 2015a. "Ancient Formulas to Strengthen the Nation: Healing the Modern Chinese Body with the Treatise on Cold Damage." *Asian Medicine: Tradition and Modernity* 8 (2): 394–422.

———. 2015b. "Slow Medicine: How Chinese Medicine Became Efficacious Only for Chronic Conditions." In *Historical Epistemology and the Making of Modern Chinese Medicine*, edited by Howard Chiang. Manchester: Manchester University Press.

Karchmer, Eric, Nick Driver, and Arthur Kroeber. 1998. *Healthcare in China into the 21st Century.* Edited by Richard Latker. London: Ecnomist Intelligence Unit.

Kleinman, Arthur. 1981. *Patients and Healers in the Context of Culture: An Exploration of the Borderland between Anthropology, Medicine, and Psychiatry.* Berkeley: University of California Press.

———. 1986. *Social Origins of Distress and Disease: Depression, Neurasthenia, and Pain in Modern China.* New Haven and London: Yale University Press.

Kuhn, Thomas S. 1970. *The Structure of Scientific Revolutions.* 2nd ed. Chicago: University of Chicago Press.

Kuriyama, Shigehisa. 1999. *The Expressiveness of the Body and the Divergence of Greek and Chinese Medicine.* New York: Zone.

Lampton, David M. 1977. *The Politics of Medicine in China: The Policy Process, 1949–1977.* Boulder, Colo.: Westview.

Lancy, David F. 2012. "'First You Must Master Pain': The Nature and Purpose of Apprenticeship." *Anthropology of Work Review* 33 (2): 113–26.

———. 2015. *The Anthropology of Childhood: Cherubs, Chattel, Changelings.* 2nd ed. Cambridge: Cambridge University Press.

Langford, Jean M. 2002. *Fluent Bodies: Ayurvedic Remedies for Postcolonial Imbalance.* Durham, N.C., and London: Duke University Press.

Langwick, Stacey. 2011. *Bodies, Politics, and African Healing: The Matter of Maladies in Tanzania.* Bloomington and Indianapolis: Indiana University Press.

Latour, Bruno. 1987. *Science in Action: How to Follow Scientists and Engineers through Society.* Cambridge, Mass.: Harvard University Press.

———. 1993. *We Have Never Been Modern.* Cambridge, Mass.: Harvard University Press.

———. 1999. "Circulating Reference: Sampling the Soil in the Amazon Forest." In *Pandora's Hope: Essays on the Reality of Science Studies.* Cambridge, Mass.: Harvard University Press.

Lee, Sing. 1999. "Diagnosis Postponed: Shenjing Shuairuo and the Transformation of Psychiatry in Post-Mao China." *Culture, Medicine, and Psychiatry* 23: 349–80.

Lei, Sean Hsiang-lin. 2002. "How Chinese Medicine Became Experiential: The Polticial Epistemology of *Jingyan*." *Positions: East Asia Cultures Critique* 10 (2): 333–64.

———. 2014. *Neither Donkey nor Horse: Medicine in the Struggle over China's Modernity.* Chicago: University of Chicago.

Leung, Angela Ki-Che (梁其姿). 2017. "近代中國醫院的誕生" (The Birth of

the Modern Chinese Hospital). In 健康與社會：華人衛生新史 *(Health and Society: A New History of Public Health in Chinese Society)*, edited by Zhu Pingyi (祝平一). Taipei: Linking Publishing Company.

Li Jingwei (李经纬), and Yan Liang (鄢良). 1990. *The Eastern Spread of Western Learning and China's Early Modern History of Medical Thought* (西学东渐与中国近代医学思潮). Wuhan: Hubei Science and Technology Publishing House.

Li Keguang (李克光), and Zhang Jiali (张家礼), eds. 1993. *Interpretation and Explication of the Essentials of the Golden Casket* (金匮要略译释). Shanghai: Shanghai Scientfic and Technical Publishers.

Li Zhiyong (李志庸), ed. 1999. *The Complete Medical Writings of Zhang Jingyue* (张景岳医学全书). Beijing: Chinese Medicine Publishing House.

Library of the China Academy of Chinese Medicine (中国中医研究院图书馆), and Xue Qinglu (薛清录), eds. 1991. *The National Chinese Medicine United Library Catalog* (全国中医图书联合目录). Beijing: Chinese Medicine Ancient Books.

Lin Lin (林琳), Yang Zhimin (杨志敏), and Deng Tietao (邓铁涛). 2004. "Clinical Research on the Chinese Medicine Treatment of SARS" (中医药治疗SARS的临床研究). In *Research on the Academic Thought of Deng Tietao (II)* (邓铁涛学术思想研究)*(II)*, edited by Xu Zhiwei (徐志伟), Peng Wei (彭炜), and Zhang Xiaojuan (张孝娟). Beijing: Huaxia Press.

Litzinger, Ralph A. 2000. *Other Chinas: The Yao and the Politics of National Belonging*. Durham, N.C., and London: Duke University Press.

Liu Bichen (刘弼臣). 2006. "Reflections on the Chinese Medicine Treatmens for Infectious Atypical Pneumonia" (对中医防治传染性非典型肺炎的探讨). *Journal of Chinese Medicine Pediatrics* (中医儿科杂志) 2 (3): 18–21.

Liu Gengsheng (刘更生), ed. 1997. *Collection of Famous Case Records, Medical Discourses, and Medical Treatises* (医案医话医论名著集成). Edited by Gao Wentao (高文铸). Beijing: Huaxia Press.

Liu, Michael Shiyung. 2009. *Prescribing Colonization: The Role of Medical Practices and Policies in Japan-ruled Taiwan, 1895–1945*. Ann Arbor: Association for Asian Studies.

Liu, Xun. 2009. *Daoist Modern: Innovation, Lay Practice, and the Community of Inner Alchemy in Republican Shanghai*. Cambridge, Mass.: Harvard University Asia Center.

Luesink, David. 2017. "Anatomy and the Reconfiguaration of Life and Death in Republican China." *Journal of Asian Studies* 76 (4): 1,000–34.

Lu Renhe, and Gao Jing. *Practical Clinical Reference Textbook for Graduate Students (in Nephrology)* (研究生 [肾病] 临床实用参考教材). Beijing University of Chinese Medicine Dongzhimen Hospital.

Lu Yuanlei (陆渊雷). 2008a. *Two Medical Books of Lu Yuanlei* (陆渊雷医书二种). Edited by Zhang Yuping (张玉萍). Fujian: Fujian Science and Technology Press.

——— . 2008b (1931). *A Modern Interpretation of The Treatise on Cold Damage* (伤寒论今释). Edited by Bao Yanju (鲍艳举), Hua Baojin (花宝金), and Hou Wei (侯炜) Beijing: Academy Press.

————. 2010a. "Chinese Formulas Have Special Efficacy for the Presentation but Not for the Disease" (中醫方藥對於証有特效對於病無特效). In *Lu Yuanlei's Collected Medical Works* (陸淵雷醫書合集). Tianjin: Tianjin Science and Technology Press.

————. 2010b. *Lu Yuanlei's Collected Medical Works* (陸淵雷醫書合集). Tianjin: Tianjin Science and Technology Press.

Mao Zedong (毛澤東). 1917. "A Study on Physical Education" (體育之研究). *New Youth* (新青年) 3 (2).

Mayanagi Makoto (真柳誠). 2013. 「證・ 証・ 症という漢字」 (The Characters 證, 証 and 症). 『漢方の臨床』 (*Clinical Kampo*) 60 (3): 431–32.

Meng Jingchun (孟景春), and Zhou Zhongying (周仲瑛), eds. 1994. *Overview of Chinese Medicine*, Revised Edition (中医学概论修订本). Beijing: People's Medical Publishing House.

Mol, Annemarie. 2002. *The Body Multiple: Ontology in Medical Practice*. Durham, N.C.: Duke University Press.

Morris, Andrew. 2004. *Marrow of the Nation: A History of Sport and Physical Culture in Republican China*. Berkeley: University of California Press.

Mote, F. W. 1999. *Imperial China, 900–1800*. Cambridge, Mass.: Harvard University Press.

Moxham, Bernard J., and Odile Plaisant. 2014. "The History of the Teaching of Gross Anatomy—How We Got to Where We Are!" *European Journal of Anatomy* 18 (3): 219–44.

Nanjing College of Chinese Medicine (南京中医学院), 1992 (1959). *The Interpretation and Explication of the Treatise on Cold Damage* (伤寒论译释). Shanghai: Shanghai Scientific and Technical Publisher.

Nanjing Zhongyi Xueyuan (南京中医学院), 1958. *Overview of Chinese Medicine* (中医学概论). Beijing: People's Medical Publishing House.

Ochs, Shelley, and Thomas Avery Garran. 2020. *Chinese Medicine and COVID-19: Results and Reflections from China*. Passiflora Press, www.passiflora-press.com.

Ōtsuka, Keisetsu (大塚敬節). 1934. "Key to Classifying and Discriminating Presentations in Kampo Medicine" (類證鑒別漢醫要訣). *Suzhou Journal of National Medicine* (蘇州國醫雜誌), 2: 4.

Pigg, Stacy Leigh. 1996. "The Credible and the Credulous: The Question of 'Villager's Beliefs' in Nepal." *Cultural Anthropology* 11 (2): 160–201.

Porkert, Manfred. 1974. *The Theoretical Foundations of Chinese Medicine: Systems of Correspondence*. Cambridge, Mass.: MIT Press.

————. 1976. "The Intellectual and Social Impulses Behind the Evolution of Traditional Chinese Medicine." In *Asian Medical Systems: A Comparative Study*, edited by Charles Leslie. Berkeley: University of California Press.

Pu Fuzhou (蒲辅周), and Gao Huiyuan (高辉远). 1960. *The Pattern Recognition and Treatment Determination for the Chinese Medicine Treatment of Several Acute Infectious Diseases* (中医对几种急性传染病的辨证论治). Beijing: People's Medical Press.

Qin Bowei (秦伯未). 1955 (1931). *Principles of Diagnosis* (診斷大綱). Shanghai: Chinese Medicine Publishing House.

———. 1957. "Overview of Chinese Medicine 'Pattern Discrimination and Treatment Determination'" (中医"辨证论治"概说). *Jiangsu Chinese Medicine* (江苏中医) 1: 2–6.

Qiu Shiting (裘诗庭). 2006. *Collection of Medical Essays by the Famous Early Modern Physician Qiu Jisheng* (近代名医裘吉生医文集). Beijing: People's Medical Publishing House.

Ren Xiaofeng (任小风). 1955. "Criticizing Comrade He Cheng's Mistaken Policies towards Chinese Medicine" (批判贺诚同志在对待中医的政策上的错误). *People's Daily* (人民日报), December 20, 1955.

Ren Yingqiu (任应秋). 1955. "The Chinese Medicine System of Pattern Discrimination and Treatment Determination" (中医的辨证论治体系). *Journal of Chinese Medicine* (中医杂志) 4: 19–24.

———. 1984. *Collected Medical Writings of Ren Yingqiu* (任应秋论医集). Beijing: People's Medical Publishing House.

Said, Edward W. 1978. *Orientalism*. New York: Pantheon.

Scheid, Volker. 2002. *Chinese Medicine in Contemporary China: Plurality and Synthesis*. Durham, N.C.: Duke University Press.

———. 2007. *Currents of Tradition in Chinese Medicine 1626–2006*. Seattle: Eastland.

———. 2014. "Convergent Lines of Descent: Symptoms, Patterns, Constellations, and the Emergent Interface of Systems Biology and Chinese Medicine." *East Asian Science, Technology, and Society: An International Journal* 8 (1): 107–39.

Scheid, Volker, Dan Bensky, Andrew Ellis, and Randall Barolet, eds. 2009 (1990). *Chinese Herbal Medicines: Formulas and Strategies*. 2nd ed. Seattle: Eastland.

Scheid, Volker, and Eric I. Karchmer. 2016. "The History of Chinese Medicine, 1890–2010." In *Modern Chinese Religion*, vol. 2, *1850–2015*, edited by Vincent Goossaert, Jan Kiely, and John Lagerway. Leiden: Brill.

Shanghai College of Chinese Medicine (上海中医学院). 1979. *Internal Medicine* (内科学). *Provisional Textbooks for National Higher Education Medical Institutions* (全国高等医药院校试用教材). Shanghai: Shanghai Science and Technology Press.

Shapiro, Hugh. 1998. "The Puzzle of Spermatorrhea in Republican China." *Positions* 6 (3): 551–96.

———. 2003. "How Different Are Western and Chinese Medicine? The Case of Nerves." In *Medicine Across Cultures*, edited by Helaine Selin, 351–72. Dordrecht, Boston, and London: Kluwer Academic.

Sidel, Victor W. 1973. "Medical Personnel and Their Training." In *Medicine and Public Health in the People's Republic of China*, edited by Joseph R. Quinn. Washington, D.C.: National Institutes of Health.

Sivin, Nathan. 1987. *Traditional Medicine in Contemporary China: A Partial Translation of Revised Outline of Chinese Medicine (1972) with an Introductory*

Study on Change in Present Day and Early Medicine. Ann Arbor: University of Michigan Center for Chinese Studies.

Smith, Hilary A. 2017. *Forgotten Disease: Illnesses Transformed in Chinese Medicine*. Stanford: Stanford University Press.

State Administration of Traditional Chinese Medicine (国家中医药管理局). 2000. *Chinese Medical Record Standards* (中医病案规范). Beijing.

State Administration of Traditional Chinese Medicine (国家中医药管理局), and Hu Ximing (胡熙明), eds. 1989. *Scientific and Technological Achievements of Chinese Medicine in the Forty Years since the Founding of the Nation* (建国四十年中医药科技成就). Beijing: Ancient Literature of Chinese Medicine Press.

Stengers, Isabelle. 1997. *Power and Invention: Situating Science*. Translated by Paul Bains. Minneapolis: University of Minnesota Press.

Suh, Soyoung. 2017. *Naming the Local: Medicine, Language, and Identity in Korea since the Fifteenth Century*. Cambridge, Mass.: Harvard University Asia Center.

Suzhou Hospital of National Medicine (蘇州國醫醫院). 1939. *Journal of the Suzhou Hospital of National Medicine* (蘇州國醫醫院院刊): 1(1).

Taylor, Kim. 2004. *Chinese Medicine in Early Communist China, 1945–1963: A Medicine of Revolution*. London: Routledge Curzon.

Turner, Victor. 1967. *The Forest of Symbols: Aspects of Ndembu Ritual*. Ithaca, N.Y.: Cornell University Press.

Wan Yousheng (万友生). 1988 (1983). *On the Unification of Warm and Cold* (寒温统一论). Shanghai: Shanghai Science and Technology Press.

Wang Mimi (王咪咪), and Li Lin (李林), eds. 1999. *The Complete Medical Works of Tang Rongchuan* (唐荣川医学全书). Beijing: Chinese Medicine Publishing House.

Wang, Mingming. 2005. "Anthropology in Mainland China in the Past Decade: A Brief Report." *Asian Anthropology* 4 (1): 179–86.

Wang Yongyan (王永炎), and Han Xiao (寒啸), eds. 2000. *Handbook of Standards for the Writing of Chinese Medicine Case Records* (中医病案规范书写手册). Changsha: Hunan Science and Technology Press.

Wang Yongyan (王永炎), Li Mingfu (李明富), and Dai Ximeng (戴锡孟), eds. 1997. *Chinese Internal Medicine* (中医内科学). *Standardized Textbooks for General Higher Learning in Chinese Medicine* (普通高等教育中医药类规划教材). Shanghai: Shanghai Science and Technology Publishing House.

Wang Yuchuan (王玉川). 1999. "My Thoughts on 'Pattern Recognition and Treatment Determination'" (关于"辨证论治"之我见). *Chinese Medicine Education* (中医教育) 18 (3): 9–10.

Wang Zhiying (王志英), Zhou Xueping (周学平), Ye Fang (叶放), and Ye Lihong (叶丽红), eds. 2008. *Getting to Know the Great Chinese Medicine Master Zhou Zhongying* (走近中医大家周仲英). Beijing: Chinese Medicine Press of China.

Wittgenstein, Ludwig. 2009 (1953). *Philosophical Investigations*. Rev. 4th ed. Translated by G. E. M. Anscombe, P. M. S. Hacker, and Joachim Schulte. West Sussex: Wiley-Blackwell.

Wu Dunxu (吴敦序), Liu Yanchi (刘燕池), and Li Dexin (李德新), eds. 1995. *Basic Theory of Chinese Medicine* (中医基础理论). *Standardized Textbooks for General Higher Education in Chinese Medicine* (普通高等教育中医药类规划教材). Shanghai: Shanghai Science and Technology Publishing House.

Wu Keqian (吴克潜). 1933. *National Medicine Practical Diagnosis* (國醫實用診斷學). Shanghai: Popular Publishing House.

———. 1937. *Physiology and Public Health* (生理衛生講義). Edited by Wu Keqian (吴克潜). *Lecture Notes for Fourteen Courses at China Institute of Medicine* (中國醫學院講義十四種). Shanghai: China Institute of Medicine.

Wu, Yi-Li. 2015. "Bodily Knowledge and Western Learning in Late Imperial China: The Case of Wang Shixiong (1808–1868)." In *Historical Epistemology and the Making of Modern Chinese Medicine*, edited by Howard Chiang. Manchester: University of Manchester.

———. 2017. "A Trauma Doctor's Practice in Nineteenth Century China: The Medical Cases of Hu Tingguang." *Social History of Medicine* 30 (2): 299–322.

Xie Guan (谢观), ed. 1994 (1921). *Comprehensive Dictionary of Chinese Medicine* (中国医学大词典). Beijing: Chinese Medicine Publishing House.

Xu Lingtai (徐灵胎). 2008 (1757). *Treatise on the Origin and Development of Medicine* (医学源流论). Beijing: China Press of Traditional Chinese Medicine.

Yakazu, Dōmei (矢数道明), ed. 1988. *Tōa igaku kyōkai sōritsu 50 shūnen kinen bunshū* (東亜医学協会創立50周年記念文集). Commemorative Collection for the Fiftieth Anniversary of the Founding of the Association of East Asian Medicine. Tokyo: Tōa igaku kyōkai.

Yan Zhenguo (严振国), Zhu Peichun (朱培纯), and Wei Dajin (尉大金), eds. 1995. *Normal Human Anatomy* (正常人体解剖学). *Standardized Textbooks for General Higher Education in Chinese Medicine* (普通高等教育中医药类规划教材). Shanghai: Shanghai Science and Technology Press.

Yang Jizhou (楊繼洲). 1955 (1601). *Compendium of Acupuncture and Moxibustion* (針灸大成). Beijing: People's Medical Publishing House.

Yang Nianqun (杨念群). 2005. *Reconstructing Patients* (再造病人). Beijing: China People's University Press.

Yang, Taoyu. 2019. "Redefining Semi-Colonialism: A Historiographical Essay on British Colonial Presence in China." *Journal of Colonialism & Colonial History* 20 (3).

Ye Juquan (叶橘泉). 2014 (1958). "The Crux of Pattern Recognition and Treatment Determination—Presentation and Formula" (辨证论治的关键—证与方). In *Ye Juquan's Medical Discourses on Formula Presentation and Drug* (叶橘泉方证药证医话), edited by Ye Jianan (叶加南). Beijing: China Chinese Medicine Press.

Yin Huihe (印会河), and Zhang Bo'ne (张伯讷), eds. 1984. *Basic Theory of Chinese Medicine* (中医基础理论). *Textbooks for Higher Education Medical Institutions* (高等医药院校教材). Shanghai: Shanghai Science and Technology Publishing House.

Yu Yunxiu (余云岫). 1932 (1928). *Collected Essays on the Medical Revolution* (医学革命论集). Shanghai: Great East.

Yumoto Kyūshin (湯本求真). 1939. "Xu (序) (Preface)." *Journal of the Suzhou Hospital of National Medicine* (蘇州國醫醫院院刊): 1 (1).

———. 1983 (1927). *Kōkan igaku* (皇漢醫學) (*Sino-Japanese Medicine*). Tokyo: Ryōgen.

———. 2007 (1930). *Sino-Japanese Medicine* (皇汉医学). Translated by Zhou Zixu (周子敘). Beijing: Chinese Medicine Press of China.

Yun Tieqiao (惲鐵樵). 1948. *A Record of Insights from the Canons* (群經見智錄). Shanghai: Chinese Medicine Press.

———. 2007 (1924). *Research on the Treatise of Cold Damage* (伤寒论研究). Beijing: Academy Press.

———. 2008. *Selected Chinese Medicine Correspondence Textbooks of Yun Tieqiao* (恽铁樵中医函授讲义[选编]). Beijing: Academy Press.

Zhan, Mei. 2009. *Other Worldly: Making Chinese Medicine through Transnational Frames*. Durham, N.C.: Duke University Press.

Zhang Gongyao (张功耀). 2006. "Farewell to Chinese Medicine and Chinese Herbs" (告别中医中药). *Medicine and Philosophy (Humanistic and Social Science Edition)* (医学与哲学) (人文社会医学版) 27 (4): 14–17.

Zhang Shouyi (张寿颐). 2008. *Two Medical Books by Zhang Shanlei* (张山雷医书二种). Edited by Zhang Yuping (张玉萍). Fuzhou: Fujian Science and Technology Press.

Zhang Taiyan (章太炎). 2009. *Mr. Zhang Taiyan's Discourse on Cold Damage* (章太炎先生论伤寒). Edited by Wu Yue (伍悦) and Lin Lin (林霖). Beijing: Academy Press.

Zhang, Xudong. 1997. *Chinese Modernism in the Era of Reforms: Cultural Fever, Avant-Garde Fiction, and the New Chinese Cinema*. Durham, N.C.: Duke University Press.

Zhang, Yanhua. 2007. *Transforming the Emotions with Chinese Medicine: An Ethnographic Account from China*. Albany: State University of New York Press.

Zhao Hongjun (赵洪钧). 1982. *The History of the Early Modern Controversy Between Chinese Medicine and Western Medicine* (近代中西医论争史). Shijiazhuang: Hebei Branch of the Integrated Medicine Research Center.

Zhen Zhiya (甄志亚), and Fu Weikang (傅维康), eds. 1984. *The History of Medicine in China* (中国医学史). *Textbooks for Higher Education Medical Institutions* (高等医药院校教材). Shanghai: Shanghai Science and Technology Publishing House.

Zhong Jiaxi (钟嘉熙), Chen Yinhuan (陈银环), Huang Yong (黄勇), Yan Xianwei (杨贤卫), Zhu Min (朱敏), Wu Zhibing (吴智兵), Zuo Junling (左俊岭), Liu Nan (刘南), Ye Zhizhong (叶志中), Tian Ping (田平), and Zhu Dan (朱丹). 2005. "Image Tacking Survery of Recovered SARS Patients One Year after Primary Treatment with Traditional Chinese Drugs" (中医药为主治疗非典"患

者康复一年后影像学追踪). *Journal of Shaanxi College of Traditional Chinese Medicine* (陕西中医学院学报) 28 (5): 9–10.

Zhu Jiayong (朱家勇), and Zhu Shengshan (朱盛山). 2003. "The Effects of Chinese Medicine on the Prevention and Treatment of SARS" (中医药在防治非典中的作用). *Journal of the Guangdong Pharmaceutical College* (广东药学院学报) 19 (3).

Zhu Liangchun (朱良春), ed. 1980. *Medical Cases of Zhang Cigong.* Nanjing: Jiangsu Science and Technology Press (江苏科学技术出版社).

———, ed. 2005. *Famous Masters and Top Apprentices* (名师与高徒): *Selected Essays from the First High Level Forum on Academic Apprenticeships with Famous Specialists of Chinese Medicine* (首届著名中医药学家学术传承高层论坛选粹). Changsha: South Central University Press.

Zhu Weiju (祝味菊). 2005. *Interrogating Difficulties Concerning the Treatise on Cold Damage* (伤寒质难). Fuzhou: Fujian Science and Technology Press.

Zhu Wenfeng (朱文锋), ed. 1995. *Chinese Medicine Diagnosis* (中医诊断学). *Standardized Textbooks for General Higher Education in Chinese Medicine* (普通高等教育中医药类规划教材). Shanghai: Shanghai Science and Technology Publishing House.

Zhu Yan (朱颜). 1954. "The General Rules of Pattern Treatment in China's Classical Medicine" (中国古典医学症候治疗的一般规律). *Chinese Journal of Medicine* (中华医学杂志) 9, 11: 734–36, 865–67.

Index

Note: Illustrations and tables are indicated by page numbers in *italics*.

Eric I. Karchmer, Ph.D., M.D. (China), L.Ac. is Visiting Assistant Professor at China Medical University in Taichung, Taiwan.

Lightning Source UK Ltd.
Milton Keynes UK
UKHW011818050822
406910UK00003B/383